AF386397

Current Topics in Pathology

Ergebnisse der Pathologie

56

Edited by

H.-W. Altmann, Würzburg · K. Benirschke, La Jolla · A. Bohle, Tübingen

K. M. Brinkhous, Chapel Hill · P. Cohrs, Hannover · H. Cottier, Bern

M. Eder, München · P. Gedigk, Bonn · W. Giese, Münster · Chr. Hedinger, Zürich

S. Iijima, Hiroshima · W. H. Kirsten, Chicago · I. Klatzo, Bethesda

K. Lennert, Kiel · H. Meessen, Düsseldorf · W. Sandritter, Freiburg

G. Seifert, Hamburg · H. C. Stoerk, New York · H. U. Zollinger, Basel

With 36 Figures

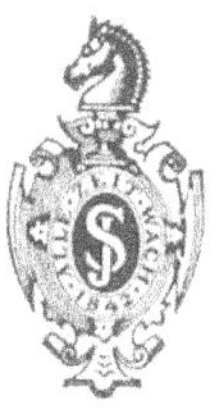

Springer-Verlag Berlin · Heidelberg · New York 1972

ISBN-13: 978-3-642-65326-1   e-ISBN-13: 978-3-642-65324-7
DOI: 10.1007/978-3-642-65324-7

Softcover reprint of the hardcover 1st edition 1972

Contents

List of Contributors

EBERHARD ALTENÄHR, Pathologisches Institut der Universität,
D-2000 Hamburg 20, Martinistr. 52, Germany

KONSTANTIN CHRISTOV, Pathologisches Institut der Universität.
D-7800 Freiburg, Albertstr. 19, Germany

FRIEDHELM HUTH, Pathologisches Institut der Universität.
D-4000 Düsseldorf, Moorenstr. 5, Germany

WILHELM KLEIN, Chirurgische Universitätsklinik,
D-4000 Düsseldorf, Moorenstr. 5, Germany

RAIKO RAICHEV, Cancer Research Institute, Department of
Pathology and Carcinogenesis, Sofia, Bulgaria

DANIEL G. SHEAHAN, Department of Pathology, Yale University,
School of Medicine, 310 Cedar Street, New Haven, CT 06510, USA

ARNOLD SOREN, New York University Medical Center,
550–560 First Avenue, New York, NY 10016, USA

Department of Pathology, University of Hamburg
Head: Professor Dr. G. Seifert

Ultrastructural Pathology of Parathyroid Glands*

EBERHARD ALTENÄHR

With 18 Figures

Contents

* Supported by DFG, Sonderforschungsbereich 34 Endokrinologie.

A. Introduction

The normal and pathological anatomy of the parathyroid glands (PTG) as seen by light microscopy is well known (BARGMANN, 1939; CASTLEMAN, 1952; ROTH, 1962; ALTENÄHR *et al.*, 1969; SEIFERT and ALTENÄHR, 1969). However, the cellular mechanisms of hormone production and secretion have not yet been clarified to any great extent. Therefore the aim of ultrastructural studies of PTG was primarily to analyse in more detail the function of PTG under different physiological and pathological conditions. In addition, a more refined cytological diagnosis of PTG would offer new prospects regarding clinical, diagnostic, and therapeutical questions, by determining whether a primary change in the PTG causes the disturbance in calcium metabolism or whether the altered PTG ultrastructure is secondary to calcium metabolism disturbances of other aetiology.

B. Functional Cytology and Ultrastructural Pathology of Parathyroid Glands in Animal Experiments

The electron microscopic studies of animal PTG in different species published so far are summarized in Table 1. There are observations under normal conditions, special physiological conditions (growth, pregnancy, lactation, laying hens, hibernation, metamorphosis of amphibians), as well as under pathological and experimental conditions.

Knowledge of the morphological equivalents of cellular hormone synthesis, storage, and secretion is an essential prerequisite for diagnostic conclusions. In addition, there is the problem of morphologic definition and staining of parathyroid hormone. To solve these questions, comparative experimental studies of stimulated and suppressed PTG were performed.

The dominating cell in PTG of all species is the *chief cell*. Detailed descriptions of their nuclei have only been published by MONTSKO *et al.* (1963) and ZAWISTOWSKI (1966). Ultrastructural changes in the nuclei, dependent on functional activity, have not been satisfactorily investigated. As in other glands synthesizing protein hormones, it can be assumed that ribosomes, rough endoplasmic reticulum and Golgi complex are involved in hormone synthesis and storage. The hormone or its precursors are synthesized by ribosomes, transported to the Golgi complex via the endoplasmic reticulum and packed into hormone-containing vesicles and granules in the Golgi complex (Fig. 1a). The morphological indications for this process are the proliferation of ribosomes and the increased size of the rough endoplasmic reticulum and Golgi complex when PTG are overactive or experimentally stimulated (Figs. 2 and 3). A corresponding reduction and involution of these cellular components is observed in experimental suppression or inactivity (Fig. 4) (LEVER, 1959; ROTH and RAISZ, 1964, 1966; CAPEN *et al.*, 1965a; STOECKEL and PORTE, 1966b; NAKAGAMI, 1967; MAZZOCCHI *et al.*, 1967b; ALTENÄHR, 1970; and others). MELSON

(1966), LEVER (1958), and NAKAGAMI (1967) have described proliferation of mitochondria following stimulation of the PTG and MAZZOCCHI *et al.* (1967b) observed an increase in mitochondrial size. Following stimulation, the number of lipid bodies is reduced (ROTH and RAISZ, 1964; MAZZOCCHI *et al.*, 1967b) while it is increased following suppression (MURAKAMI, 1970) (Fig. 2).

The cytoplasm of active chief cells appears dark due to an increase in cell organelles. As a result, stimulated PTG mainly consist of dark chief cells, rich in cell organelles (Fig. 3). The cytoplasm of inactive chief cells, especially when suppressed, is light and shows fewer organelles (Fig. 4) (LEVER, 1958; CAPEN *et al.*, 1965a; NAKAGAMI, 1967; MAZZOCCHI *et al.*, 1967b; HARA and NAGATSU, 1968; ALTENÄHR, 1970; ALTENÄHR and LIETZ, 1970). STOECKEL and PORTE (1966a) consider the different electron density of the ground plasma to be a fixation artefact. We, however, think the electron density of the ground plasma may depend on differences in the fixation lability caused by different functional cell activity.

The described findings in animal PTG are somewhat more complex in the individual species because of differences in cell type differentiation. Apart from chief cells, monkey PTG also contain oxyphil cells (TRIER, 1958; NAKAGAMI, 1965), characterized by a special prevalence of mitochondria. Cell type differentiation of equine PTG appears to be most similar to human PTG. FUJIMOTO *et al.* (1967) observed light and dark oxyphil cells, dark, light and vacuolized chief cells, as well as water-clear cells in horse PTG. Light chief cells, light vacuolized chief cells, and water-clear cells are characterized by an increased amount of glycogen in their cytoplasm. CAPEN and ROWLAND (1968b) described a glycogen increase after stimulation in cat PTG.

Vesicles with a moderately electron-dense homogeneous or loose granular content located inside or close to the Golgi complex are characteristic for protein hormone production (Fig. 1a). Their diameter is between 30 and 200 mμ, and they are generally called immature secretory or *prosecretory granules*, although they most probably contain completed parathyroid hormone ready for secretion. The cells of stimulated glands contain a significantly increased number of these prosecretory granules.

The membrane-surrounded bodies containing more densely packed fine granular material have a larger diameter (100–700 mμ) than the prosecretory granules of the corresponding species and are called *secretory granules* by most authors (Fig. 1b). They are derived from prosecretory granules by condensation of their content (NAKAGAMI, 1967; NEVALAINEN, 1969) through the fusion of several prosecretory granules, possibly via an intermediate multivesicular body (DAVIS and ENDERS, 1961). It is commonly believed that these "mature" secretory granules are hormone storage granules.

The number of secretory granules in cells of normally active PTG is species-dependent. The PTG cells of cows and mice, for example, contain relatively numerous secretory granules (CAPEN *et al.*, 1965a; STOECKEL and PORTE, 1966a) (Fig. 1b). Cat PTG show a moderate number of secretory granules (CAPEN and ROWLAND, 1968), while PTG of most other species, especially rat

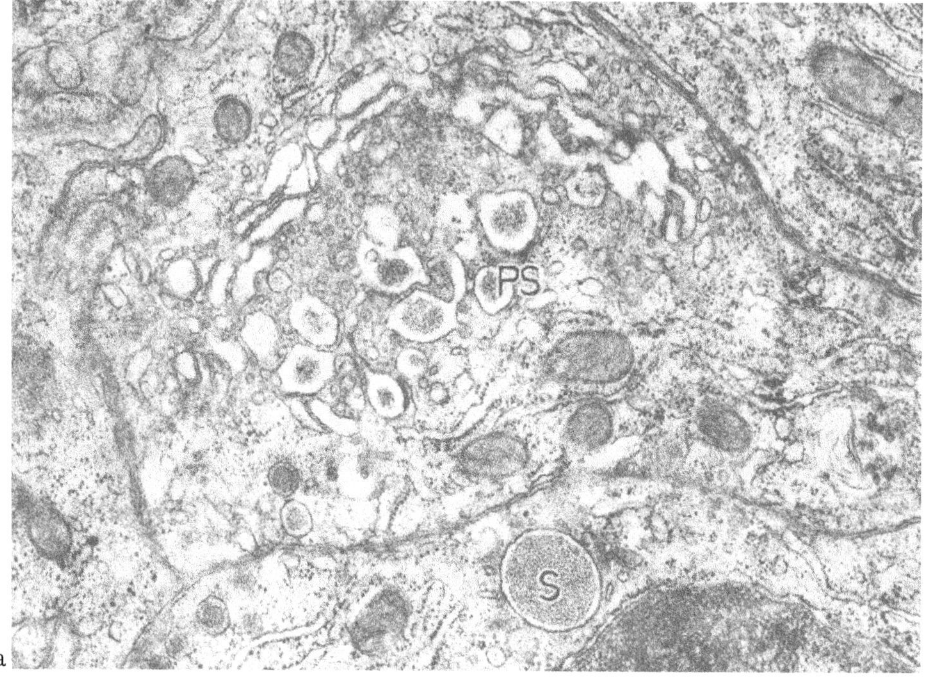

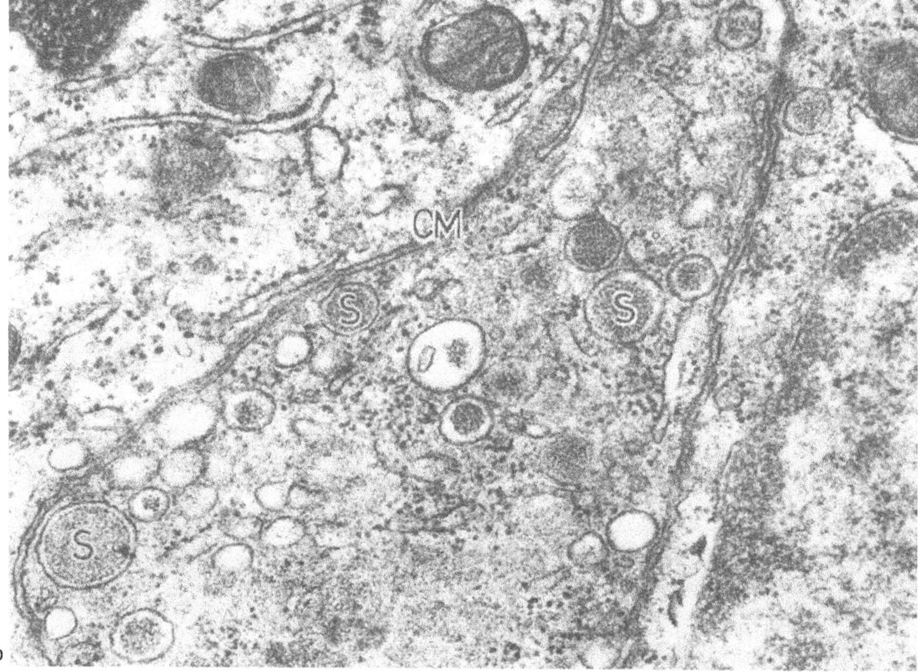

Fig. 1. Normal mouse PTG: a) Formation of prosecretory granules (*PS*) in Golgi vesicles by packing of electron-dense, fine granular material. S = secretory granule. 32000 ×. b) Secretory granules (*S*) with varying diameters, often close to the cell membrane (*CM*). 41000 ×

PTG, contain very few, their number differing even from cell to cell. The quantitative distribution of secretory granules during different functional stages is not uniform. For example, MAZZOCCHI *et al.* (1967b) described an increased number of storage granules in the stimulated PTG, while others (ROTH and RAISZ, 1964; MELSON, 1966; CAPEN and ROWLAND, 1968b) observed a degranulation. In suppressed PTG, ROTH and RAISZ (1964) and MURAKAMI (1970) found an increased amount of storage granules, while NAKAGAMI (1967) observed a reduced number. Other authors have not found significant differences in the number of storage granules (ALTENÄHR, 1970) or have not commented on this problem at all. There seems to be a lysosomal digestion of storage granules (HARA and NAGATSU, 1968; ROHR and KRÄSSIG, 1968; ALTENÄHR, 1970). Our own observations (ALTENÄHR, 1970) indicate that hormone storage and secretion of stored hormone do cccur, but are not an important functional principle of PTG. In this respect the PTG are quite unlike the C-cells of the thyroid gland, their most obvious functional changes being degranulation, storage in granules and phagolysis of granules (LIETZ, 1970; ALTENÄHR and LIETZ, 1970).

The assumption that the described prosecretory and storage granules in PTG cells contain hormone is based on their similarity to secretory granules of other glands producing protein hormones, and also on the changes observed under experimental conditions. L'HEUREUX and MELLIUS (1956) found parathyroid hormone activity in a corpuscular fraction of similar size obtained after differential centrifugation of bovine PTG tissue homogenate. However, they have not examined these corpuscules by electron microscopy. Immunocytochemical proof of parathyroid hormones has not so far been obtained. Cellular secretion of synthesized hormone packed by the Golgi complex to prosecretory and secretory granules has not been completely clarified morphologically in spite of numerous attempts. Often, secretory granules are located near the plasma membrane (Fig. 1b) and prosecretory granules, too, show a transfer from the Golgi complex to the periphery of the cell, especially following stimulation. In some PTG a preferential location in peripheral areas of the cytoplasm and at cell membranes adjacent to narrow intercellular spaces is observed (e. g. mouse PTG; STOECKEL and PORTE, 1966a); in others, they are located near cell surfaces next to widened intercellular spaces or towards the interstitial space (e. g. human PTG: ALTENÄHR and SEIFERT, 1971). Most authors assume a fusion between granule membrane and plasma membrane (STOECKEL and PORTE, 1966a; MELSON, 1966; NAGAGAMI, 1967; HARA and NAGATSU, 1968; TANAKA, 1969; YOUSHAK and CAPEN, 1970). An increased incorporation of granule membranes into the cell membrane could be the reason for the enlargement of the cell surface and the increased tortuosity of plasma membranes in stimulated PTG. It is very difficult, however, to obtain an electron micrograph of such a fusion and exocytosis (Fig. 6b), which definitely excludes a tangential section. Probably, the hormone is liquified when secreted from the cell. Rarely, isolated granules have been described in the interstitial spaces (human PTG: MUNGER and ROTH, 1963; cow PTG: CAPEN *et al.*, 1965a; pig PTG: FETTER and CAPEN, 1968). The situation in pig PTG, however, is different, because cytoplasmic processes containing secretory granules reach through the basement membrane into the perivascular space. They seem to be subsequently detached from the cell.

The frequently observed widened intercellular spaces contain a moderately electron-dense colloidal homogeneous or fine granular material, and communicate with the perivascular space via a system of channels (ALTENÄHR, 1970; SETOGUTI et al., 1970; COLEMAN, 1969). Colloidal storage of hormone in such intercellular spaces would seem possible, and would be consistent with the findings of PERKIN et al. (1968) obtained by immune fluorescence microscopy.

A direct secretion of hormone from the gland cell into the capillary does not seem possible because the capillary wall and the endocrine cells have no direct contact. Therefore, the hormone must reach the blood via intercellular and perivascular spaces. The fenestrated capillary endothelium with numerous pores is especially well suited for an intense exchange of substances. The great pinocytotic activity of the endothelial cells could also be of importance for hormone transport across the capillary wall. Whether the electron-dense granules in the endothelial cells actually represent secretory granules has not yet been proved (MUNGER and ROTH, 1963; CAPEN et al., 1965a; MELSON, 1966; FETTER and CAPEN, 1968).

Because of the function-dependent change in PTG cytology, a *functional cycle* of the endocrine cells is assumed with a primarily inactive resting chief cell, which is stimulated and activated and thereafter returns to the resting phase (ROTH and RAISZ, 1966; MAZZOCCHI et al., 1967b). This cycle is supposed to be essentially the same in all species (Fig. 2). In the modified and summarized scheme the tortuous cell membranes with numerous indentations following stimulation have been considered, as well as the fact that active cells secrete mainly "immature" prosecretory granules. The described reduction of glycogen after stimulation (ROTH and RAISZ, 1966) does not occur in all species (cat PTG: CAPEN and ROWLAND, 1968; horse PTG: FUJIMOTO et al., 1967; human PTG: ALTENÄHR and SEIFERT, 1971). In addition, the scheme shows cells of human PTG during chronic secondary hyperparathyroidism (activated light chief cell, small water-clear cell, transitional oxyphil cell) and the extreme cell types of human PTG (large water-clear cell, oxyphil cell) (Fig. 2).

The experimental ultrastructural investigations have confirmed that the calcium concentration of serum or culture medium is the essential factor regulating the endocrine activity of the PTG.

A *reduction in serum calcium* results in *stimulation* of PTG cells (MONTSKO et al., 1963; ROTH and RAISZ, 1964, 1966; CAPEN and ROWLAND, 1968; ROTH et al., 1968; ALTENÄHR, 1970; ALTENÄHR und LIETZ, 1971):

A low-calcium diet produces hypocalcaemia and ultrastuructural signs of activation in the PTG (ROTH et al., 1968; CAPEN and ROWLAND, 1968b; ALTENÄHR, 1970) (Fig. 3).

Administration of phosphates also results in stimulation of PTG (LEVER, 1958; LANGE and von BREHM, 1963; MELSON, 1966; STOECKEL and PORTE,

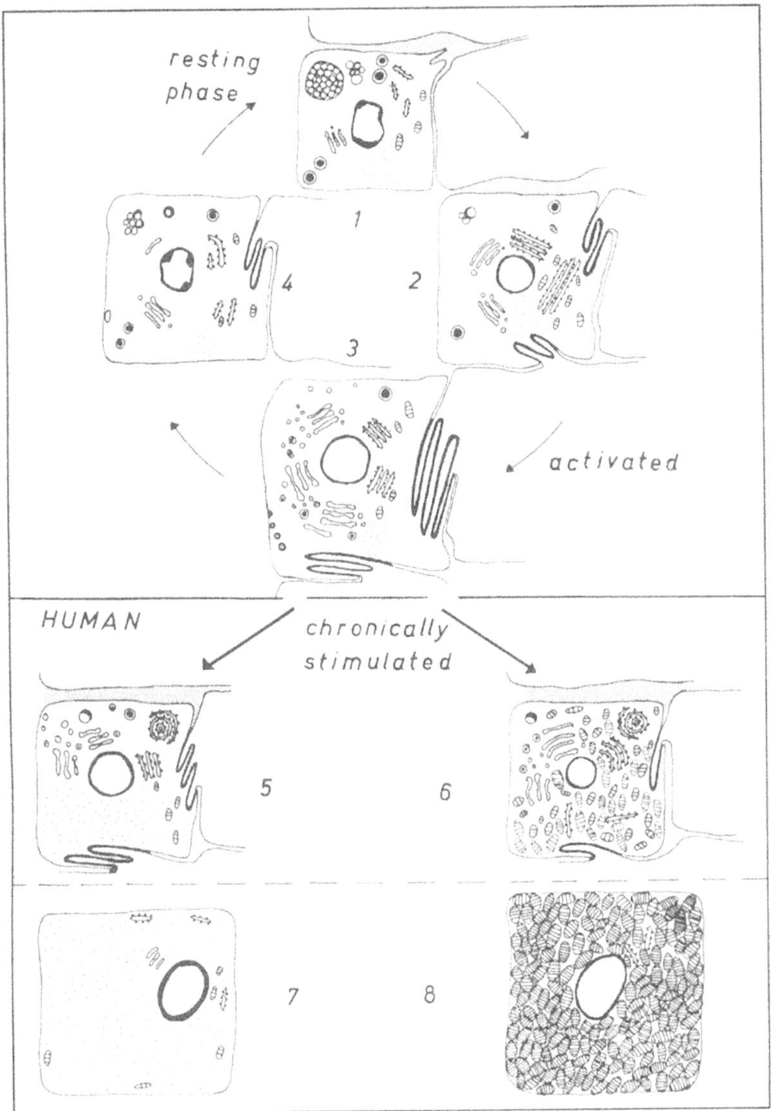

Fig. 2. Diagram demonstrating the secretory cycle and functional changes of PTG cells:
During transformation of PTG cells from the resting phase (1) to the active phase (2, 3)
the endoplasmic reticulum first increases in size, followed by an increased Golgi complex,
the number of prosecretory granules subsequently becoming more numerous. The tortuosity of cell membranes and interdigitations increases. At the same time the number of
lipid vacuoles in the cytoplasm diminishes.—During regression (4) from the active to
the resting phase (1) the size of the protein-synthesizing apparatus decreases and lipid
vacuoles become more numerous again. Tortuosity of cell membranes diminishes.—Under
conditions of chronic stimulation (secondary hyperparathyroidism), human PTG show
glycogen-rich light chief cells and small water-clear (5), containing in addition an extended
protein-synthesizing apparatus. Oxyphil chief cells or transitional oxyphil cells (6)
containing numerous mitochondria may also exhibit a prominent protein-synthesizing
apparatus in secondary hyperparathyroidism.—Extreme cell forms of human PTG are
the large water-clear cell (7) and the typical oxyphil cell (8) with an inconspicuous or
absent protein-synthesizing apparatus

1966b; Altenähr, 1970), obviously by producing hypocalcemia (Aurbach and Potts, 1969; Altenähr, 1970).

Following repeated applications of thyrocalcitonin, PTG also show ultrastructural signs of activation (Altenähr, 1970). Since no specific changes in the ultrastructure were observed, as compared to other hypocalcemic conditions, it can be concluded that calcitonin also indirectly activates the PTG by a transient hypocalcemia, and that it does not exert a direct stimulating influence on the PTG (Altenähr, 1970).

Ultrastructural studies of PTG in animals with experimental *renoprived hyperparathyroidism* demonstrated the same changes of increased cellular activity (Lever, 1958; Davis and Enders, 1961; Mazzocchi *et al.*, 1967b). The stimulus for this activation has not been definitely clarified so far.

An *elevation of serum calcium* produced by calcium infusions, oral calcium, parathyroid hormone (Fig. 4), or dihydrotachysterol causes the ultrastructural changes of inactivation of the PTG cells (Montsko *et al.*, 1963; Roth and Raisz, 1964, 1966; Stoeckel and Porte, 1966b; Hara and Nagatsu, 1968; Altenähr, 1970; Altenähr and Lietz, 1970).

Controversial results have been obtained following *vitamin D administration* and in *experimental rickets.* Capen *et al.* (1965b, 1968) describe inactivation and atrophy of the PTG, following administration of vitamin D to normal, pregnant and lactating cows. Klotz *et al.* (1966), however, did not observe any changes in dog PTG. Following administration of a rachitogenic diet to rats, Mazzocchi *et al.* (1967b) observed activation of the PTG, while Roth *et al.* (1968) could not find any influence of vitamin D or rickets on the ultrastructure of PTG.

Drinking water containing high doses of *fluoride* causes hyperplasia in sheep PTG and ultrastructural changes typical of stimulation (Faccini and Care, 1965). Faccini (1969) interprets this observation by assuming a diminished resorption of calcium from the fluoroapatite-containing bone, and thus an increased demand for parathyroid hormone. However, Raisz and Taves (1967), using biochemical methods, did not find increased PTG activity after fluoride administration.

Lupulescu *et al.* (1968) studied dog PTG in *experimental isoimmune hypoparathyroidism* following repeated injections of emulsions of dog PTG together with Freund's adjuvant over a period of four months. Using light microscopy, they observed atrophy and disorganization of the cellular pattern, lymphoplasmocytic infiltration and progressive sclerosis. Electron microscopically, these glands showed atrophy of the endoplasmic reticulum, irregular swollen and vacuolized mitochondria with ruptured cristae and an irregular ragged nuclear membrane. The number and size of secretory and prosecretory granules were reduced. These changes explain the reduction in the hormone secretion rate and the resulting disturbance of phosphate and calcium metabolism in these animals. – No morphological studies of experimental immune parathyroiditis caused by highly purified parathyroid hormone have yet been published. Experimental investigation of immune parathyroiditis will become more important, because human idiopathic hypoparathyroidism is now considered to

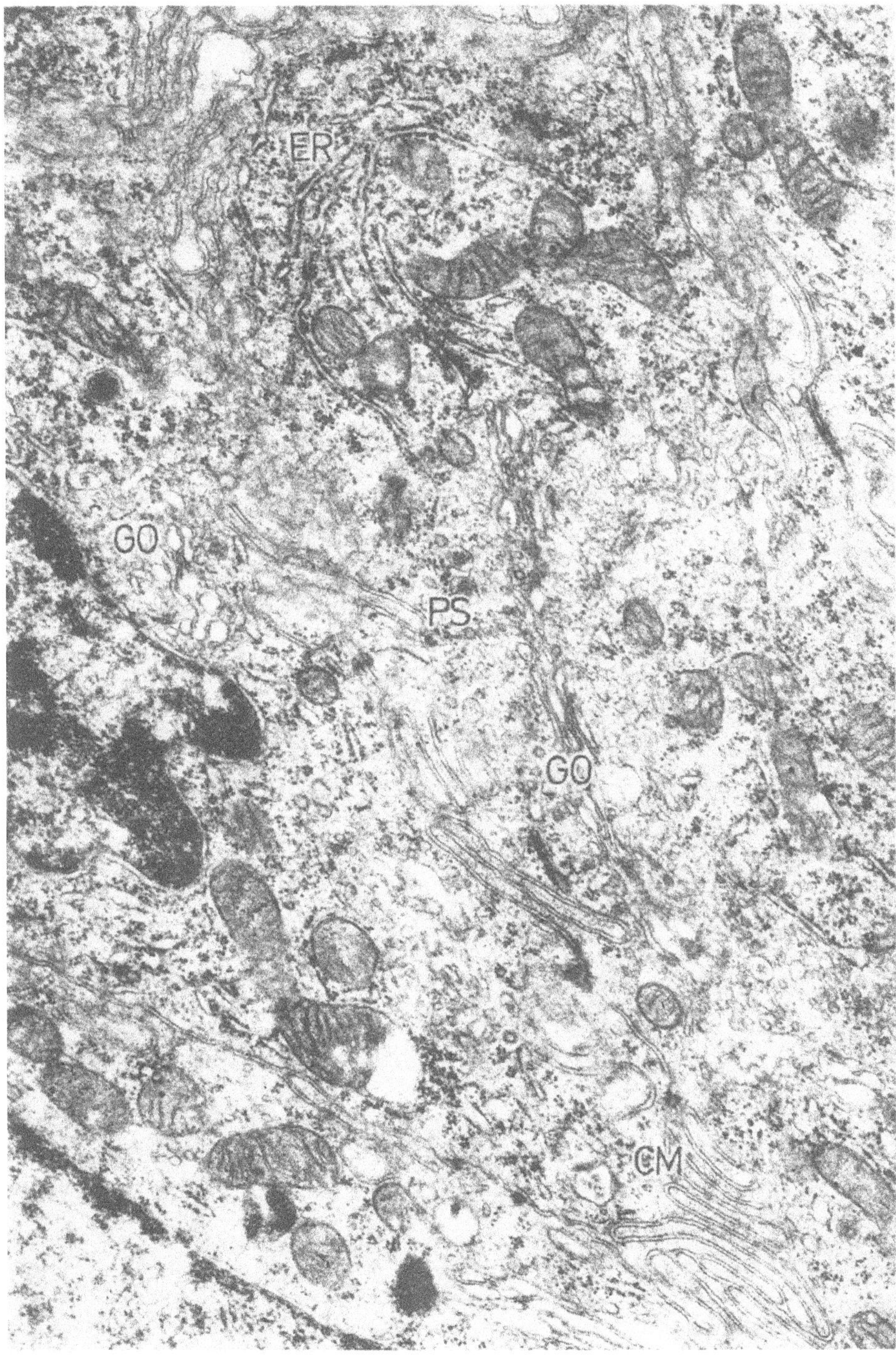

Fig. 3. Rat PTG stimulated by administration of a low-calcium, low-phosphate diet for 4 weeks: Dark cytoplasm, rich in cell organelles, with numerous ribosomes, extended rough endoplasmic reticulum (*ER*) and Golgi complex (*GO*). *PS* = prosecretory granules, *CM* = tortuous cell membrane. 32000 ×

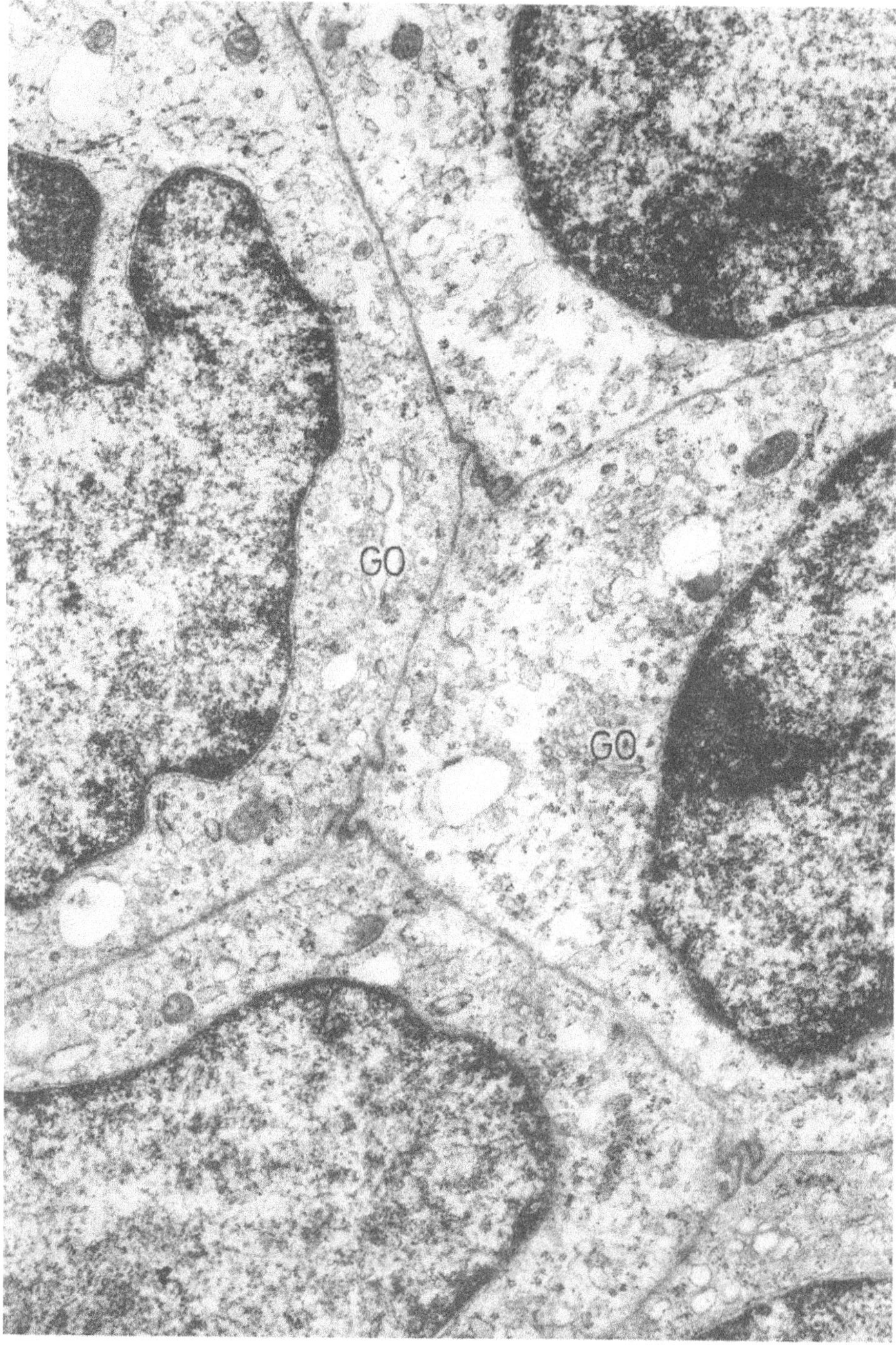

Fig. 4. Suppressed rat PTG after subcutaneous injections of parathyroid hormone for 8 days (twice daily 20 USP Units PTH Lilly): Organelle-depleted light cytoplasm, fewer ribosomes, diminished size of the rough endoplasmic reticulum and of the Golgi complex (*GO*), straight cell membranes. 17 000 ×

be an autoimmune disease (BLIZZARD, 1969). Results of ultrastructural studies of human PTG in idiopathic hypoparathyroidism are not yet available.

Nervous regulation of parathyroid function is unknown. Light microscopically, RAYBUCK (1952) observed unmyelinated nerves in close contact with endocrine cells in rat PTG. Electron microscope studies have repeatedly demonstrated nerves in perivascular spaces of PTG, but no innervation of endocrine epithelial cells has been described by other electron microscopists (ROGERS, 1963; MAZZOCCHI *et al.*, 1967b; NAKAGAMI, 1967). Apart from an innervation of arterioles, we were able to demonstrate neuroepithelial synapses of autonomous neurons with chief cells (ALTENÄHR, 1971). This makes a nervous influence on endocrine functions of PTG cells seem possible, although no corresponding experimental results are as yet available.[1]

C. Ultrastructure of Animal Parathyroid Glands under Special Physiological Conditions

Ultrastructural studies of PTG of *growing* cats (CAPEN and ROWLAND, 1968) and pigs (FETTER and CAPEN, 1970) have shown somewhat differing results. While fast-growing cats show predominantly active chief cells, rich in cell organelles, the authors found mainly inactive chief cells with transparent cytoplasm and fewer organelles in young pigs. These results do not allow any conclusion concerning endocrine function of PTG in growing animals.

At the end of *pregnancy*, immediately before the calculated date of parturition, PTG of cows show a definite activation in their ultrastructure. This continues after parturition and reaches maximum activation at the beginning of lactation, 20 hours after parturition (CAPEN *et al.*, 1965a). These authors consider the rapid calcification of fetal bones at the end of pregnancy and the increased calcium demand of the lactating glands after parturition to be the reason for the PTG activation. Serum calcium level of cows reaches the lower limit of normal at this time and obviously has to be kept at this level by increased PTG function.

Ultrastructural investigations of the PTG of *laying hens* show a special physiological activation (NEVALAINEN, 1969). This is obviously the result of the increased calcium requirement for egg shell formation.

Seasonal changes of PTG ultrastructure in Triturus pyrrhogaster (Boié) have been investigated by SETOGUTI et al. (1970a, b). They observed signs of increased activity in the spring as compared to hibernation.

COLEMAN (1969) studied and discussed PTG changes during the *metamorphosis* of Xenopus laevis (Daudin) in the larva and mature toad. There are striking changes in the ratio of light and dark cells, but the author does not come to definite conclusions in regard to endocrine activity.

---

[1] *Note added in proof:* Since completion of this article an experimental light and electron microscopical study by G. M. SALZER (Acta endocrin., Copenhagen, **68**, Suppl. 157, 1–64, 1971) appeared, which indicates some influence of pituitary gland on parathyroid glands and C-cells.

D. Ultrastructural Pathology of Animal Parathyroid Glands During Different Spontaneous Diseases

1. Parturient Paresis of Cows with Hypocalcaemia

The parturient paresis of cows with hypocalcaemia represents a spontaneous metabolic disease. It develops in lactating cows during the first few days following parturition and is characterized by hypocalcaemia, tetany, and eventually pareses and coma. The PTG cells of these cows show the morphological changes typical of increased activity and hormone production: increased tortuosity of cell membranes with multiple interdigitating cytoplasmic processes, prominent Golgi complexes with numerous prosecretory granules, lamellar aggregates of granular endoplasmic reticulum, multiplication of ribosomes, reduction in mature secretory granules (CAPEN and YOUNG, 1967a). At the same time, the parafollicular cells of thyroid gland are depleted of secretory granules, and their Golgi complexes and endoplasmic reticula are only poorly developed. The number and size of parafollicular cells are reduced and they are cytologically inactive.

CAPEN and YOUNG (1967a) therefore assume that the abrupt discharge of stored thyrocalcitonin from the parafollicular cells causes this hypocalcaemia and hypophosphataemia. Corresponding to the morphological findings, these animals show a reduction in stored thyrocalcitonin in the thyroid gland as determined by bioassay (CAPEN and YOUNG, 1967b) and an increased serum level of parathyroid hormone as demonstrated by immunoassay (SHERWOOD et al., 1966). These results allow two interpretations of the course and mechanism of this disease:

1. Unknown stimulus (?)—discharge of stored thyrocalcitonin from thyroid C-cells—hypocalcaemia and hypophosphataemia with parturient paresis—activation of PTG. or

2. Subnormal serum calcium level after delivery and during lactation—inactivity of C-cells and activation of PTG—transient hypercalcaemia (?, not demonstrated)—secretion of stored thyrocalcitonin—hypocalcaemia and hypophosphataemia with parturient paresis.

2. Osteopetrosis of Chicken

This disease is characterized by slight hypocalcaemia and irregular subperiosteal and endosteal fibrous bone formation, predominantly at the diaphyses of the long bones. The aetiological agent is considered to be a virus (SIMPSON and SANGER, 1968) which can be demonstrated in and next to osteoblasts and in cells of various endocrine glands. YOUSHAK and CAPEN (1970) electron microscopically observed in the PTG intercellular aggregates of leucosis viruses and occasionally intracellular virus particles. In addition, the PTG show the ultrastructural changes typical of hyperactivity (prominent rough endoplasmic reticulum and Golgi complex, augmented production and secretion of prosecretory granules, reduction of storage granules). The raised activity of the PTG, however, is not capable of compensating for the hypocalcaemia. The C-cells of the ultimobranchial body of these animals are activated at the same time (YOUSHAK and CAPEN, 1970), and there is a reduction in stored calcitonin (DENT and BROWN, 1969). YOUSHAK and CAPEN (1970) discuss the possibility that the observed leucosis viruses stimulate cellular activity of osteocytes as well as of the endocrine cells of the ultimobranchial body and of the PTG. The increased activity of the PTG could, of course, also be explained by the persistent hypocalcaemia, possibly a result of new bone formation.

3. Atrophic Rhinitis of Pigs

The conchae of pigs suffering from this disease are atrophic and reduced in size. Infections (PEARCE and ROE, 1966) and dietetic disturbances of calcium and phosphate metabolism (BROWN *et al.*, 1966) are discussed as causative agents. Serum calcium level is statistically reduced compared to normal controls. It is, however, within the normal range. FETTER and CAPEN (1968) have described electron microscopically a slight activation of endocrine cells in PTG. C-cells of the thyroid glands show a normal ultrastructure (FETTER and CAPEN, 1970b). Since this disease is characterized by reduced formation of organic bone matrix and not by increased resorption of bone (FETTER and CAPEN, 1971), the insignificant changes in PTG ultrastructure probably are concomitant changes of the disease and do not signify a causative role of PTG in the pathogenesis of this condition.

4. Osteodystrophy of Horses

The investigations of horse PTG by FUJIMOTO *et al.* (1967) are of special relevance for human PTG pathology because of the similarity of equine and human cell types. In diet-induced osteodystrophy FUJIMOTO *et al.* (1967) observed an increased number of light chief cells and groups of vacuolized chief cells and the presence of small and large water-clear cells. Cellular glycogen content increases progressively from the light chief cells to the large water-clear cells. The authors consider the light chief cell with prominent Golgi complex and numerous secretory and prosecretory granules in addition to glycogen to be the active cell type. The endoplasmic reticulum was partly distributed in stacked parallel or concentric arrays. Some vacuolized chief cells showed a vacuolated and cystically dilated endoplasmic reticulum and Golgi complex with fewer prosecretory granules. The authors interpret these ultrastructural changes of some vacuolized chief cells as an abnormal state of secretory overactivity. The water-clear cells, extremely rich in glycogen, contained a small Golgi complex, but with multiple vesicles and vacuoles around it, and are considered to be abnormally inactive cells, as a result of preceding overstimulation (FUJIMOTO *et al.*, 1967). These findings are similar to the results obtained in human PTG secondary renal hyperparathyroidism with osteopathy (ALTENÄHR and SEIFERT, 1971) (cf. p. 23 ff.).

E. Ultrastructure of Normal Human Parathyroid Glands

Human PTG differ cytologically from those of most other species in their different cell types: dark and light chief cells, small and large water-clear cells, transitional oxyphil cells and oxyphil cells. These light microscopic descriptions of the cytoplasm correspond to ultrastructural cell components as follows: light, vacuolized and water-clear cytoplasm represents an accumulation of glycogen granules (often solubilized during preparation) or—in special cases—numerous vesicles. Light microscopically dark cytoplasm contains less glycogen and fewer vacuoles, and the cytoplasmic components are more densely packed. A granular or oxyphil cytoplasm, as seen by light microscopy, consists of multiple, closely packed mitochondria. It is obvious from this comparison that description of the cytoplasm as light, dark, or oxyphil does not give any information about the real contents of the protein- and hormone-synthesizing apparatus, i. e. rough endoplasmic reticulum, Golgi complex, prosecretory and secretory granules. Information concerning the endocrine activity of these cell types can only be gained if there is a definite ultrastructural correlation between hormone-synthesizing apparatus and cell contents of glycogen, vacuoles, and mitochondria.

1. Chief Cells

The ultrastructure of human PTG from patients without disturbance of calcium metabolism has been described most extensively by MUNGER and ROTH (1963) and MAZZOCCHI et al. (1967a). Both groups differentiate between active and inactive chief cells.

Active chief cells (Fig. 5) contain an overall dark cytoplasm with numerous cell organelles, a Golgi complex and a well-developed endoplasmic reticulum, sometimes located in parallel or concentrically arranged, stacked arrays. Prosecretory granules or vesicles (50–150 mμ) can be seen next to the Golgi coplex and secretory granules (100–500 mμ) in the cell periphery. They are mostly round (Fig. 6), partly elongated or dumbbell shaped. The morphological variability does not seem to exclude an identical functional, i. e. hormonal nature of these granules (HOLZMANN and LANGE, 1963; ALTENÄHR and SEIFERT, 1971). We classified the electron-dense bodies in normal human PTG cells morphologically and assume the following development: Golgi vesicles—prosecretory granules—fusion and condensation of prosecretory granules—secretory (storage) granules—lysosomal transformation—lipid bodies. (ALTENÄHR and SEIFERT, 1971). According to this hypothesis prosecretory and secretory granules can either be secreted or converted to lipid bodies. Only a small amount of glycogen is present in active chief cells of normal PTG (MUNGER and ROTH, 1963; MAZZOCCHI et al., 1967a). Occasionally cilia are present. Generally the arrangement of their filaments is of the (9 + 0) type (ALTENÄHR and SEIFERT, 1971). MUNGER and ROTH (1963), however, observed the (8 + 1) type also.

In contrast to active chief cells, the *inactive chief cells* (Fig. 7) contain large amounts of glycogen in normal PTG. Golgi complex and endoplasmic reticulum are not prominent. Fewer prosecretory and secretory granules are visible than

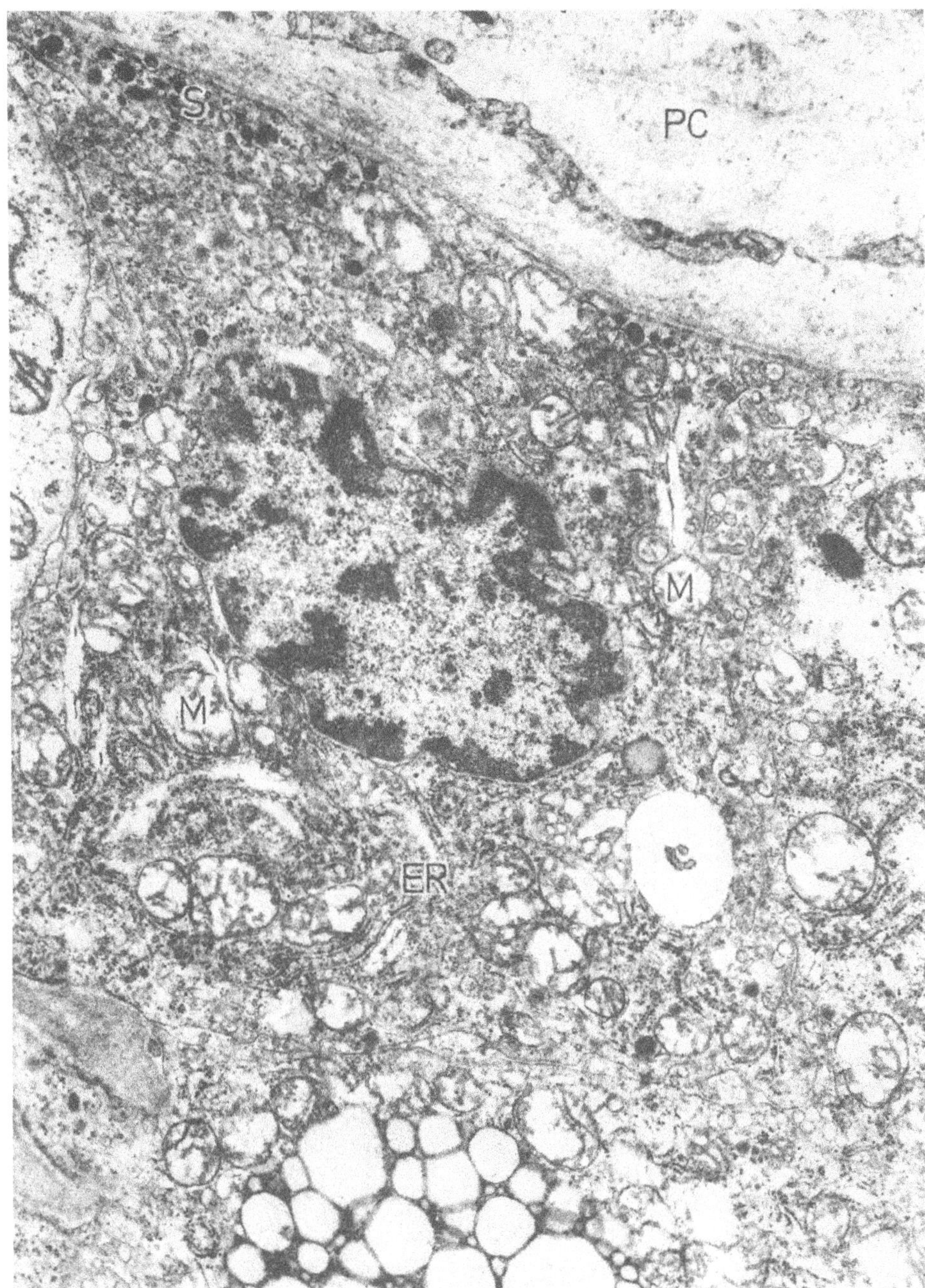

Fig. 5. Normal human PTG: Active chief cell with dark cytoplasm rich in cell organelles, prominent rough endoplasmic reticulum (*ER*), Mitochondria (*M*). *S* = secretory granules at the vascular pole of the cell; *PC* = pericapillary space. Tissue obtained 1 hour after death. 17000 ×

in active cells. MUNGER and ROTH (1963) did not observe cilia in inactive chief cells, but these cells, too, contain lipid bodies. The lipid bodies or vacuoles can aggregate and fuse. Following fusion, they sometimes are surrounded by a

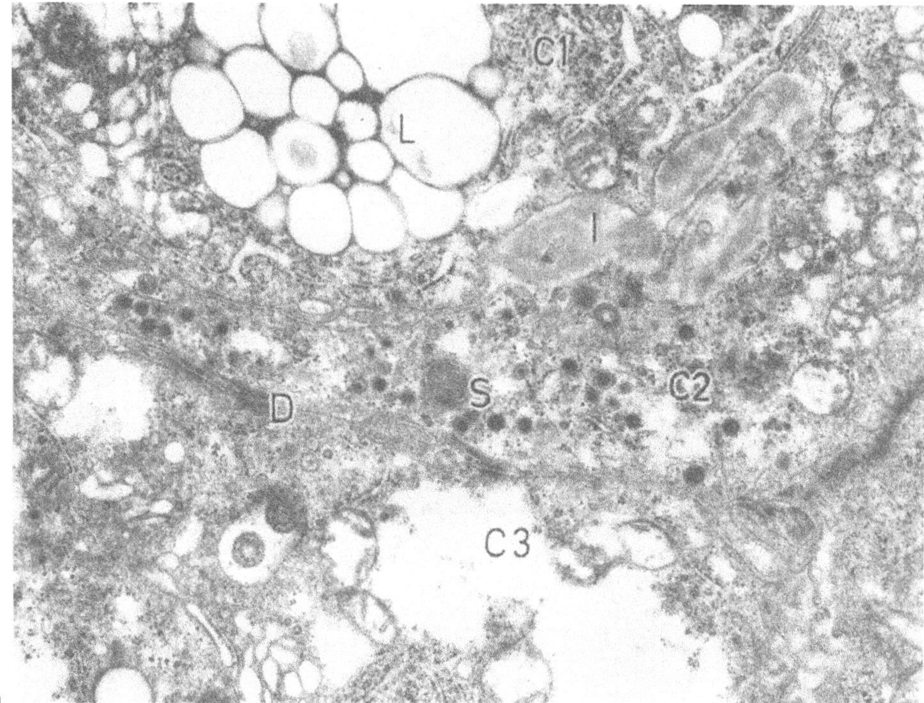

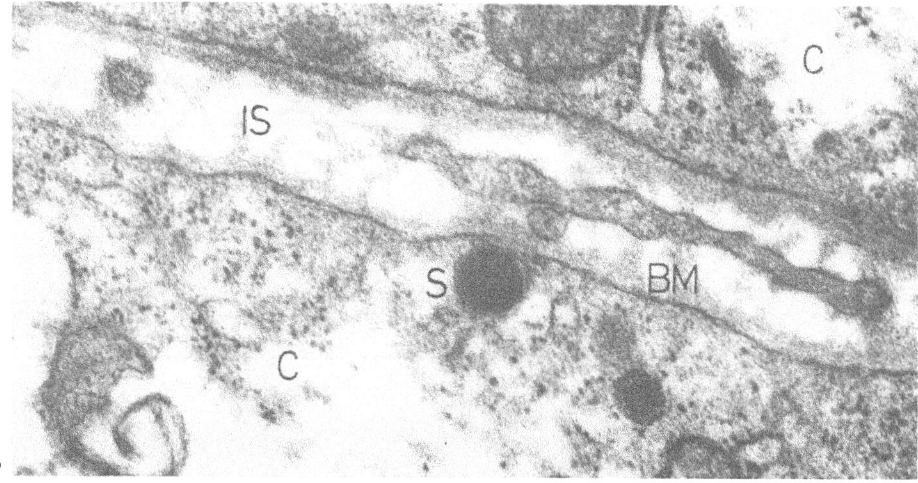

Fig. 6a and b. Normal human PTG: a) Sections of several chief cells ($C1$–$C3$); there are partly intercellular desmosomes (D), partly widened intercellular spaces (I) containing a colloidal, moderately electron-dense material. In one of the cells ($C2$) numerous membrane-bound secretory granules (S) of varying diameters. L = complex lipoid body. 19000 ×.
b) Cellular excretion of a secretory granule (S) by fusion of granule membrane and cell membrane. BM = basement membrane, C = chief cell, IS = interstitial space. 48000 ×

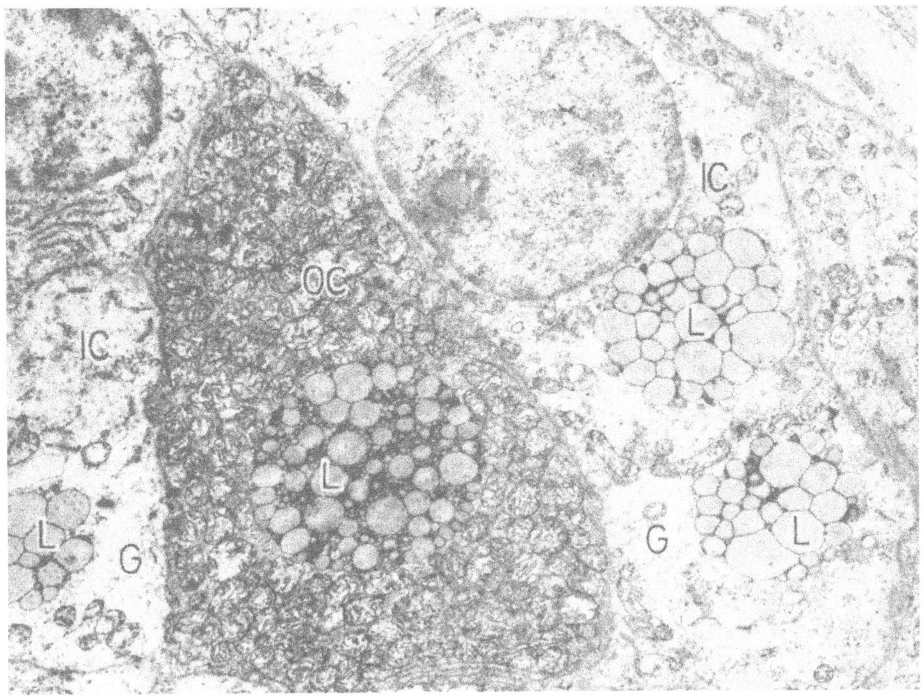

Fig. 7. Normal human PTG: Inactive light chief cells (*IC*) rich in glycogen (*G*) and complex lipid bodies (*L*); oxyphil cell (*OC*) with densely packed mitochondria and a big lipid body (*L*). 7000 ×

delicate one-layer membrane. ALTENÄHR and SEIFERT (1971) generally found relatively numerous lipid bodies and complex lipid vacuoles in cells from PTG of patients with normal calcium metabolism. They consider this among others a criterion for normal activity, as compared to secondary hyperplastic PTG. However, since these PTG investigated by us were obtained from patients aged 57 to 62 years and since the cells only contained a small Golgi complex, the presence of multiple lipid vacuoles could indicate an age-related inactivation of the PTG (cf. "Atrophy", p. 22). Obviously the lipid bodies correspond to the wear-and-tear pigment described by HAMPERL (1934).

The functional correlation of MUNGER and ROTH (1963) and MAZZOCCHI *et al.* (1967b)—dark chief cells with little glycogen and rich in cell organelles = endocrine activity; light chief cells rich in glycogen and with few cell organelles = endocrine inactivity—is valid for normal PTG. It is, however, not applicable to secondary (renal) hyperparathyroidism (ALTENÄHR and SEIFERT, 1971; FRIES *et al.*, 1967; BLACK *et al.*, 1970) (cf. "Secondary Hyperparathyroidism, p. 23 ff.).

Nuclei with loose homogeneously distributed chromatin display a smooth round nuclear surface, while others with dense chromatin are somewhat more irregular and show indentations of the nuclear membrane. The cell membranes

show some tortuosity, which is most prominent in places where several cells
come into contact.

2. Water-Clear Cells

Water-clear cells are rare and their ultrastructure has not yet been described in normal human PTG.

3. Oxyphil Cells and Transitional Oxyphil Cells

PTG cells are oxyphil when they contain numerous mitochondria (Fig. 7).
The same applies to oncocytes of other organs. Mitochondria cause the oxyphil
granulation of cytoplasm, observed by light microscopy, and they contain the
oxidative enzymes which are prevalent in oxyphil cells. In typical oxyphil cells
mitochondria are packed so closely that there is only room for a few glycogen
granules. A Golgi complex is not present in typical oxyphil cells and only
occasionally can short narrow cisterns of the endoplasmic reticulum be seen
(MUNGER and ROTH, 1963; MAZZOCCHI *et al.*, 1967a). Very rarely, electron-
dense (secretory?) granules are observed. In contrast to chief cells and transitional oxyphil cells, it has not been possible to demonstrate a nucleolus in
nuclei of typical oxyphil cells of normal human PTG (MAZZOCCHI *et al.*, 1967a).
The cell membrane is extended and does not show any tortuosity.

Some of the closely packed mitochondria show structural abnormalities.
They are frequently enlarged and giant mitochondria, up to 3 mμ in length,
can be seen. The mitochondrial matrix is strikingly electron-dense. Cristae
mitochondriales are numerous and frequently elongated. MAZZOCCHI *et al.*
(1967a) consider the following changes in mitochondria to be an indication of
oxyphil cell degeneration, apart from nuclear alterations: mitochondrial swelling, reduced electron density of the matrix, storage of a finely granular material,
large osmiophilic matrix droplets, fusion of the external and internal mitochondrial membranes, onion-like disposition of the cristae mitochondriales.

The absence of a typical protein-synthesizing, i. e. hormone-producing
apparatus makes hormone production in fully developed typical oxyphil cells
of human PTG improbable. It has not been possible to classify these cells
functionally, even by electron microscopy. There have been discussions as to
whether oxyphil cells have any regulatory influence on neighbouring chief cells
or oxyphil chief cells, or whether they can be transformed back to transitional
oxyphil cells or chief cells. Cell division of oxyphil cells seems to be possible.

Cells less rich in mitochondria than oxyphil cells and containing more mitochondria than chief cells are called transitional oxyphil cells. In contrast to
typical fully developed oxyphil cells, the transitional oxyphil cells contain, in
addition to the numerous mitochondria, a well-developed endoplasmic reticulum and Golgi complex, as well as prosecretory and secretory granules. Their
nuclei show nucleoli, like chief cells. Mitochondria of transitional cells can,
however, show the same changes as those of typical oxyphil cells. Since transitional oxyphil cells do not necessarily develop into oxyphil cells and since their
hormone-producing apparatus resembles that of chief cells, the term oxyphil
chief cell seems appropriate for this cell type.

4. Interstitial and Perivascular Space

The interstitial and perivascular spaces of normal human PTG are similar to those of animal PTG (MUNGER and ROTH, 1963; MAZZOCCHI *et al.*, 1967a; ALTENÄHR and SEIFERT, 1971). Microvilli protrude into widened intercellular fissures and into lumina of acini containing a colloidal material which is moderately electron-dense (Fig. 6a). The hormone can obviously be secreted into these intercellular spaces and partly be stored here (MAZZOCCHI *et al.*, 1967a; ALTENÄHR and SEIFERT, 1971). Secretion is also possible across the basement membrane covering the cell surface into the pericapillary space (Fig. 6b). Electron-dense granules, similar to the secretory granules of the endocrine cells, can be seen in endothelial and Schwann cells. Only MUNGER and ROTH (1963), however, describe these granules in the perivascular space of normal human PTG. It is uncertain whether they really are hormonal secretory granules.

Also in human PTG capillary endothelium is characterized by multiple cell pores. The pericapillary space contains fibrocytes, collagen fibres and occasionally unmyelinated autonomous nerves, generally along blood vessels. The axons are often unfolded within the interstitial space without coming into contact with other cells. We have been able to demonstrate an innervation of blood vessels and neuroepithelial synapses with chief cells in human PTG. (ALTENÄHR, 1971). This indicates the possibility of partial nervous control of hormone secretion.

5. Ultrastructure of Normal Human Parathyroid Glands During Embryonal, Fetal and Neonatal Period

NAKAGAMI et al. (1968) studied the PTG of two human fetuses weighing 500 and 730 g respectively. They described two cell types. The dominating type is the "inactive chief cell" with extended glycogen fields, small Golgi complex, little developed granular endoplasmic reticulum, and few secretory granules. More infrequent are "intermediary chief cells" with relatively well developed Golgi complex and endoplasmic reticulum, numerous ribosomes and mitochondria. These cells also contain glycogen. Active chief cells and oxyphil cells have not been demonstrated by these authors. They assume that PTG are in a resting phase during this developmental stage, while the production of secretory granules has already commenced. They also consider the relative thickness of capillary walls a sign of low endocrine activity.

Our own extensive studies of embryonal, fetal human and rat PTG (ALTENÄHR and WÖHLER, 1971) have basically confirmed the results of NAKAGAMI et al. (1968). A definite differentiation of "intermediary chief cells" and "inactive chief cells", however, is difficult. Almost all epithelial cells contain glycogen from the embryonal to the neonatal period. This glycogen causes the light cytoplasm, seen by light microscopy in PTG of human fetuses and neonates. The differentiation and amount of cytoplasmic organelles increase with the developmental stage. Rough endoplasmic reticulum, Golgi complex,

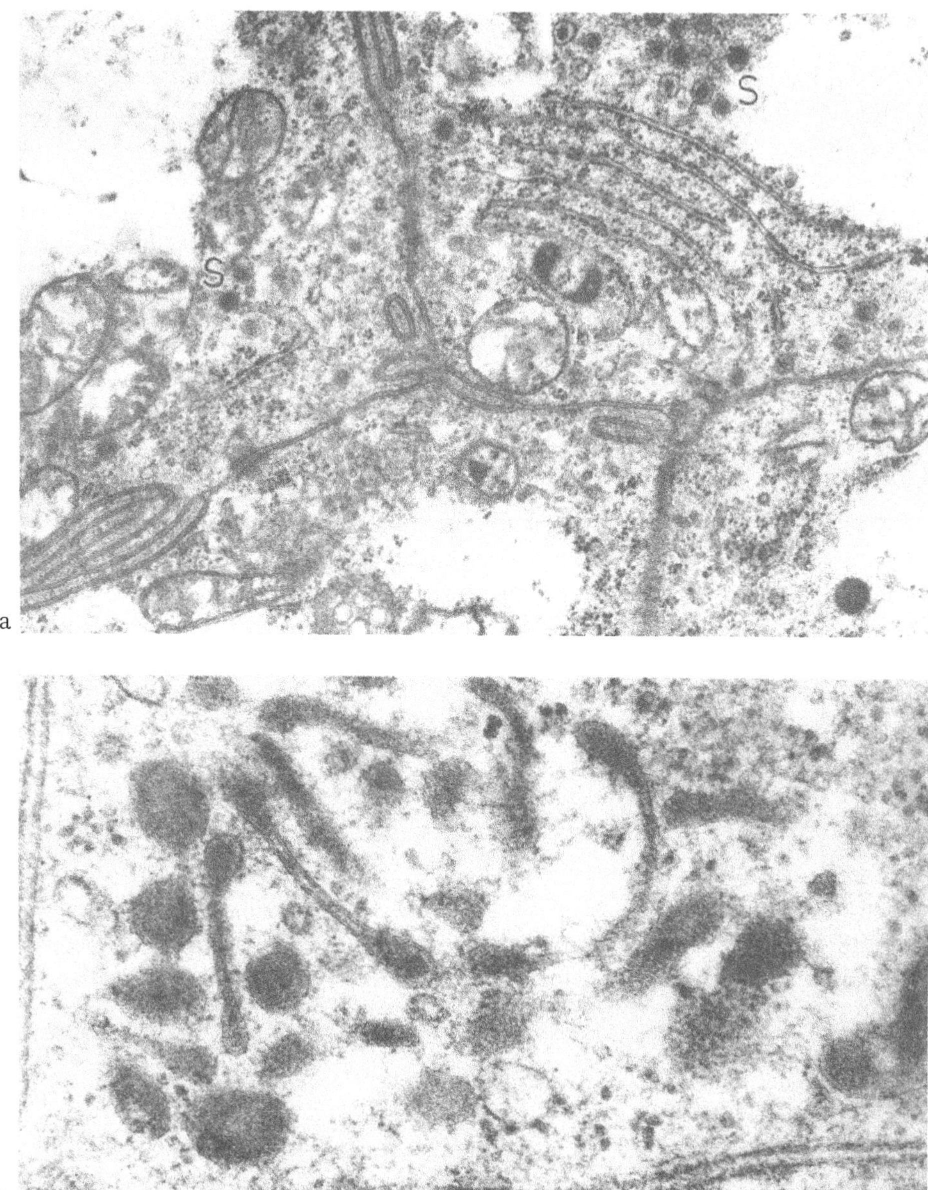

Fig. 8. a) PTG of a human neonate (48 cm, 2800 g, 7 days old): Sections of chief cells with prominent rough endoplasmic reticulum and numerous small secretory granules (S). 25000 ×. b) PTG of a human fetus (30 cm, 700 g): Membrane-bound electron-dense granules, round, oval, or dumbbell shaped. 74000 ×

mitochondria, prosecretory and secretory granules increase in size and number. Embryos, 6 cm in length, already contain sporadic secretory granules. Later the granules accumulate next to the plasma membrane. They are membrane-

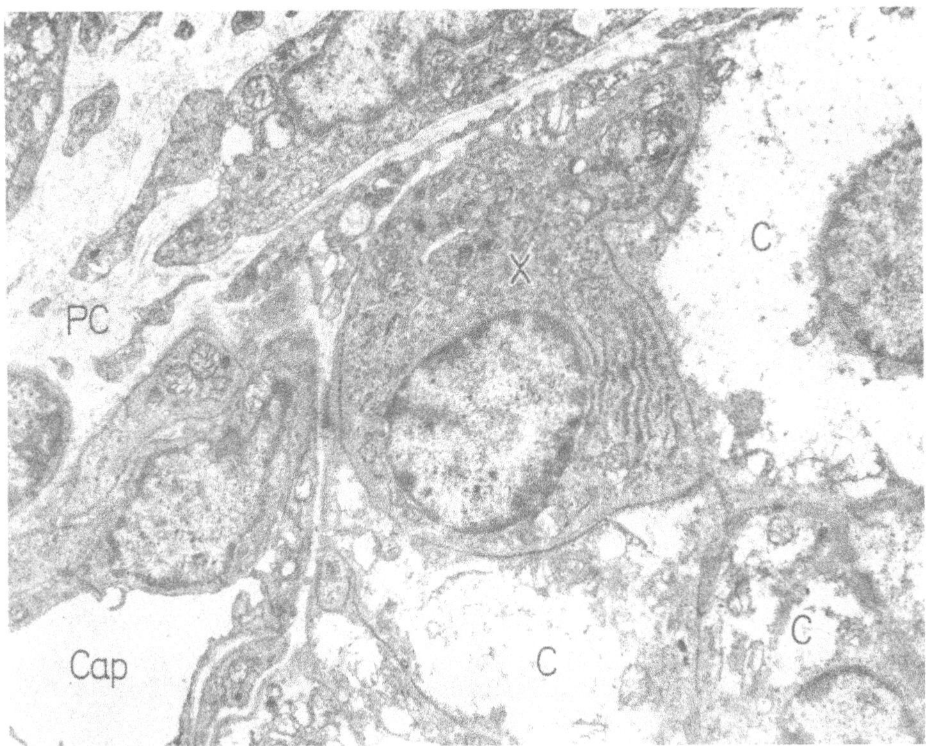

Fig. 9. PTG of a human fetus (42 cm, 1 740 g): Glycogen-free dark epithelial cell (*X*) in between light chief cells (*C*) rich in glycogen; this cell is located next to the pericapillary space (*PC*) and is covered by a basement membrane. *Cap* = capillary. 6 100 ×

bound, round to oval, more often longish or dumbbell shaped (Fig. 8b). In rat experiments, GAREL (1971) has demonstrated that fetal parathyroid hormone contributes to fetal calcium homeostasis.

A few days after parturition the PTG of human neonates, as well as those of newborn rats, show a proliferation of the Golgi complex and the rough endoplasmic reticulum, which is arranged in parallel or concentric lamellae, and an increased number of prosecretory vesicles and granules (Fig. 8a). This indicates ultrastructurally an endocrine PTG activation (ALTENÄHR and WÖHLER, 1971). A cytologic functional insufficiency at this stage is probably the reason for the transitory hypocalcaemia of some low-birth-weight infants and for the transitory hypoparathyroidism of children born to mothers with primary hyperparathyroidism (TSANG and OH, 1970; FANCONI, 1969).

We also found in human PTG of the late fetal period a special interepithelially located rare cell type, differing from the neighbouring chief cells in its glycogen-free dark cytoplasm (Fig. 9) (ALTENÄHR and WÖHLER, 1971). Judging by the differentiation of its cytoplasm, this cell does not represent one of the known functional types of human chief cells. The cells show ramification and resemble the "Adventitiazellen" described light microscopically by BARG-

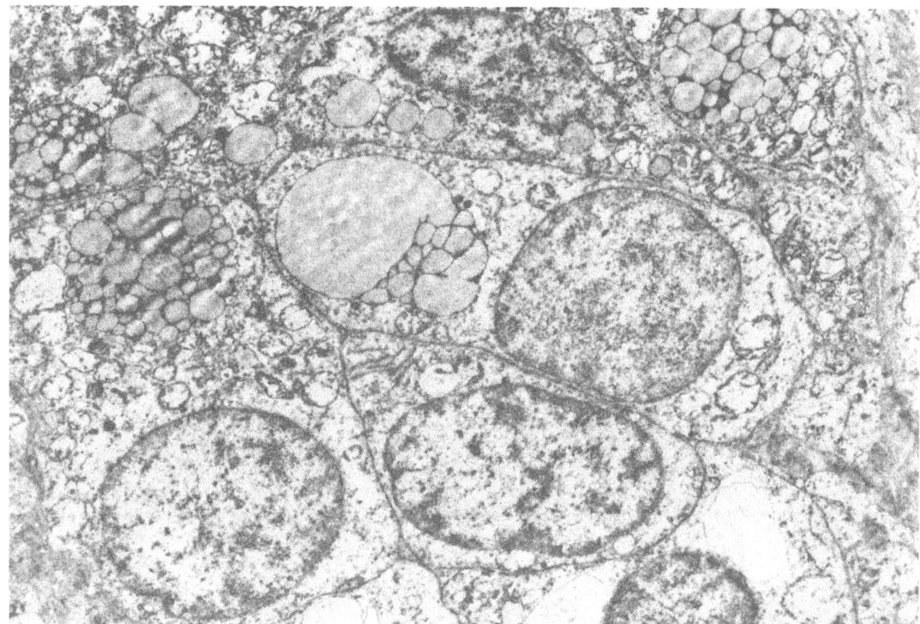

Fig. 10. Atrophic human PTG as a result of hypercalcaemia secondary to multiple myeloma: The glandular tissue mainly consists of inactive light chief cells with multiple complex lipoid bodies. 5100 ×

MANN (1939). His figures show these cells in an interepithelial position too. Since we were unable to demonstrate any relationship to perivascular cell types and since these cells are separated from the perivascular space by a basement membrane, we consider them a special type of epithelial cell of so far unknown function.

F. Ultrastructural Pathology of Human Parathyroid Glands

1. Atrophic Parathyroid Glands

In patients with a PTG adenoma, the other PTG are inactive or atrophic. The same applies to hypercalcaemias of different aetiology (Fig. 10). They show an increased number of fat cells in the light microscope, chief cells being small and dark. By electron microscopy a decrease of cytoplasmic organelles can be seen. Rough endoplasmic reticulum and hormone-producing apparatus are inconspicuous, and prosecretory and secretory granules are rare (ROTH and MUNGER, 1962; MARSHALL *et al.*, 1967; BLACK, 1969; FACCINI, 1970). The number of mitochondria varies. There is a striking increase of lipid vacuoles in cells of atrophic glands, which often aggregate to large complex lipid bodies (BLACK, 1969; BARTSCH, 1970; FACCINI, 1970; own unpublished observations). The accumulation of intracellular fat in atrophic glands supports the assumption that lipid vacuoles represent the residual bodies of lysosomal digestion of non-secreted hormone granules (HARA and NAGATSU, 1968; ROHR and KRÄSSIG, 1968; ALTENÄHR and SEIFERT, 1971). The cell membrane is straight and the nuclei are irregularly shaped, containing dense, clumped chromatin in the nuclear periphery.

2. Secondary Parathyroid Gland Hyperplasia

a) Secondary Hyperparathyroidism

Secondary hyperparathyroidism is the reaction of the PTG to another disease causing a derangement of calcium metabolism, i. e. chronic renal insufficiency, malabsorption, C-cell carcinoma (?) (BARTELHEIMER and KUHLENCORDT, 1967). At first, this hyperfunction is regulatory and suppressible (KUHLENCORDT, 1968). Stimulation and function of PTG, in the fully developed PTG hyperplasia, however, are no more in the physiological range and have to be considered pathological. Endocrine hyperactivity of secondarily hyperplastic PTG can be demonstrated cytologically by the increased size of structures active in hormone synthesis, i. e. rough endoplasmic reticulum and Golgi complex, and by the numerous prosecretory vesicles and granules near the Golgi complex (FRIES *et al.*, 1967; ROTH and MARSHALL, 1969; BLACK *et al.*, 1970; ALTENÄHR and SEIFERT, 1971). The rough endoplasmic reticulum is arranged in parallel cisterns or in concentric systems (Fig. 11). The increased tortuosity of cell membranes in human secondary hyperparathyroidism (BLACK *et al.*, 1970; ALTENÄHR and SEIFERT, 1971) corresponds to results obtained in animal experiments with different species after PTG stimulation.

Further characteristics of secondary hyperparathyroidism are the reduced number of lipid bodies and vacuoles and the more homogeneous distribution of chromatin in the nucleus (ALTENÄHR and SEIFERT, 1971). The number of mature secretory storage granules does not allow of any conclusion as regards endocrine hyperfunction (ALTENÄHR and SEIFERT, 1971). BLACK *et al.* (1970) report a diminution, others present varying results. The number of secretory granules also varies from cell to cell.

The increased amount of glycogen (Fig. 11) and/or mitochondria (Fig. 12) is also typical of cells of secondarily hyperplastic human PTG. This increased glycogen content causes the light cytoplasm of chronically stimulated light or "vacuolized" chief cells (ROTH and MARSHALL, 1969) as well as of small and large water-clear cells in secondary PTG hyperplasia (SEEMANN, 1967). It has to be pointed out that these light vacuolized chief cells, and small water-clear cells in secondary hyperparathyroidism, often contain in addition to glycogen a prominent protein-synthesizing apparatus for hormone production (Fig. 11). (ALTENÄHR and SEIFERT, 1971; FRIES *et al.*, 1967), in contrast to glycogen-containing—inactive—chief cells of normal human PTG (MUNGER and ROTH, 1963; MAZZOCCHI *et al.*, 1967). The same changes have been observed in activated PTG cells of horses with osteodystrophy (FUJIMOTO *et al.*, 1967; cf. p. 14) and in activated cat PTG following administration of a calcium-deficient diet (CAPEN and ROWLAND, 1968b). These results indicate increased activity and

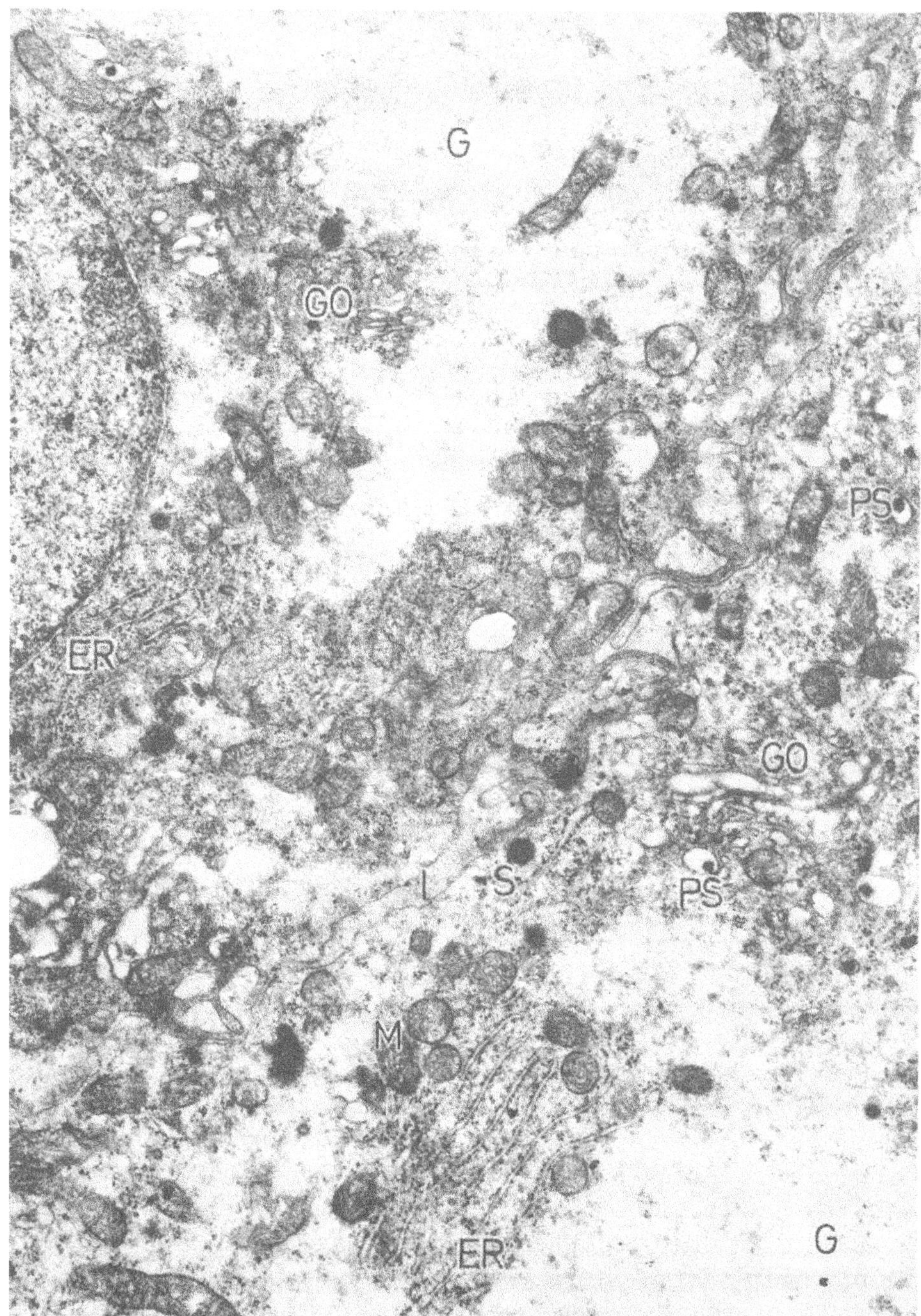

Fig. 11. Secondarily hyperplastic human PTG: Sections of activated chief cells with extended glycogen stores (*G*) and numerous cell organelles. *GO* = Golgi complex, *M* = mitochondria, *ER* = endoplasmic reticulum, *PS* = prosecretory granule, *S* = secretory granule, *I* = intercellular space. 20000 ×

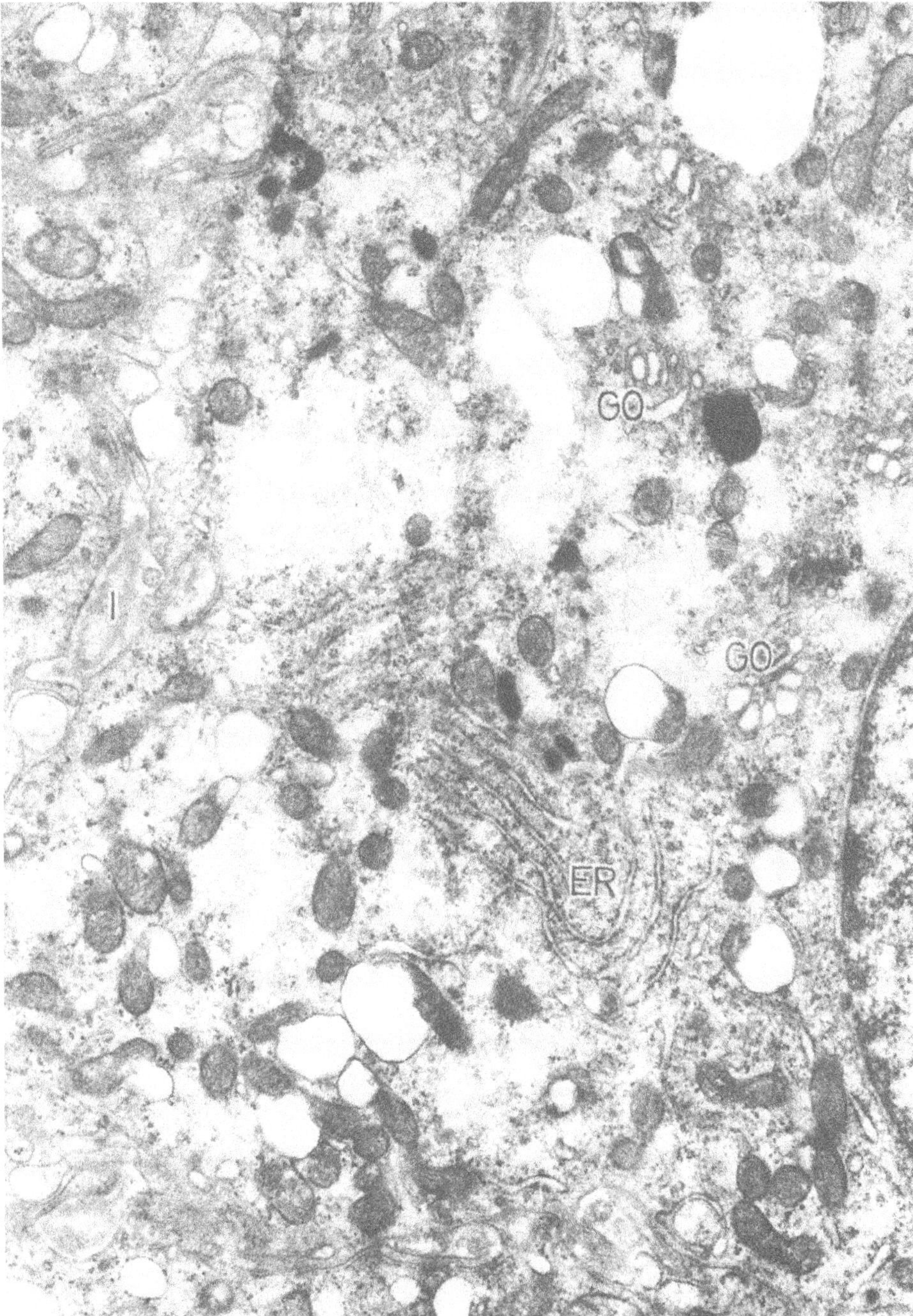

Fig. 12. Secondarily hyperplastic human PTG: Section of a transitional cell with moderate glycogen content and a moderate increase of mitochondria in addition to a prominent rough endoplasmic reticulum (*ER*) and Golgi complex (*GO*). *I* = intercellular space.
20000 ×

hormone production of these glycogen-rich cells in secondary hyperparathyroidism. It is not clear whether this increased glycogen is of functional importance relative to energy storage and production for the increased hormone synthesis (ALTENÄHR and SEIFERT, 1971), or whether it is a sign of abnormal overstimulation of these cells (FUJIMOTO *et al.*, 1967). The large water-clear cells, extremely rich in glycogen, are rare. They contain few organelles and appear to be inactive.

Secondarily hyperplastic PTG also show an increased number of transitional oxyphil cells (ROTH and MARSHALL, 1969; ALTENÄHR and SEIFERT, 1971) and oxyphil chief cells, respectively (BLACK *et al.*, 1970). Both terms describe the same type of cell: cells with numerous mitochondria occupying about 50% of the cytoplasm. In addition, these cells contain a prominent rough endoplasmic reticulum, Golgi complex, and prosecretory and secretory granules. Some of these mitochondria, however, do show changes (Fig. 13b): swelling, incorporation of fine granular material, large matrix granules, increased size up to giant mitochondria, structural changes of cristae with formation of lamellar and myelin-like structures. MAZZOCCHI *et al.* (1967a) considered similar changes in some oxyphil cells of normal PTG degenerative. Typical fully developed oxyphil cells with a cytoplasm completely filled with mitochondria and no protein-synthesizing apparatus are rare in secondarily hyperplastic PTG (Fig. 13a); they too may show changes in mitochondrial structure.

It can be summarized that in secondarily hyperplastic PTG light vacuolized chief cells rich in glycogen, small water-clear cells and oxyphil transitional cells rich in mitochondria (= oxyphil chief cells) are active endocrinically, while the extremely large water-clear and fully developed oxyphil cells do not show endocrine activity. It still has to be elucidated whether the increased content of glycogen and of mitochondria in the active cells provides energy for the increased hormone synthesis (the extreme content of glycogen or mitochondria being pathological), or whether the increase of glycogen in vacuolized chief cells and the increase of mitochondria in transitional oxyphil cells are the first indications of degenerative changes, as a result of chronic overstimulation.

b) Tertiary Hyperparathyroidism

In long-standing secondary hyperparathyroidism the regulatory character of overactivity can be lost. Hyperfunction becomes autonomous and can no longer be suppressed. This condition is called "tertiary hyperparathyroidism" (ST. GOAR, 1963; KUHLENCORDT, 1968; KUHLENCORDT and KRACHT, 1968; SEIFERT and SEEMANN, 1967). Four of the six cases described by BLACK *et al.* (1970) belong to this group of tertiary hyperparathyroidism. These authors did not observe any structural differences by light or electron microscopy between suppressible (secondary) and non-suppressible (tertiary) hyperparathyroidism. Since PTG function was again suppressible following subtotal parathyroidectomy, they assume that the autonomy in these cases is dependent on the total mass of hyperplastic gland tissue.

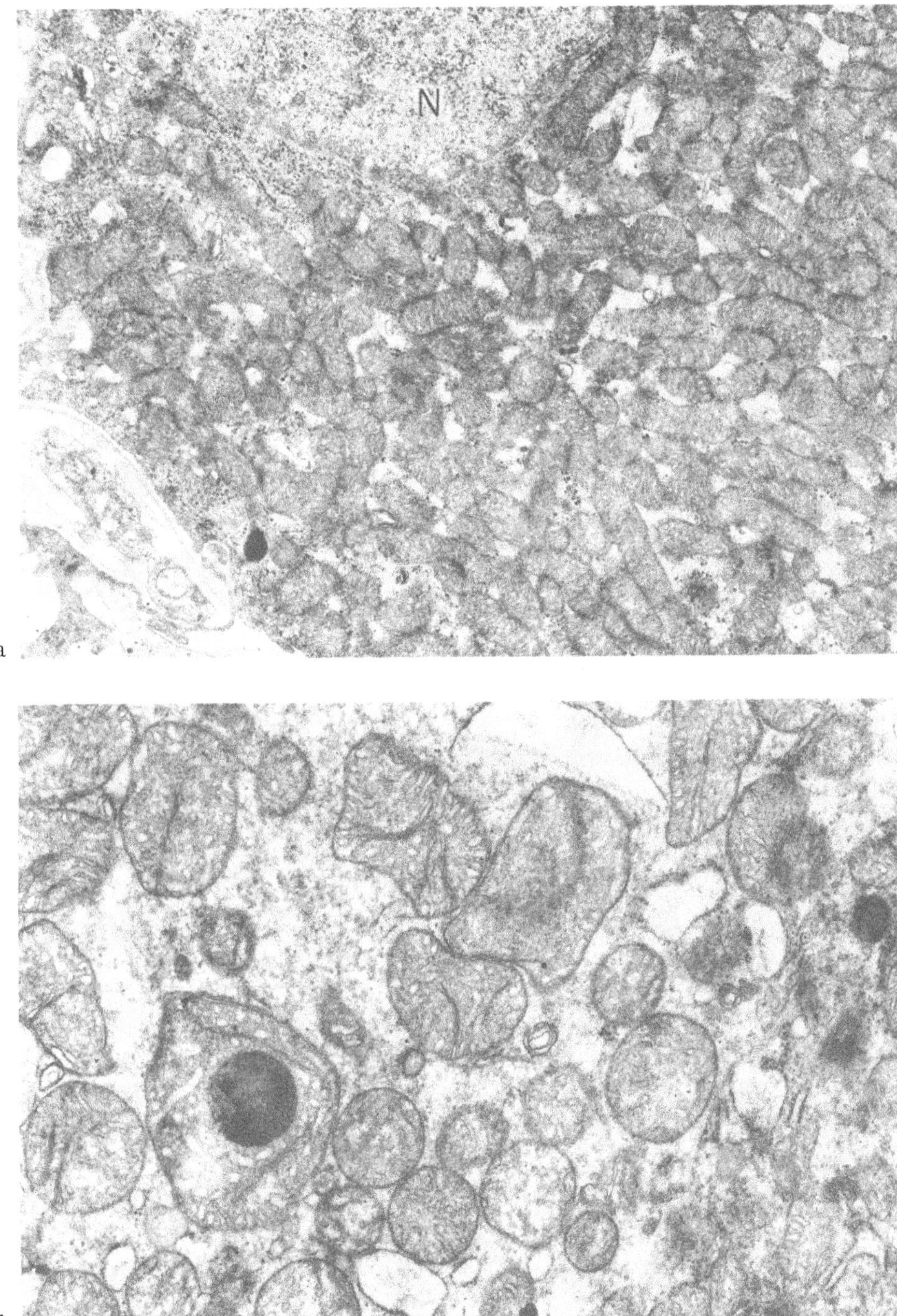

Fig. 13a and b. Secondarily hyperplastic human PTG: a) Oxyphil cell with densely packed mitochondria; an inconspicuous Golgi field can be seen in the upper left corner. N = nucleus. 15000 ×. b) Area of an oxyphil transitional cell with degenerative changes of mitochondria: increased size of the mitochondria, elongation and vacuolization of cristae mitochondriales, big electron-dense intramitochondrial body. 19000 ×

3. Primary Parathyroid Gland Hyperplasia

a) Primary Chief Cell Hyperplasia

According to older statistics, primary chief cell hyperplasia is the cause of primary hyperparathyroidism in 12% of cases (Cope, 1960; Roth, 1962; Altenähr *et al.*, 1969). According to these statistics, 6% show primary chief cell hyperplasia and 6% primary water-clear cell hyperplasia. The ultrastructural findings in primary chief cell hyperplasia correspond almost completely to those in secondary hyperplasia: increased tortuosity of cell membranes, prominent rough endoplasmic reticulum and Golgi complex, numerous prosecretory granules, presence of light cells rich in glycogen, and of oxyphil chief cells containing numerous mitochondria (Roth and Munger 1962; Weymouth and Sheridan, 1966; Weymouth and Seibel, 1969; Black and Haff, 1970; Bartsch, 1970). These ultrastructural signs of cell activation, in addition to the increase in cell number, are indications of a real PTG stimulation. The nature of the underlying stimulus is, however, unknown in primary chief cell hyperplasia.

In comparison to the more monotonous distribution of cells in secondarily hyperplastic PTG, the distribution of cells in primary chief cell hyperplasia seems more variable (Black *et al.*, 1970). Ultrastructural criteria for diagnostic differentiation between primary chief cell hyperplasia and secondary PTG hyperplasia have not yet been developed.

Electron microscopy, however, is of help for differential diagnosis of solitary PTG adenomas and primary chief cell hyperplasia. The studies of Black (1969), Black and Haff (1970), and Haff *et al.* (1970) have demonstrated differences in relation to the size of PTG in primary chief cell hyperplasia. Black and Haff (1970), therefore, differentiate between a "classical type" (enlargement of all PTG) and a "pseudoadenomatous type" (adenomatous hyperplasia of one PTG; other PTG of approximately normal size) and an "occult type" (all PTG of approximately normal size, with definite primary hyperparathyroidism). In these cases, electron microscopy is better able than light microscopy to help decide whether the glands of approximately normal size are activated in the form of primary chief cell hyperplasia, or whether the glands are normal or atrophic. Investigations of this kind have demonstrated chief cell hyperplasia in one quarter of all cases of primary hyperparathyroidism (Haff *et al.*, 1970). These results, however, have to be confirmed. Consequently a biopsy specimen of one of the "normal" PTG should be taken during exstirpation of PTG adenomas, and should be investigated by light or–if possible–electron microscopy, in order to exclude pseudoadenomatous hyperplasia.

b) Primary Water-Clear Cell Hyperplasia

In contrast to secondary hyperparathyroidism, the light cytoplasm in primary water-clear cell hyperplasia is not due to glycogen, but to numerous vacuoles (HOLZMANN and LANGE, 1963; SHELDON, 1964; ROTH, 1970; FACCINI, 1970). Their diameter is 0,2—0,5μ. The wall of these vacuoles is a triple-layered unit membrane (HOLZMANN and LANGE, 1963; ROTH, 1970). The function and formation of these vacuoles is unknown. They are considered to be lipoid vacuoles (HOLZMANN and LANGE, 1963), extended Golgi cisterns (ROTH, 1970) or extended degranulated cisterns of rough—or smooth—endoplasmic reticulum (FACCINI, 1970). Since fine granular material can be observed on occasion in these vacuoles, a possible relationship to secretory granules is discussed (SHELDON, 1964; ROTH, 1970). The water-clear cells contain varying amounts of mitochondria, rough and smooth endoplasmic reticulum, Golgi complex and normal secretory granules.

The water-clear cell, rich in vacuoles, is of diagnostic significance because this cell type has not yet been observed in normal or secondarily hyperplastic PTG. Among the numerous ultrastructurally documented PTG adenomas, this type of cell has been described only once (MITROVIC *et al.*, 1967).

In addition to the typical water-clear cells containing numerous vacuoles, several authors also found chief cells (ROTH, 1970), oxyphil cells (HOLZMANN and LANGE, 1963) and intermediate forms with fewer and smaller vacuoles (ROTH, 1970; FACCINI, 1970) in primary water-clear cell hyperplasia.

4. Parathyroid Gland Adenomas

a) Chief Cell Adenomas and Mixed Adenomas

Chief cell adenomas consist predominantly of cells similar to chief cells. That means that the number of mitochondria, as well as the content of glycogen, is limited. None of these cytoplasmic constituents dominates the character of the cell. They are well mixed with the other cytoplasmic components. The details of the adenomas described by different authors, however, vary to such an extent that it is difficult to extract common criteria for the ultrastructure of PTG adenomas (Figs. 14–17).

There are also prosecretory granules and vesicles near the Golgi region in adenoma cells. In addition, the cytoplasm contains electron-dense secretory granules of such different size and form that HOLZMANN and LANGE (1963) have tried to classify these granules. According to ALTENÄHR and SEIFERT (1971), the form and size of the granules in adenoma cells only partly correspond to those of normal PTG cells. A close association and fusion of granules with lipid vacuoles can often be observed (Fig. 14). We consider it improbable that the large intramitochondrial granules represent secretory material (WEYMOUTH and SHERIDAN, 1966; WEYMOUTH and SEIBEL, 1969). Electron-dense query secretory granules can also be observed in endothelial cells, and rarely in the perivascular space (Fig. 14 Inset) (ROTH and MUNGER, 1962; WEYMOUTH and SHERIDAN, 1966). We observed in one of our adenomas cell processes protruding into the perivascular space containing electron-dense granules (Fig. 14) (ALTENÄHR and SEIFERT, 1971). These cell protrusions

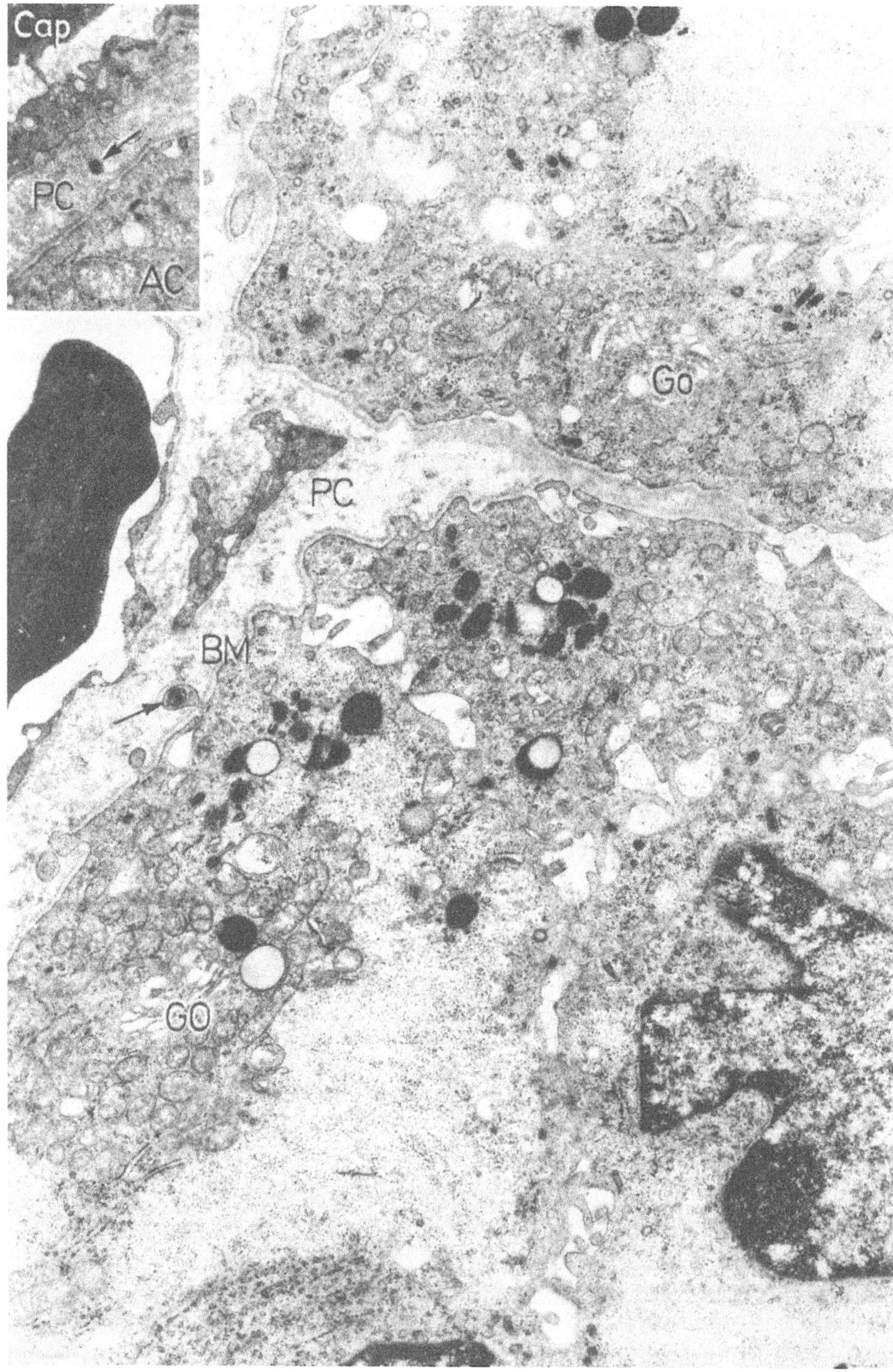

Fig. 14. Human PTG adenoma: Adenoma cells with glycogen-rich areas and other areas rich in mitochondria or secretory granules; small Golgi fields (*GO*); indented nucleus; protrusion of cytoplasmic processes into the pericapillary space (*PC*), partly containing an electron-dense granule (arrow). *BM* = basement membrane. 14000 ×. Inset: Free electron-dense granule (arrow) in the pericapillary space (*PC*) between capillary (*Cap*) and adenoma cell (*AC*). 12000 ×

seem to be detached from the cell body with the granules. This corresponds to the mode of secretion observed in pigs (FETTER and CAPEN, 1968, 1970).

In comparison to normal PTG, some adenomas show a prominent rough endoplasmic reticulum, either in all cells or in individual cells only (Fig. 17). It is often arranged in parallel rows or concentric rings (LANGE, 1961; ROTH and MUNGER, 1962; MARSHALL et al., 1967; ELLIOTT and ARHELGER, 1967; BLACK, 1969; FACCINI, 1970; ALTENÄHR and SEIFERT, 1971). The Golgi complex, too, often is increased in size (ROTH and MUNGER, 1962; WEYMOUTH and SHERIDAN, 1966; ELLIOTT and ARHELGER, 1967; BLACK, 1969). Sometimes an increased number of prosecretory and secretory granules (ROTH and MUNGER, 1962; WEYMUTH and SHERIDAN, 1966) and an increased tortuosity of cell membranes (BLACK, 1969; FACCINI, 1970) are described as further signs of cell activation.

Therefore, some authors consider the adenomatous cell to be endocrinically activated (ROTH and MUNGER, 1962; WEYMOUTH and SHERIDAN, 1966; WEYMOUTH and SEIBEL, 1969; BLACK, 1969; FACCINI, 1970). On the other hand, complex lipid bodies consisting of a conglomeration of lipid vacuoles can be observed, as in normal and atrophic PTG (ROTH and MUNGER, 1962; WEYMOUTH and SHERIDAN, 1966; ELLIOTT and ARHELGER, 1967; MARSHALL et al., 1967; BLACK, 1969; ALTENÄHR and SEIFERT, 1971). The glycogen content and number of mitochondria vary to a great extent and are increased predominantly in the clear and oxyphil cells, respectively, of mixed adenomas. The cells of PTG adenomas show such a great variation in their contents of different cell organelles that any generalization regarding their endocrine activity does not seem possible. The adenomas reported by us (ALTENÄHR and SEIFERT, 1971) contained, for example, a prominent rough endoplasmic reticulum, but a less well-developed Golgi complex. It seems possible that there may be adenomas with normal or even reduced endocrine activity of the individual cells. Apart from the highly variable serum level of parathyroid hormone in primary hyperparathyroidism (BERSON and YALOW, 1966; MELICK and MARTIN, 1968; POTTS et al., 1969), hyperparathyroidism also seems possible, in spite of normal or reduced hormone secretion by the individual cell, because of the absolute increase in cell number (ALTENÄHR and SEIFERT, 1971; MARSHALL et al., 1967). No investigations relating ultrastructure of adenomas and clinical severity of primary hyperparathyroidism and serum level of parathyroid hormone have been performed so far. FACCINI (1970) only reports that PTG adenomas were larger and appeared ultrastructurally more active in patients with clinically manifest bone involvement, than in patients with nephrolithiasis only.

Some PTG adenomas are characterized by the presence of annulate lamellae (Fig. 15). So far, they have been described in six PTG adenomas (ELLIOTT and ARHELGER, 1967; MARSHALL et al., 1967; BOQUIST, 1970; ALTENÄHR and SEIFERT, 1971). Since they have not been found in other

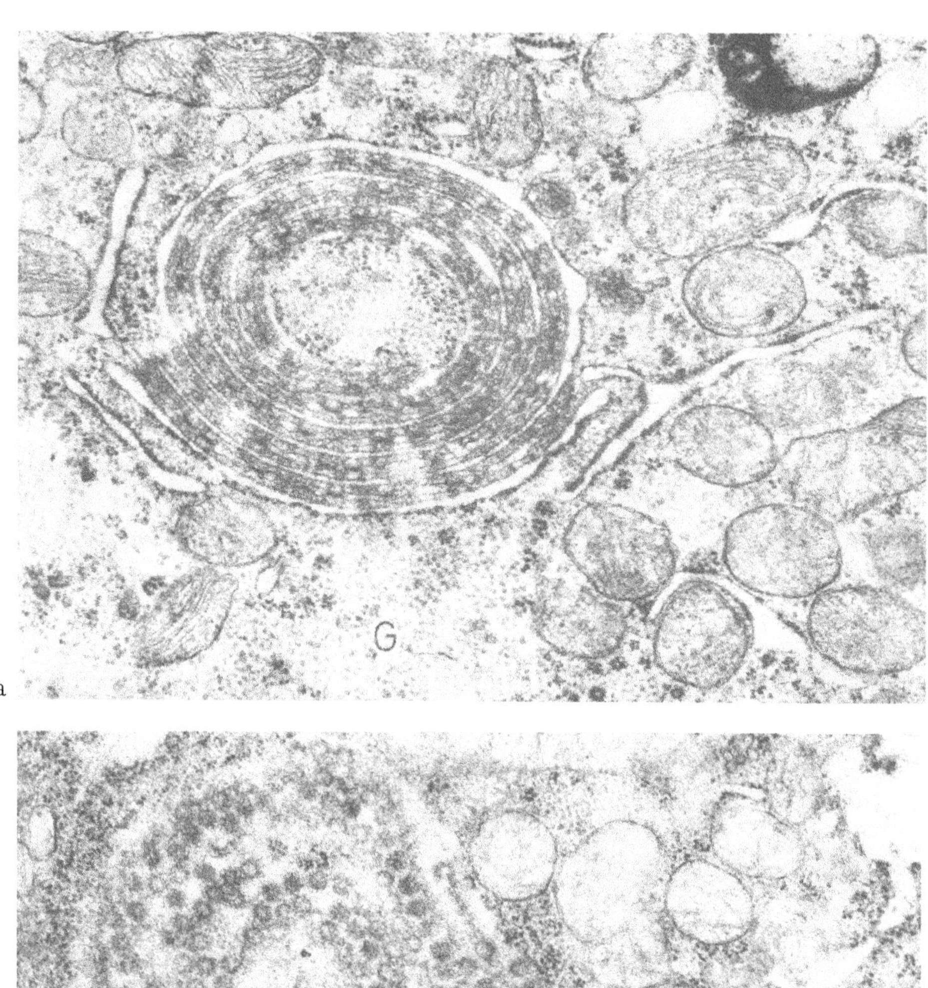

Fig. 15a and b. Human PTG adenoma with annulate lamellae: a) Section through whorl-like annulate lamellae with extension into the rough endoplasmic reticulum and near mitochondria. G = Glycogen. 28000 ×. b) Tangential section of annulate lamellae; view of the sieve-like pattern of pores. 28000 ×

pathological conditions of the PTG, they could be a specific criterion for diagnosis of an adenoma. Annulate lamellae are mainly seen in parallel lamellar systems, interrupted by numerous pores. These pores give a sieve-like pattern (Fig. 15 b). Sometimes there are light fissures between lamellae, and the annulate lamellae can open on to cisterns of the rough endoplasmic reticulum. Similar to the parallel systems of the rough endoplasmic reticulum, the annulate lamellae are extended, wound, arranged concentrically, whorl-like (Fig. 15 a), or in a semicircle. They are located close to mitochondria.

Therefore, some authors consider the annulate lamellae a pathological form or precursor of the endoplasmic reticulum, or a product derived from endoplasmic reticulum. Others discuss the nuclear membrane as the origin of annulate lamellae, with mitochondria participating in their formation (BOQUIST, 1970). We consider the annulate lamellae of PTG adenomas a sign of fast, accelerated or pathological cell proliferation (ALTENÄHR and SEIFERT, 1971) because annulate lamellae can be observed in other organs and species in immature cells, as a result of chemical alterations, or in tumour cells. MARSHALL *et al.* (1967) also suggest induction by the [75]selenium methionine used in PTG scintigraphy. Because of their similarity and position relative to the rough endoplasmic reticulum, annulate lamellae may play a role in protein and hormone synthesis in these adenoma cells.

As in normal and hyperplastic PTG, many authors also describe occasional cilia in adenoma cells. The arrangement of their filaments is of the $(9 + 0)$ type. They mostly lie within the cells and rarely extend above the cell surface. They are, however, mostly surrounded by an invaginated plasmalemma and therefore do protrude into the extracellular space. Real intracellular cilia are assumed to be present in adenomas only (POLYZONIS, 1970). The finding of an increased number of cilia in adenomas as compared to normal PTG (POLYZONIS, 1970) cannot be generalized.

The form, size, and chromatin distribution of nuclei in PTG adenoma cells vary to a great extent between adenomas and between different cells of the same adenoma, as can also be observed by light microscopy (CASTLEMAN, 1952; ALTENÄHR and DAMMANN, 1971). The chromatin in some nuclei is evenly distributed, forming a loose structure; in others it is condensed near the nuclear membrane (ROTH and MUNGER, 1962; MARSHALL *et al.*, 1967; FACCINI, 1970; ALTENÄHR and SEIFERT, 1971). The nuclear membrane shows pores. The size of the nucleoli varies, displaying a prominent pars amorpha of variable size. The nucleonema is more compact in some nuclei (LANGE, 1961; FACCINI, 1970). Mitoses have not been described in adenoma cells electron microscopically. If mitoses are seen by light microscopy, their presence is highly suggestive of carcinoma (BLACK, 1954; ALTENÄHR and DAMMANN, 1971).

Mixed PTG adenomas contain, in addition to the described types of chief cells, light and water-clear cells (Fig. 16) and/or oxyphil cells with all transitional forms (Fig. 17). The cytoplasm of light and water-clear adenoma cells

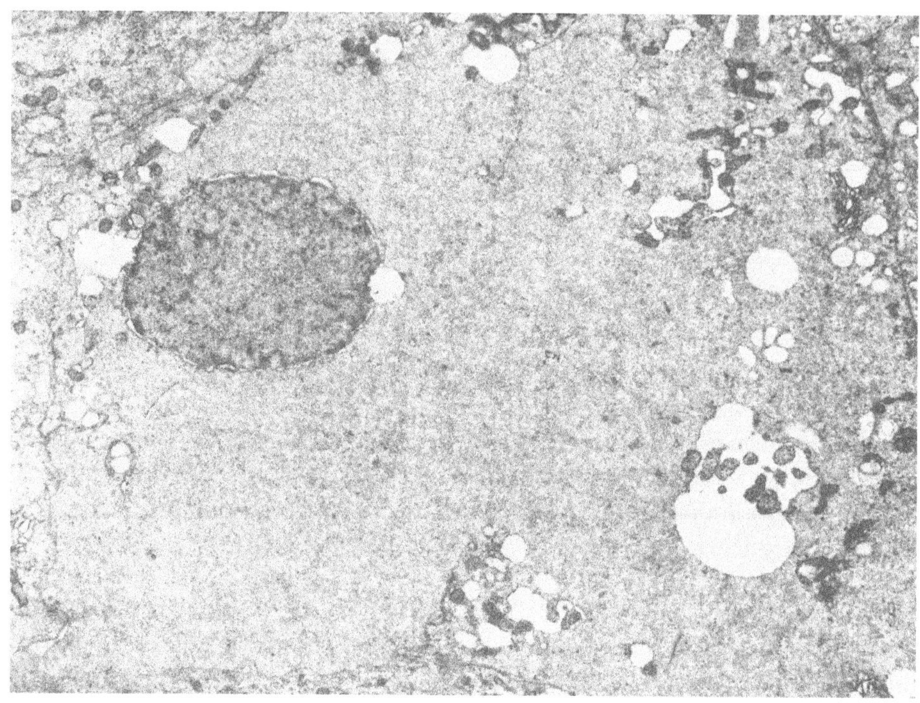

Fig. 16. Human PTG adenoma with mixed cell types: Water-clear adenoma cell. The cytoplasm is almost completely filled with glycogen. Some vacuoles are apparently of mitochondrial origin. 5700 ×

is characterized by an increased glycogen content (LANGE, 1961; ROTH and MUNGER, 1962; BLACK, 1969). The relative and absolute content of other cell components varies, resulting in transitional cell types intermediate between water-clear cells, chief cells, and oxyphil cells. MITROVIC *et al.* (1967) describe, in addition, clear adenoma cells containing numerous vesicles and vacuoles, resembling the cells in water-clear cell hyperplasia.

Large numbers of mitochondria in the cytoplasm cause the typical eosinophilic granulation of oxyphil cells observed in the light microscope in normal glands, as well as in hyperplastic and adenomatous PTG. Changes in mitochondrial structure are similar, too, in the oxyphil cells of mixed PTG adenomas (LANGE, 1961; ALTENÄHR and SEIFERT, 1971). The nuclei of oxyphil cells in adenomas sometimes show a nucleolus, in contrast to normal PTG. A further difference is the fact, that rough endoplasmic reticulum, Golgi complex and secretory granules, although not prominent, can be observed in the oxyphil cells of adenomas in between mitochondria and glycogen (Fig. 17) (ROTH and MUNGER, 1962; BLACK, 1969). Typical fully developed oxyphil cells without Golgi complex and endoplasmic reticulum seem to be very rare in adenomas. The greater the content of other organelles, relative to the mitochondria, the more these cells resemble transitional oxyphil cells or oxyphil chief cells.

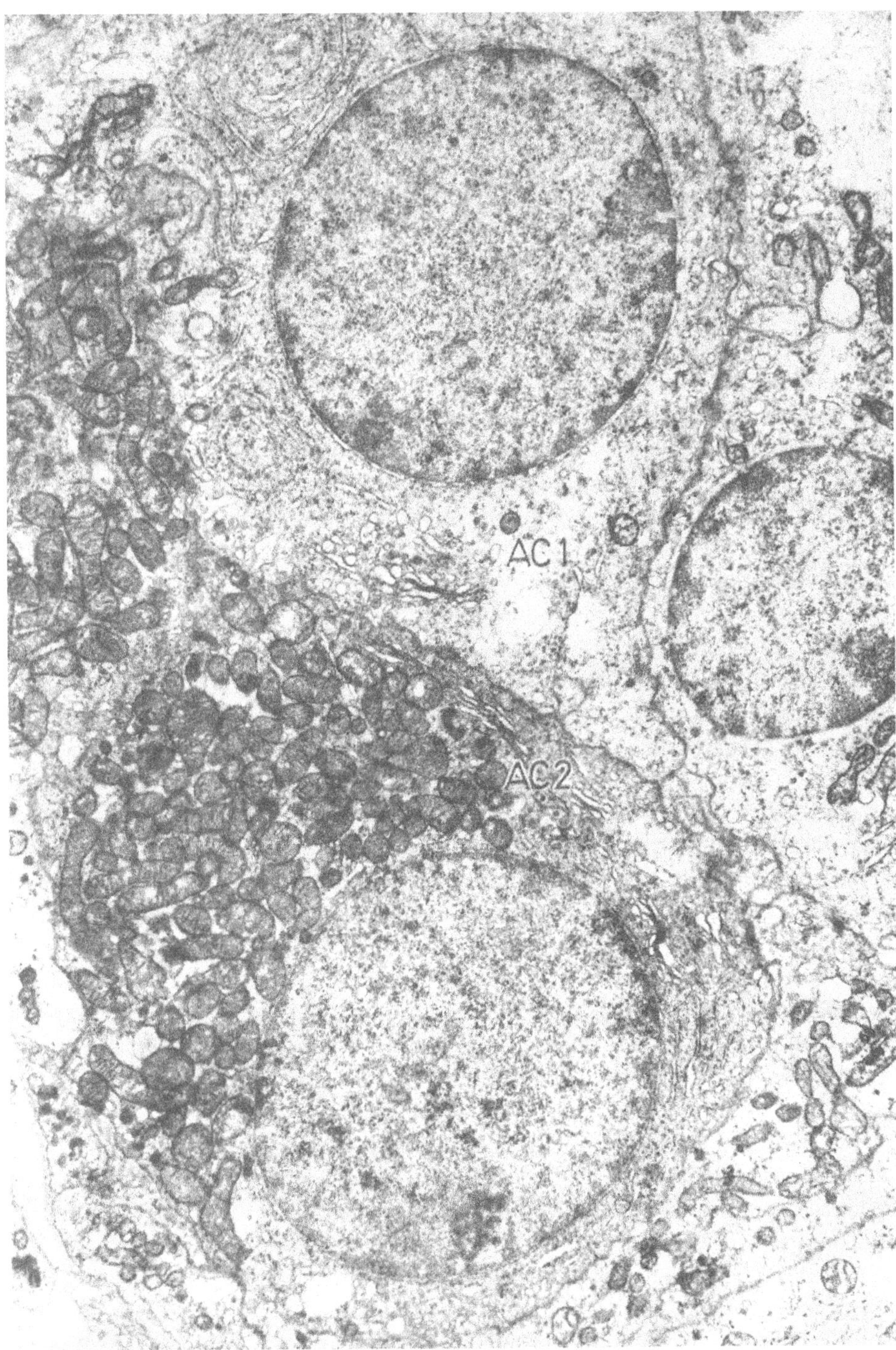

Fig. 17. Human PTG adenoma with mixed cell types: Adenoma cells with varying distribution of cytoplasmic organelles, AC 1 containing a prominent endoplasmic reticulum and a moderately developed Golgi complex, AC 2 containing an oxyphil area with closely packed mitochondria, and an area with Golgi complex and moderately developed rough endoplasmic reticulum. 10000 ×

The varying cell structure in PTG adenomas possibly reflects neoplastic growth and absence of regulation. Although there exists a specific relationship between light microscopic cell type and ultrastructurally demonstrable cell activity in normal or secondarily stimulated PTG, these rules cannot be applied to adenomatous cells (Holzmann and Lange, 1963; Altenähr and Seifert, 1971). The varying cell structure of adenomas and their range of variation might also be related to the age and size of adenomas, possibly because of disturbed nutrition (Lange, 1961). Marshall *et al.* (1967) discuss the possibility that the differences between adenomas observed by these authors are caused by earlier [75]selenium methionine scintigraphy of the PTG. They observed the greatest alteration of cell structure 9 to 10 days following [75]selenium methionine administration. Most of their observations relate to the endoplasmic reticulum, Golgi complex, mitochondria, and the presence of annulate lamellae. The basis for their assumption is the fact that the γ-ray-emitting [75]selenium methionine is incorporated into PTG cells and into parathyroid hormone. According to our observations, however, these multiple variations in organelle distribution in adenomatous cells are also present where scintigraphy has not been performed.

The intercellular contacts between adenoma cells and the interstitial spaces in adenomas resemble those of normal PTG. The areas of contact between two cells often show interdigitations and desmosomes. While only desmosomes of the macula adhaerens type have been described by most authors, Elliott and Arhelger (1967) also observed septate desmosomes which normally only occur in invertebrates. They therefore suggest, that septate desmosomes are immature precursors of desmosomes of the macula adhaerens type. Acini of adenoma cells with intraluminal microvilli are described by Lange (1961), Weymouth and Sheridan (1966), Black (1969) and Altenähr and Seifert (1971). Adenoma cells, too, are covered by a basement membrane towards the blood-vessel-containing interstitial space. The pericapillary space is widened in some adenomas. It contains collagen fibres, fibroblasts and fibrocytes, and occasionally mast cells. Roth and Munger (1962) and Elliott and Arhelger (1967) described unmyelinated nerve fibres in the pericapillary space. We did not observe nerves in the adenomas (Altenähr and Seifert, 1971) but it is possible of course that vegetative nerves grow along proliferated vessels into the adenomas.

PTG adenomas can partly resemble secondarily and primarily hyperplastic PTG (Altenähr and Seifert, 1971; Black, 1969). This specially applies to adenomas with fa fairly constant cell type and cytological signs of cell activation. Specific ultrastructural criteria for differential diagnosis of PTG adenomas have not yet been developed. Therefore it is still necessary to look histologically for an atrophic rim in PTG tumors. Furthermore, all other PTG need to be checked macroscopically during operation. To confirm the diagnosis, histological and/or ultrastructural investigation of biopsy specimens from the other PTG is recommended (cf. p. 26f). It can generally be concluded that some adenomas are characterized by their more varied structure of nuclei

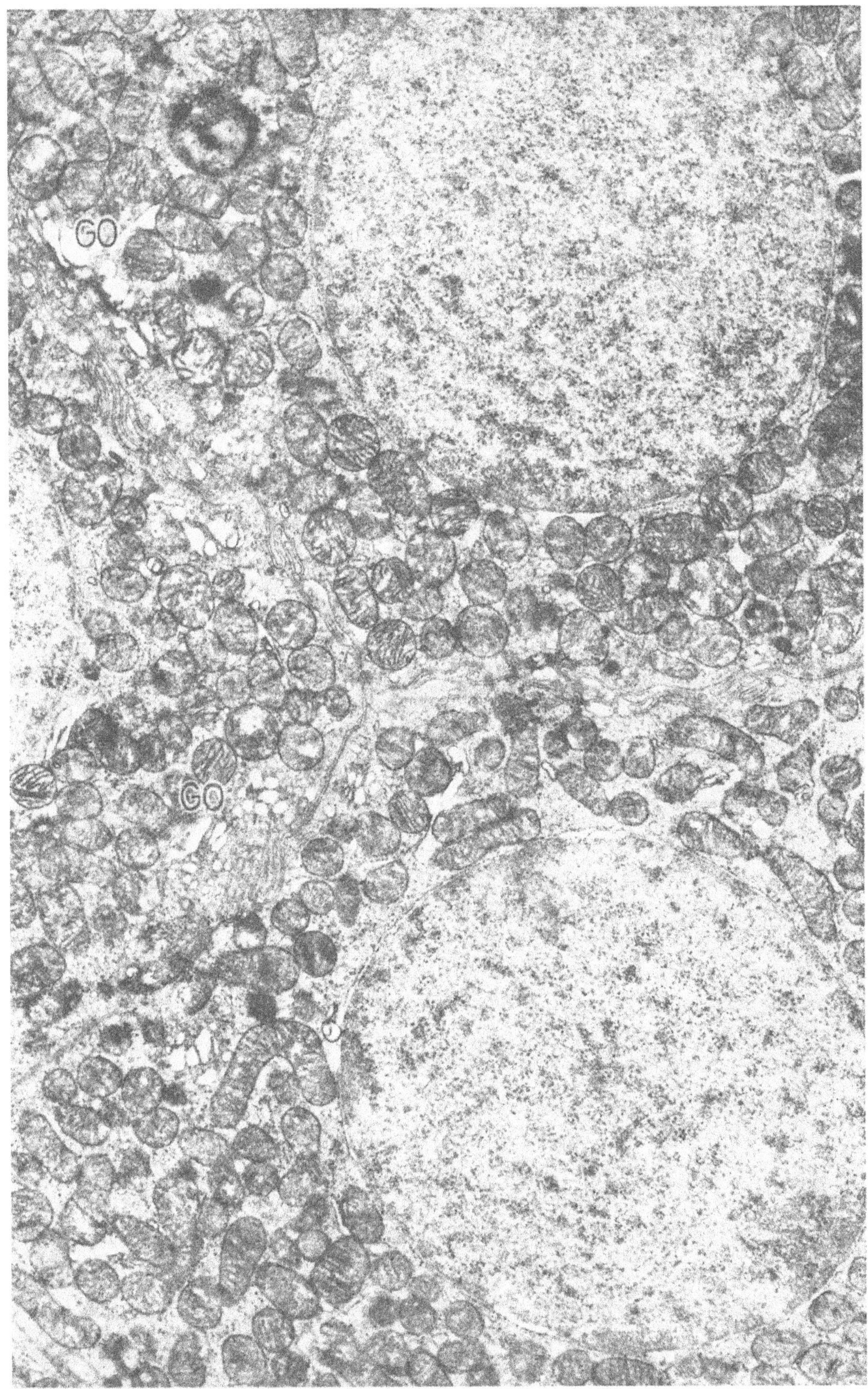

Fig. 18. Human oxyphil PTG adenoma: Oxyphil cells with densely packed mitochondria and small areas with a Golgi complex (*GO*), probably related to hormone synthesis in endocrinically active oxyphil adenomas. 11 500 ×

and distribution of cell organelles as against the more homogeneous hyperplastic PTG (BLACK, 1969; ALTENÄHR and SEIFERT, 1971).

b) Oxyphil Parathyroid Adenomas

Oxyphil PTG adenomas occupy a special position because many adenomas of this group do not show endocrine activity (BLACK and ACKERMANN, 1950). They are detected only by chance or because of their size. However, other oxyphil adenomas show endocrine activity, and cause primary hyperparathyroidism (SOMMERS and YOUNG, 1952). No ultrastructural studies of oxyphil adenomas without endocrine activity have been carried out so far, but the ultrastructure of five oxyphil adenomas associated with primary hyperparathyroidism has been studied (ROTH *et al.*, 1962; SELZMAN and FECHNER, 1967; FACCINI, 1970; HEIMANN *et al.*, 1971; own unpublished observation). These tumours consist of oxyphil cells rich in mitochondria (Fig. 18). None of these adenomas, however, contained exclusively typical fully developed oxyphil cells. Even by light microscopy it was possible to observe transitional oxyphil cells. Electron microscopic demonstration of rough endoplasmic reticulum, Golgi complex, prosecretory and secretory granules confirmed the light microscopic observation. The presence of hormone-producing apparatus explains the endocrine activity of these tumours. Possibly, oxyphil PTG adenomas without endocrine activity consist of typical oxyphil cells without other cell organelles than mitochondria.

5. Parathyroid Gland Carcinoma

Electron microscope studies of PTG carcinomas have been published only by FACCINI (1970; 4 cases). The organelle distribution resembled cellular activation. The endoplasmic reticulum was extended and often dilated, the Golgi complex very prominent and there were numerous secretory granules in the cell periphery. The agranular reticulum was augmented, too, and partly difficult to separate from the Golgi complex. Centrioles and cilia were not observed by FACCINI (1970). Plasma membranes showed increased tortuosity and interdigitations. Strikingly rare were desmosomes between adjacent cells.

The most prominent changes were present in nuclei and nucleoli of carcinoma cells: extreme differences in nuclear size and form, frequent lack of nuclear membrane, irregularly condensed chromatin, hypertrophy and increased electron density of nucleoli, condensation of nucleonemata, enlarged and duplicated pars amorpha with microtubular structures. Striking changes of nuclear structure and atypical nuclei have also been observed in benign adenomas (FACCINI, 1970; ALTENÄHR and DAMMANN, 1971; ALTENÄHR and SEIFERT, 1971). Further studies are necessary in order to evaluate the significance of alterations in nucleoli structure for the diagnosis of carcinomas. Since mitoses can only be observed in carcinomas and not in adenomas by means of light microscopy (BLACK, 1954; ALTENÄHR and DAMMANN, 1971), the frequently noted absence of the nuclear membrane (FACCINI, 1970), corresponding to a prophase, could be of relevance for carcinoma diagnosis.

G. Prospects

PTG in idiopathic human hypoparathyroidism have not yet been studied electron microscopically. It can be assumed that cytological analysis by electron microscopy will contribute a great deal to studies of its aetiology. No ultrastructural investigations of endocrinically inactive oxyphil adenomas have been done, either, nor have PTG carcinomas been satisfactorily studied by electron microscopy. The aim must be to develop definite cytological criteria for differential diagnosis of primary chief cell hyperplasia, PTG adenomas and PTG carcinomas.

Cytochemical studies will be necessary in the future to correlate ultra-structural analysis and endocrine activity of cells to a further extent. In this respect, the intracellular enzyme pattern is of interest, as well the incorporation of substrates by the cell and their metabolism and catabolism. Immunocyto-chemical methods seem to be of special importance for the study of cellular production, storage and secretion of parathyroid hormone. The function-dependent cytological characteristics of the endocrine PTG cells favour further ultrastructural investigation of nerve function in PTG.

H. Summary

Ultrastructural investigation of PTG in animal experiments has established criteria allowing cytological evaluation of the endocrine activity of single cells and of the whole gland. This evaluation is based on the varying development of the protein- and proteohormone-synthesizing apparatus. The endocrine activity of PTG has been studied in different experimental models and it has been ultrastructurally confirmed that the calcium level of serum or culture media is the most important factor in the endocrine regulation of PTG. A nervous regulation seems possible, because of the demonstrated nerve fibres and neuroepithelial synapses; it has, however, not been experimentally con-firmed as yet.

Basically, human PTG show corresponding function-dependent ultra-structural changes. In addition, there are characteristic differences in the glycogen, mitochondria and lipid contents which are not found in most animal species, and which allow differentiation of cell types. The cells of human PTG show a quantitative distribution of cell organelles which is typical of either normal, atrophic or secondarily hyperplastic PTG. Findings obtained in tertiary hyperparathyroidism and primary chief cells hyperplasia are similar to those in secondary hyperparathyroidism. The distribution of cell organelles in PTG adenomas is so variable that it has not been possible to find any definite quantitative criteria common to all adenomas. This appears to be the result of neoplastic, non-regulated tumour growth. Oxyphil adenomas seem to be active only when oxyphil cells contain a protein-synthesizing apparatus or when transitional oxyphil cells are present.

Human PTG in idiopathic hypoparathyroidism have not yet been studied and human PTG carcinomas only inadequately.

Table 1. *Electron microscopic communications on Parathyroid Glands (PTG) in various animal species and under various conditions. (Summarized review of the literature)*

Authors	Species	Conditions (normal, physiologically different, experimental, pathological)	Endocrine Activity of PTG (cytologically)
ALTENÄHR (1970)	rat	normal controls	normal
		parathyroid hormone injections (acute, chronic)	suppressed
		dihydrotachysterol per os	suppressed
		low calcium and low phosphorus diet	stimulated
		low calcium diet	stimulated
		ferric-glycerophosphate injections	stimulated
		thyrocalcitonin injections (chronic)	stimulated
ALTENÄHR and LIETZ (1970)	rat	(same as ALTENÄHR, 1970) comparison with thyroid C-cell ultrastructure	
ALTENÄHR and WÖHLER (1971)	rat	fetal period (16th-22nd day)	low activity
		neonatal period	raised activity
CAPEN ct al. (1965 a)	cow	normal, nonpregnant, nonlactating	normal
		pregnant, at calculated date of parturition, non lactating	activated
		20 hours after parturition, lactating	activated
CAPEN et al. (1965 b)	cow	nonpregnant, nonlactating; high dosage of vitamin D per os	atrophic
CAPEN et al. (1968)		pregnant, at calculated date of parturition, non-lactating; high dosage of vitamin D per os	inactive
		20 hours after parturition, lactating high dosage of vitamin D per os	inactive
CAPEN and ROWLAND (1968 a)	young cat	normal, rapidly growing	active
CAPEN and ROWLAND (1968 b)	young cat	normal rapidly growing controls	active
		calcium-deficient diet	stimulated

Table 1 (Continued)

Authors	Species	Conditions (normal, physiologically different, experimental, pathological)	Endocrine Activity of PTG (cytologically)
CAPEN and YOUNG (1967)	cow	postpartum controls parturient paresis with hypocalcemia	active even more activated
COLEMAN (1969)	Xenopus laevis (DAUDIN)	larvae young, mature toads young, mature toads living in 1 % CaCl$_2$ solution	active normal inactive
CORTELYOU and McWHINNIE (1967)	Rana pipiens	normal, mature frogs	normal
DAVIS and ENDERS (1961)	rat	normal controls bilateral nephrectomy	normal stimulated
DUNAY *et al.* (1969)	rat	accessory PTG within the thymus	normal
EKHOLM (1957)	mouse	normal	normal
FACCINI and CARE (1965)	sheep	normal controls high fluoride concentration of drinking water	normal stimulated (hyperplasia)
FETTER and CAPEN (1968)	pig	normal controls atrophic rhinitis	normal slightly activated
FETTER and CAPEN (1970)	pig	normal, rapidly growing	relatively inactive
FUJIMOTO *et al.* (1967)	horse	normal, with immature bone normal, with mature bone osteodystrophia fibrosa	normal normal activated
HARA and NAGATSU-ISHIBASHI (1964)	mouse	normal	normal
HARA and NAGATSU (1968)	rat	normal controls parathyroid hormone injections (various doses)	normal suppressed

Table 1 (Continued)

Authors	Species	Conditions (normal, physiologically different, experimental, pathological)	Endocrine Activity of PTG (cytologically)
HATAKEYAMA *et al.* (1970)	rat	dihydrotachysterol and calcium acetate per os	formation of parathyroid cysts
KAYSER *et al.* (1961)	hamster	seasonal comparison: June	relatively inactive
		September	active
		November	active
KLOTZ *et al.* (1966)	dog	normal controls	normal
		vitamin D injections	normal
		sodium phytate per os	normal
LANGE and VAN BREHM (1965)	Rana temporaria	normal	normal
	Bufo vulgaris	normal	normal
		phosphate injections	stimulated
LEVER (1957)	rat	normal	normal
LEVER (1958)	rat	normal controls	normal
		unilateral parathyroidectomy	sligthly activated
		unilateral parathyroidectomy plus parathyroid hormone	normal
		phosphate injections	stimulated
		bilateral nephrectomy	stimulated
LUPULESCU *et al.* (1968)	dog	normal controls	normal
		iso-immune-hypoparathyroidism by injection of para-thyroid-iso-antibody containing serum	structure of glands and cells damaged
MAZZOCCHI *et al.* (1967b)	rat	normal controls	normal
		rachitogenic diet	stimulated
		bilateral nephrectomy	stimulated

Table 1 (Continued)

Authors	Species	Conditions (normal, physiologically different, experimental, pathological)	Endocrine Activity of PTG (cytological)
MELSON (1968)	rabbit	normal controls ferric-glycerophosphate injections	normal stimulated
MENEGHELLI and MAZZOCCHI (1966)	rat monkey human	normal (presence of cilia) normal (presence of cilia) normal (presence of cilia)	
MIZUOCHI (1958)	dog	normal	normal
MONTSKO *et al.*	Rana esculenta	normal dihydrotachysterol per os EDTA injections	normal suppressed stimulated
MUNGER and ROTH (1963)	Virginia deer	normal	normal
MURAKAMI (1970)	rat	normal controls vitamin D_2 injections and $CaCl_2$ per os	normal suppressed
NAKAGAMI (1965)	monkey dog	normal normal	normal normal
NAKAGAMI *et al.* (1968)	mouse	normal controls $CaCl_2$ injections	normal suppressed
NEVALAINEN (1968)	hen	laying hen	active
PORTE and PETROVIC (1961)	hamster	normal in vitro cultures (14 and 20 days)	normal
ROGERS (1965)	Rana clamitans	normal (december)	
ROHR and KRÄSSIG (1968)	rat	normal controls (comparison of inclusion bodies) EDTA injections (comparison of inclusion bodies)	

Table 1 (Continued)

Authors	Species	Conditions (normal, physiologically different, experimental, pathological)	Endocrine Activity of PTG (cytologically)
ROTH *et al.* (1968)	rat	*dietetic experiments regarding rickets and PTG:*	
		low Ca:P diet; vitamin D-deficient	stimulated
		low Ca:P diet; plus vitamin D	stimulated
		normal Ca:P diet; vitamin D-deficient	stimulated
		normal Ca:P diet; plus vitamin D (= normal controls)	normal
		high Ca:P diet; vitamin D-deficient	stimulated
		high calcium/low phosphorus, vitamin D-free diet	normal
		high Ca:P diet; plus vitamin D	suppressed
		high calcium/low phosphorus, vitamin D free diet plus phosphorus	normal
		high calcium/low phosphorus, vitamin D-free diet; plus vitamin D	normal
		high calcium/low phosphorus; vitamin D-free diet; plus phosphorus plus vitamin D	partly suppressed, partly normal
ROTH and RAISZ (1964)	rat	*organ cultures in vitro*	
		medium with low calcium content	stimulated
		medium with normal calcium content	normal
		medium with high calcium content	suppressed
		medium with low calcium content plus magnesium or plus strontium	stimulated
ROTH and RAISZ (1966)	rat	*organ cultures in vitro*	
		medium with low calcium content; and reversal	reversibility of stimulation and suppression
		medium with high calcium content; and reversal	
SETOGUTI *et al.* (1970a)	Triturus pyrrhogaster (Boie)	spring season (April/May)	activated (in relation to hibernation)

Table 1 (Continued)

Authors	Specis	Conditions (normal, physiologically different, experimental, pathological)	Endocrine Activity of PTG (cytologically)
Setoguti *et al.* (1970b)	Triturus pyrrhogaster (Boie)	natural hibernation (January)	moderate
Stoeckel and Porte (1966a)	mouse	normal	normal
Stoeckel and Porte (1966b)	mouse	phosphate injections calcium acetate per os calcium acetate per os, plus vitamin D injections calcium acetate per os, plus parathyroid hormone injections parathyroid hormone injections	stimulated suppressed suppressed suppressed suppressed
Tanaka (1969)	rabbit	normal (details on secretory granules) EDTA injections (details on secretory granules)	
Tanaka *et al.* (1969)	rabbit	long-term administration of calcium and vitamin D_2	suppressed (afterwards restitution)
Tanaka *et al.*)1969b)	rabbit	EDTA administration	stimulated
Trier (1958)	monkey	normal	normal
Youshak and Capen (1970)	chicken	normal controls osteopetrosis	normal activated
Welsch and Pearse (1969)	rabbit	normal (demonstration of C-cells in PTG)	
Zawistowski (1966)	rat	normal	normal

Table 2. *Electron microscopic communications on human Parathyroid Glands (PTG). (Summarized review of the literature)*

Authors	Number of Cases								
	normal PTG	atrophic PTG in adenoma cases	second-ary PTG-hyper-plasia	primary PTG-hyperplasia		PTG-Adenomas		PTG-carci-nomas	other conditions
				chief cell hyper plasia	water clear hyper-cell plasia	chief cell Ade-nomas	oxyphil Adenomas		
ALTENÄHR and SEIFERT (1971)	3		3			3			
ALTENÄHR and WÖHLER 1971)									17 embryonal, fetal and neonatal PTG
BARTSCH (1970)		?	2			6			
BLACK (1969)		4	4			4			3 cases uncertain
BLACK and HAFF (1970)				17					
BLACK *et al.* (1970)			6						4 of these 6 cases tertiary Hyperpara-thyroidism
BOQUIST (1970)						2			
ELLIOTT and ARHELGER (1966)						3			
ENGFELDT *et al.* (1959)						11			
FACCINI (1970)		5		1	1	33	1	4	
FRIES *et al.* (1967)			1						
HEIMANN *et al.* (1971)							1		
HOLZMANN and LANGE (1963)					1	3			

Table 2 (Continued)

Authors	Number of Cases								
	normal PTG	atrophic PTG in aderoma cases	second-ary PTG-hyper-plasia	primary PTG-hyperplasia		PTG-Adenomas		PTG-carci-nomas	other conditions
				chief cell hyper-plasia	water-clear cell hyper-plasia	chief cell Ade-nomas	oxyphil Ade-nomas		
Lange (1961)						4			
Marshall *et al.* (1967)	1	1				7			
Mazzocchi *et al.* (1967 a)	15								
Mitrovic *et al.* (1967)						1			
Munger and Roth (1963)	6								
Nakagami *et al.* (1968)									2 fetal PTG
Polyzonis (1970)	1					1			
Roth (1970)					1				
Roth and Marshall (1969)			1						
Roth and Munger (1962)		2		2		2			
Roth *et al.* (1962)							1		
Selzman and Fechner (1967)							1		
Sheldon (1964)					1				
Szilagyi *et al.* (1967)						1			multiple adenomas
Weymouth and Seibel (1969)				1		3			
Weymouth and Sheridan (1966)	1			1		1			

Acknowledgements

Patients, whose parathyroid glands have been studied ultrastructurally in connection with the present investigation, were clinically examined and treated by Prof. Dr. F. Kuhlencordt and colleagues (Abteilung für Klinische Osteologie der I. Medizinischen Universitätsklinik Hamburg, Head: Prof. Dr. H. Bartelheimer). His detailed clinical studies made it possible to correlate ultrastructural characteristics and clinical disease. Operations on parathyroid glands were carried out in the Chirurgische Universitätsklinik Hamburg (Head: Prof. Dr. F. Stelzner). Further material for our investigation was kindly supplied by Prof. Dr. W. Janssen (Institut für Gerichtliche Medizin und Kriminalistik, Hamburg), Prof. Dr. K.-H. Schäfer (Universitätskinderklinik Hamburg) and Prof. Dr. K. Thomsen (Universitäts-Frauenklinik, Hamburg).

References

Altenähr, E.: Zur Ultrastruktur der Rattenepithelkörperchen bei Normo,- Hyper- und Hypocalcämie. Application von Parathormon, Thyreocalcitonin, Dihydrotachysterin, Glycerophosphat und verschiedener Diät. Virchows Arch. Abt. A. Path. Anat. 351, 122—141 (1971).
— Electron microscopical evidence for innervation of chief cells in human parathyroid gland. Experientia (Basel) 27, 1077 (1971).
— Dammann, H. G.: Über Beziehungen zwischen Zelltyp und Kernstruktur in Epithelkörperchen-Tumoren. Virchows Arch. Abt. A Path. Anat. 352, 111—121 (1971).
— Lietz, H.: Vergleichende experimentelle Untersuchungen zur Ultrastruktur von Epithelkörperchen und C-Zellen der Schilddrüse bei verschiedenen Funktionszuständen. Verh. dtsch. Ges. Path. 54, 360–367 (1970).
— Seemann, N., Seifert, G.: Pathologische Anatomie der Epithelkörperchen. In: Bay, V. (ed.), Der autonome und regulative Hyperparathyreoidismus, S. 1–61. Stuttgart: Ferdinand Enke 1969.
— Seifert, G.: Ultrastruktureller Vergleich menschlicher Epithelkörperchen bei sekundärem Hyperparathyreoidismus und primärem Adenom. Virchows Arch. Abt. A Path. Anat. 353, 60–86 (1971).
— Wöhler, J.: Ultrastrukturelle Untersuchungen zur funktionellen Epithelkörperchendifferenzierung während der Embryonal-, Fetal- und Neonatalperiode. Verh. dtsch. Ges. Path. 55, 160–166 (1971).
Aurbach, G. D., Potts, J. T. Jr.: Radioimmunoassay of parathyroid hormone. Arch. intern. Med. 124, 413–416 (1969).
Bargmann, W.: Die Epithelkörperchen. In: v. Möllendorff, W. (ed.), Handbuch der mikroskopischen Anatomie des Menschen, Bd. VI/2, S. 137–196. Berlin: Springer 1939.
Bartelheimer, H., Kuhlencordt, F.: Primärer, sekundärer und tertiärer Hyperparathyreoidismus. Med. Klin. 62, 821–825 (1967).
Bartsch, G.: Elektronenmikroskopische Untersuchungen von Epithelkörperchen bei primärem Hyperparathyreoidismus. Verh. dtsch. Ges. Path. 54, 682–683 (1970).
Berson, S. A., Yalow, R. S.: Parathyroid hormone in plasma in adenomatous hyperparathyroidism, uremia, and bronchogenic carcinoma. Science 154, 907–909 (1966).
Black, B. K.: Carcinoma of the parathyroid. Amer. Surg. 139, 355–363 (1954).
Ackermann, L. V.: Tumors of the parathyroid: Review of 23 cases. Cancer 3, 415–444 (1950).
Black, W. C.: Correlative light and electron microscopy in primary hyperparathyroidism. Arch. Path. 88, 225–241 (1969).

BLACK, W. C., HAFF, R. C.: The surgical pathology of parathyroid chief cell hyperplasia. Amer. J. clin. Path. **53**, 565–579 (1970).
— SLATOPOLSKY, E., ELKAN, J., HOFFSTEIN, P.: Parathyroid morphology in suppressible and nonsuppressible renal hyperparathyroidism. Lab. Invest. **23**, 497–509 (1970).
BLIZZARD, R. M.: Idiopathic hypoparathyroidism: a probable autoimmune disease. In: Miescher, P. A., Müller-Eberhard, H. J. (eds.), Textbook of immunopathology, vol. II, p. 547–550. New York and London: Grune & Stratton 1969.
BOQUIST, L.: Annulate lamellae in human parathyroid adenoma. Virchows Arch. Abt. B Zellpath. **6**, 234–246 (1970).
BROWN, W. R., KROOK, L., POND, W. G.: Atrophic rhinitis in swine. Etiology, pathogenesis, and prophylaxis. Cornell Vet. **56**, Suppl. 1, 1–107 (1966).
CAPEN, C. C., COLE, C. R., HIBBS, J. W.: Influence of vitamin D on calcium metabolism and the parathyroid glands of cattle. Fed. Proc. **27**, 142–152 (1968).
— KOESTNER, A., COLE, C. R.: The ultrastructure and histochemistry of normal parathyroid glands of pregnant and non-pregnant cows. Lab. Invest. **14**, 1673–1690 (1965 a).
— — — The ultrastructure, histopathology, and histochemistry of the parathyroid glands of pregnant and non-pregnant cows fed a high level of vitamin D. Lab. Invest. **14**, 1809–1825 (1965 b).
— ROWLAND, G. N.: The ultrastructure of the parathyroid glands of young cats. Anat. Rec. **162**, 327–340 (1968 a).
— — Ultrastructural evaluation of the parathyroid glands of young cats with experimental hyperparathyroidism. Z. Zellforsch. **90**, 495–506 (1968 b).
— YOUNG, D. M.: The ultrastructure of the parathyroid glands and thyroid parafollicular cells of cows with parturient paresis and hypocalcemia. Lab. Invest. **17**, 717–737 (1967 a).
— — Thyrocalcitonin: evidence for release in spontaneous hypocalcemic disorder. Science **157**, 205–206 (1967 b).
CASTLEMAN, B.: Tumors of the parathyroid glands. Atlas of tumor pathology, IV, 15. Washington, D. C.: Armed Forces Inst. Path. 1952.
COLEMAN, R.: Ultrastructural observations on the parathyroid glands of Xenopus laevis Daudin. Z. Zellforsch. **100**, 201–214 (1969).
COPE, O.: Hyperparathyroidism: Diagnosis and management. Amer. J. Surg. **99**, 394–403 (1960).
CORTELYOU, J. R., McWHINNIE, D. J.: Parathyroid glands of amphibians I. Parathyroid structure and function in the amphibian, with emphasis on regulation of mineral ions in body fluids. Amer. Zoologist **7**, 843–855 (1967).
DAVIS, R., ENDERS, A. C.: Light and electron microscopic studies of the parathyroid gland. In: R. O. Greep and R. V. Talmage (eds.), The parathyroids, p. 76–92. Springfield (Ill.): Ch. C. Thomas 1961.
DENT, T. B., BROWN, D. M.: Calcitonin in avian osteopetrosis. Fed. Proc. **28**, 368 (1969).
DUNAY, C., OLAH, I., KISS, J.: Accessory parathyroid tissue in the rat thymus. Electron- and light-microscopic autoradiographic studies. Acta biol. Acad. Sci. hung. **20**, 193–203 (1969).
EKHOLM, R.: Some observations on the ultrastructure of the mouse parathyroid gland. J. Ultrastruct. Res. **1**, 26–37 (1957).
ELLIOTT, R. L., ARHELGER, R. B.: Fine structure of parathyroid adenomas. With special reference to annulate lamellae and septate desmosomes. Arch. Path. **81**, 200–212 (1966).
ENGFELDT, A. B., HELLSTRÖM, J., IVEMARK, B., RHODIN, J.: Elektronmikroskopi och histokemi vid parathyreoideaadenom. Nord. Med. **61**, 558–559 (1959).
FACCINI, J. M.: Fluoride-induced hyperplasia of the parathyroid glands. Proc. Roy. Soc. Med. **62**, 241 (1969).

Faccini, J. M.: The ultrastructure of parathyroid glands removed from patients with primary hyperparathyroidism: A report of 40 cases, including four carcinomata. J. Path. **102**, 189–199 (1970).
— Care, A. D.: Effect of sodium fluoride on the ultrastructure of parathyroid glands of the sheep. Nature (Lond.) **207**, 1399–1401 (1965).
Fanconi, A.: Hypoparathyreoidismus im Kindesalter. Ergebn. inn. Med. Kinderheilk. **28**, 54–119 (1969).
Fetter, A. W., Capen, C. C.: Ultrastructural evaluation of the parathyroid glands of pig with naturally occuring atrophic rhinitis. Path. Vet. **5**, 481–503 (1968).
— — The ultrastructure of the parathyroid glands of young pig. Acta anat. (Basel) **75**, 359–372 (1970a).
— — Ultrastructural evaluation of thyroid parafollicular cells of pig with naturally occuring atrophic rhinitis. Path. Vet. **7**, 171–185 (1970b).
— — Fine structure of bone cells in the nasal turbinates of pig with naturally occuring atrophic rhinitis. Amer. J. Path. **62**, 265–282 (1971).
Fries, D., Feroldi, J., Lesbros, F., David, M., Brunat, N., Banssillon, N., Saubier, E., Traeger, J.: Hyperparathyroidisme secondaire au cours de l'insuffisance rénale chronique traité par parathyroidectomie subtotale; ultrastructure des parathyroids. Rev. lyon. Méd. **1967**, 1–12
Fujimoto, Y., Matsukawa, H., Inubushi, M., Nakamatsu, H., Satoh, H., Yamagiwa, S.: Electron microscopic observations of the equine parathyroid glands with particular reference to those of equine osteodystrophia fibrosa. Jap. J. vet. Res. **15**, 37–52 (1967).
Garel, J. M.: Fetal calcemia and fetal parathyroids. Israel J. med. Sci. **7**, 349–350 (1971).
Haff, R. C., Black, W. C., Ballinger, W. F.: Primary hyperparathyroidism. Changing clinical, surgical and pathologic aspects. Amer. Surg. **171**, 85–92 (1970).
Hamperl, H.: Die Fluoreszenzmikroskopie menschlicher Gewebe. Virchows Arch. path. Anat. **292**, 1–51 (1934).
Hara, J., Nagatsu, I.: Ultrastructural changes in the parathyroid glands by the injection of parathormone in rats. Okajimas Folia anat. jap. **44**, 99–133 (1968).
— Nagatsu-Ishibashi, J.: Electron microscopic study of the parathyroid glands of the mouse. Nagoya J. med. Sci. **26**, 119–124 (1964).
Hatakeyama, S., Tuchweber, B., Blaschek, J. A., Garg, B. D., Kovacs, K.: Parathyroid cyst formation by dihydrotachysterol and calcium acetate. An electron microscopic study. Endocr. jap. **17**, 355–364 (1970).
Heimann, P., Hansson, G., Nilsson, O.: Primary hyperparathyroidism in a case of oxyphilic adenoma. Acta path. microbiol. scand., Sect. A **79**, 10–14 (1971).
Holzmann, K., Lange, R.: Zur Zytologie der Glandula parathyreoidea des Menschen. Weitere Untersuchungen an Epithelkörperchenadenomen. Z. Zellforsch. **58**, 759–789 (1963).
Kayser, C., Petrovic, A., Porte, A.: Variations ultrastructurales de la parathyroide du Hamster ordinaire (Cricetus cricetus) au cours du cycle saisonnier. C. R. Soc. Biol. (Paris) **155**, 2178–2181 (1961).
Klotz, H. P., Stancou, H., Hennion, R.: Experimental study of parathyroid cytology in dogs after a hypocalcemic or a hypercalcemic diet. Sem. Hôp. Paris **42**, 3264–3270 (1966).
Kuhlencordt, F.: Der Hyperparathyroidismus. Standpunkt des Klinikers. In: Kracht, J. (Hrsg.), Nebenschilddrüse und endokrine Regulation des Calciumstoffwechsels. 14. Symp. Dtsch. Ges. Endokrinologie, S. 7–15. Berlin-Heidelberg-New York: Springer 1968.
— Kracht, J.: Chronischer Hyperparathyroidismus mit C-Zellen-Hyperplasie der Schilddrüse. Dtsch. med. Wschr. **50**, 2411–2415 (1968).

LANGE, R.: Zur Histologie und Zytologie der Glandula parathyreoidea des Menschen. Licht- und elektronenmikroskopische Untersuchungen an Epithelkörperchen-adenomen. Z. Zellforsch. **53**, 765–828 (1961).

— BREHM, H. VON: On the fine structure of the parathyroid gland in the toad and the frog. In: P. J. Gaillard, R. V. Talmage, and A. M. Budy (Hrsg.), The parathyroid glands, p. 19–26. Chicago: Chicago Univ. Press 1965.

LEVER, J. D.: Fine structural appearances in the rat parathyroid. J. Anat. (Lond.) **91**, 73–81 (1957).

— Cytological appearance in the normal and activated parathyroid of the rat. A combined study by electron and light microscopy with certain quantitative assessments. J. Endocr. **17**, 210–217 (1958).

L'HEUREUX, M. V., MELIUS, P.: Differential centrifugation of bovine parathyroid tissue. Biochem. biophys. Acta (Amst.) **20**, 447–448 (1956).

LIETZ, H.: Zur Ultrastruktur der C-Zellen in der Rattenschilddrüse bei gestörtem Calciumstoffwechsel. Virchows Arch. Abt. A Path. Anat. **350**, 136–149 (1970).

LUPULESCU, A.: Electron microscopic observations on the parathyroid gland in experimental hypoparathyroidism. Experientia (Basel) **24**, 62–63 (1968).

MARSHALL, R. B., ROBERTS, D. K., TURNER, R. A.: Adenomas of the human parathyroid. Light and electron microscopic study following selenium 75 methionine scan. Cancer (Philad.) **20**, 512–524 (1967).

MAZZOCCHI, G., MENEGHELLI, V., FRASSON, F.: The human parathyroid glands: An optical and electron microscopic study. Lo Sperimentale **117**, 383–447 (1967a).

— — SERAFINI, M. T.: The fine structure of the parathyroid glands in the normal, the rachitic and the bilaterally nephrectomized rat with special interest to their secretory cycle. Acta anat. (Basel) **68**, 550–566 (1967b).

MELICK, R., MARTIN, T. J.: Immunoassay of parathyroid hormone in human plasma. In: R. V. Talmage, L. F. Belanger (eds.), Parathyroid hormone and thyrocalcitonin (calcitonin), p. 440–441. Amsterdam: Excerpta Medica Foundation 1968.

MELSON, G. L.: Ferric glycerophosphate-induced hyperplasia of the rabbit parathyroid gland. An ultrastructural study. Lab. Invest. **15**, 818–835 (1966).

MENEGHELLI, V., MAZZOCCHI, G.: Sulla presenza di ciglia nelle cellule della ghiandola paratiroide di alcuni Mammiferi (Ratto, Scimmia, Uomo). Atti Ist. Veneto Sci. Lett. Arti. **124**, 37–41 (1966).

MITROVIC, D., MAZABRAND, A., RYCKEWAERT, A., HIOCO, D., DESEZE, S.: Adenome parathyroidien a cellules sombres et claires. Deux aspects ultrastructuraux de la cellule claire. Etudes cytochimiques et au microscope electronique. Arch. Anat. path. **15**, 225–230 (1967).

MIZUOCHI, Y.: Histological studies on parathyroid. III. Electron microscopie observations on parathyroid of a dog. Med. J. Kagoshima Univ. **10**, 1079–1092 (1958).

MONTSKO, T., TIGYI, I., BENEDECZKY, I., LISSAK, K.: Electron microscopy of parathyroid secretion in Rana esculenta. Acta biol. Acad. Sci. hung. **14**, 81–94 (1963).

MUNGER, B. L., ROTH, S. I.: The cytology of the normal parathyroid glands of man and virginia deer. A light and electron microscopic study with morphologic evidence of secretory activity. J. Cell Biol. **16**, 379–400 (1963).

MURAKAMI, K.: Electron microscopic studies on the effect of long-term hypercalcemia on the thyroid parafollicular cell and the parathyroid cell of rats. Arch. Histol. Jap. **32**, 155–178 (1970).

NAKAGAMI, K.: Comparative electron microscopic studies of the parathyroid gland. I. Fine structure of monkey and dog parathyroid glands. Arch. Histol. Jap. **25**, 435–465 (1965).

— Comparative electron microscopic studies of the parathyroid glands II. Fine structure of the parathyroid gland of the normal and the calcium chloride treated mouse. Arch. Histol. Jap. **28**, 185–205 (1967).

Nakagami, K., Yamazaki, Y., Tsunoda, Y.: An electron microscopic study of the human fetal parathyroid gland. Z. Zellforsch. 85, 89–95 (1968).

Nevalainen, T.: Fine structure of the parathyroid gland of the laying hen (Gallus domesticus). Gen. comp. Endocr. 12, 561–567 (1969).

Pearce, H. G., Roe, C. K.: Infectious porcine atrophic rhinitis: A review. Canad. vet. J. 7, 243–251 (1966).

Perkin, A. B., Bader, H. J., Tashjian, A. A., Jr., Goldhaber, P.: Immunofluorescent localization of parathyroid hormone in extracellular spaces of bovine parathyroid gland. Proc. Soc. exp. Biol. (N. Y.) 128, 218–221 (1968).

Polyzonis, M. B.: Ultrastructural study of human parathyroid adenoma and the occurrence of abnormal cilia in the adenoma cells. Path. europ. 5, 454–469 (1970).

Porte, A., Petrovic, A.: Etude au microscope électronique de la parathyroide de Hamster ordinaire (Cricetus cricetus) en culture organotypique. C. R. Soc. Biol. (Paris) 155, 2025–2027 (1961).

Potts, J. T., Reitz, R. E., Deftos, L. J., Kaye, M. B., Richardson, J. A., Buckle, R. M., Aurbach, G. D.: Secondary hyperparathyroidism in chronic renal disease. Arch. intern. Med. 124, 408–412 (1969).

Raisz, L. G., Taves, D. R.: The effect of fluoride on parathyroid function and responsiveness in the rat. Calcif. Tiss. Res. 1, 219–228 (1967).

Raybuck, H. E.: The innervation of the parathyroid glands. Anat. Rec. 112, 117–123 (1952).

Rogers, D. C.: An electron microscope study of the parathyroid gland of the frog (Rana clamitans). J. Ultrastruct. Res. 13, 478–499 (1965).

Rohr, H. P., Krässig, B.: Elektronenmikroskopische Untersuchungen über den Sekretionsmodus des Parathormons. Beitrag zu einer lysosomalen Mitbeteiligung bei Sekretionsvorgängen in endokrinen Drüsen. Z. Zellforsch. 85, 271–290 (1968).

Roth, S. I.: Pathology of the parathyroids in hyperparathyroidism. Arch. Path. 73, 495–510 (1962).

— The ultrastructure of primary water-clear cell hyperplasia of the parathyroid glands. Amer. J. Path. 61, 233–248 (1970).

— Au, W. Y. W., Kunin, A. S., Krane, S. M., Raisz, L. G.: Effect of dietary deficiency in vitamin D, calcium, and phosphorus on the ultrastructure of the rat parathyroid gland. Amer. J. Path. 53, 631–650 (1968).

— Marshall, R. B.: Pathology and ultrastructure of the human parathyroid glands in chronic renal failure. Arch. intern. Med. 124, 397–406 (1969).

— Munger, B. L.: The cytology of the adenomatous, atrophic, and hyperplastic parathyroid glands of man. A light and electron-microscopic study. Virchows Arch. path. Anat. 335, 389–410 (1962).

— Olen, E., Hansen, L. S.: The eosinophilic cells of the parathyroid (oxyphil cells), salivary (oncocytes), and thyroid (Hürthle cells) glands. Light and electron microscopic observations. Lab. Invest. 11, 933–941 (1962).

— Raisz, L. G.: Effect of calcium concentration on the ultrastructure of the rat parathyroid in organ culture. Lab. Invest. 13, 331–345 (1964).

— — The course and reversibility of calcium effect on the ultrastructure of the rat parathyroid gland in organ culture. Lab. Invest. 15, 1187–1211 (1966).

Seemann, N.: Über Vorkommen und funktionelle Bedeutung wasserheller Zellen in menschlichen Epithelkörperchen. Med. Welt 18, 2336–2339 (1967).

Seifert, G., Altenähr, E.: Pathologie des primären, sekundären und tertiären Hyperparathyreoidismus. Lebensversicher.-Med. 21, 125–132 (1969).

SEIFERT, G., SEEMANN, N.: Tertiärer Hyperparathyreoidismus. Dtsch. med. Wschr. 92, 1943–1946 (1967).

SELZMAN, H. H., FECHNER, R. E.: Oxyphil adenoma and primary hyperparathyroidism: Clinical and ultrastructural observations. J. Amer. med. Ass. 99, 359–361 (1967).

ʲTOGUTI, T., ISONO, H., SAKURAI, S.: Electron microscopic study on the parathyroid gland of the newt Triturus pyrrhogaster (Boie) in natural hibernation. J. Ultrastruct. Res. 31, 46–60 (1970a).

— — — YONEMOTO, Y., HAGIHARA, A.: Ultrastructure of the parathyroid gland of the newt, Triturus pyrrhogaster (Boie) in the spring season. Okajimas Folia anat. jap. 47, 1–17 (1970b).

SHELDON, H.: On the water-clear cell in the human parathyroid gland. J. Ultrastruct. Res. 10, 377–383 (1964).

SHERWOOD, L. M., MAYER, G. P., RAMBERG, C. F., KRONFELD, D. S., AURBACH, G. D., POTTS, J. T., JR.: Regulation of parathyroid secretion: Proportional control by calcium, lack of effect of phosphate. Endocrinology 83, 1043–1051 (1969).

— POTTS, J. T., CARE, A. D., MAYER, G. P., AURBACH, G. D.: Evaluation by radioimmunoassay of factors controlling the secretion of parathyroid hormone. Intravenous infusions of calcium, and ethylene diamine tetraacetic acid in the cow and goat. Nature (Lond.) 209, 52–55 (1966).

SIMPSON, C. F., SANGER, V. L.: A review of avian osteopetrosis: Comparisons with other bone diseases. Clin. Orthop. 58, 271–281 (1968).

SOMMERS, S. C., YOUNG, TH. L.: Oxyphil parathyroid adenomas. Amer. J. Path. 28, 673–689 (1952).

ST. GOAR, L. T.: Comment to: NICHOLS, G., JR., ROTH, S. I.: Case Records of the Massachusetts General Hospital Case 29, 1963. New Engl. J. Med. 268, 943–953 (1963).

STOECKEL, M. E., PORTE, A.: Observations ultrastrucurales sur la parathyroide des souris. I. Etude chez la souris normale. Z. Zellforsch. 73, 488–502 (1966a).

— — Observations ultrastructurales sur la parathyroide des souris. II. Etude expérimentale. Z. Zellforschung 73, 503–520 (1966b).

SZILAGYI, G., BENEDECZKY, J., LAPIS, K.: Multiple parathyroid adenoma. Clinical, histological and electron microscopical studies. Acta med. Acad. Sci. hung. 23, 125–138 (1967).

TANAKA, S.: Electron microscopic studies of the rabbit parathyroid gland. On the secretory activity of the chief cell. Folia endocr. Jap. 45, 335–338 (1969a).

— CHIN, A., TOWATARI, K., SENGA, I.: Relationship between blood calcium and the ultrastructure of the rabbit parathyroid gland following EDTA administration. Folia endocr. jap. 45, 783–786 (1969b).

— NAKAMURA, K., CHIN, A., SENGA, I.: Electron microscopic studies on restitution of the rabbit parathyroid gland following calcium and vitamin D_2. Folia endocr. jap. 45, 666–670 (1969c).

TRIER, J. S.: The fine structure of the parathyroid gland. J. biophys. biochem. Cytol. 4, 13–22 (1958).

TSANG, R. C., OH, W.: Neonatal hypocalcemia in low birth weight infants. Pediatrics 45, 773–781 (1970).

Welsch, U., Pearse, A. G. E.: Electron cytochemistry of BuChE and AChH in thyroid and parathyroid cells under normal and experimental conditions. Histochemie 17, 1–10 (1969).

Weymouth, R. J., Seibel, H. R.: An electron microscopic study of the parathyroid glands in man: evidence of secretory material. Acta endocr. (Kbh.) 61, 334–342 (1969).

— Sheridan, M. N.: Fine structure of human parathyroid glands: normal and pathological. Acta endocr. (Kbh.) 53, 529–546 (1966).

Youshak, M. S., Capen, C. C.: Fine structural alterations in parathyroid glands of chickens with osteopetrosis. Amer. J. Path. 61, 257–274 (1970).

— — Ultrastructural evaluation of ultimobranchial glands from normal and osteopetrotic chickens. Gen. comp. Endocr., in press (1970).

Zawistowski, S.: Ultrastructure of the parathyroid gland of the albino rat. Folia histochem. cytochem. 4, 273–278 (1966).

Pathologisches Institut der Universität Düsseldorf,
Direktor: Professor Dr. H. Meessen,
and Rheumatic Diseases Study Group, New York University School of Medicine

Structure of Synovial Membrane in Rheumatoid Arthritis

F. Huth, A. Soren, and W. Klein

With 16 Figures

Contents

I. The Cells of Normal Synovial Membrane

Since the investigations of Hueter (1866), Hagen-Torn (1882) and Hammar (1894) the synovial membrane has been regarded as a layer of modified connective tissue cells. Consequently, in contrast to some concepts (Bichat, 1806; Tillmann, 1877; Aschoff, 1919; Kaufman, 1922), the nature of the synovial cells as connective tissue elements is no longer disputed (Franceschini, 1930; Marquart, 1931; Sigurdson, 1956). Function of these cells regarding contribution to synovial fluid and resorption from the synovial is suggested by a dense network of blood and lymph vessels in the subsynovial tissue (Baumecker, 1932; Efskind, 1941; Hidvegi, 1954; Lang, 1958; Ruckes and Schuckmann, 1961/62; Suter and Majno, 1964).

Electron microscopic investigations disclosed various types among the synovial cells (Lever and Ford, 1958; Langer and Huth, 1960; Barland et al., 1962; Cotta, 1962; Coulter, 1962; Wyllie *et al.*, 1964; Norton and

Ziff, 1966; Ghadially and Roy, 1966; Roberts *et al.*, 1969). Barland et al. differentiated type A (Fig. 5) and type B (Fig. 7) of synovial cells. The predominant A cells contained a well developed Golgi field, numerous vacuoles, mitochondria, dense granules, pinocytotic vesicles, intracellular fibrils, and cell protrusions. The cells of type B contained ergastoplasmic tubules, smaller vacuoles, mitochondria, and pinocytotic vesicles. An intermediate type (Fig. 6) with cytoplasmic structures observed in each of these cell types was also noted. The characterization of the synovial cells as modified connective tissue cells has been corroborated by electron microscopic findings; no epithelial structure has been observed.

II. Past Studies of Rheumatoid Arthritis

1. Morphological Changes of the Synovial Membrane

Electron microscopic studies were also used to assist in the interpretation of light microscopic findings in rheumatoid arthritis.

These findings in the innermost zone of the joint capsule were characterized by proliferation of the lining cells, diffuse infiltrates of inflammatory cells, and alterations of the subsynovial vessels (Hollander et al., 1965; Grimley, 1967; Lindner, 1968; Mc Farland et al., 1968). Also focal infiltrates of neutrophil and eosinophil leukocytes in the subsynovial tissue were observed in acute stages of rheumatoid arthritis. Plasma cells constituted a special feature of the rheumatoid changes (Jordan 1938; Riddle *et al.*, 1965; Cooper, 1968). Fibrinoid necrosis of the synovial connective tissue and of the wall of subsynovial blood vessels often occurred. The vascular alterations were designated as arteriolitis or vasculitis when infiltration of the vascular wall predominated, or as obliteration of blood vessels when proliferation of intimal and medial cells predominated (Cruickshank, 1954; Sokoloff and Bunim, 1957; Norton and Ziff, 1966). Thickening of the capillary basal membrane were also noticed. According to Brånemark *et al.*, 1969), the vascular changes were very striking in light microscopy, but were partly or totally lacking in electron microscopy. Marin *et al.*, 1969 described peri- and endarteritic lesions in rheumatoid synovial membrane. The vascular changes and the composition of the concomitant inflammatory infiltrates caused several authors (Gross, 1967) to emphasize the morphologic relationship of rheumatoid changes to other collagen diseases like dermatomyositis, lupus erythematosus, and periarteritis nodosa.

Often occurring giant cells in the synovial membrane were regarded as characteristic elements in rheumatoid arthritis by Stanfield and Stephens (1963), Donald and Kerr (1968). Recurrent fibrin precipitations on the synovial cells and formation of new collagen fibrils between the proliferated synovial cells were described by Wyllie *et al.* (1966).

Special alterations of the synovial cells in rheumatoid arthritis were detected by electron microscopy. The numerical increase of the synovial cells was based according to Norton and Ziff (1968) on a proportional augmentation of A and B cells. Wyllie *et al.* (1966) noticed that the B cells were not essentially changed, whereas the A cells always contained a larger number of vacuoles and dense bodies. According to Barland et al. (1964), the A cells contained less filopodia, a smaller Golgi apparatus, and some mitochondrial changes; the lysosomal activity of the synovial cells was increased in rheumatoid arthritis.

2. Biochemical and Immunobiologic Changes

The synovial fluid contains glucose, electrolytes, enzymes and proteins among other substances. The protein concentration in rheumatoid synovial fluid is about twice as high as in normal synovial fluid; the proportion of albumin is lower than that of globulin. Also proteins of higher molecular weight like fibrinogen and lipoproteins are present (Perlmann, Ropes and Kaufman, 1954). The higher concentration of protein in synovial fluid has been correlated to the hypertrophy of ergastoplasm in B-cells and to an increased number of plasma cells. Leukocytes too are regarded as sources of higher globulin concentration. With the expansion of degenerative and regenerative processes more cells and fibrin appear in synovial fluid. Rheumatoid factors are not constantly verified in synovial fluid of rheumatoid patients. Lower glucose levels in synovial fluid of rheumatoid arthritis are presumed to be caused by greater utilization of leukocytes (Ropes, Muller and Bauer, 1960). The content of hyaluronic acid increases in synovial fluid of rheumatoid patients and accounts for higher viscosity (Blau *et al.*, 1965). Among the enzymes, acid and alkaline phosphatase, β-glucuronidase, pepsin, trypsin, and transaminases play important roles (Hamerman, Sandson, and Schubert, 1963; Thomas and Dingle, 1958; Campbell, 1968; Gugelberger, 1970).

After fixation with lead phosphate Mellors, Nowoslawsky and Korngold (1961) demonstrated phosphatase activity in vacuolar and membranous cytoplasmic structures of A-cells. Enzymes were probably liberated from the lysosomes of synovial cells and from leukocytes. Lysosomes, in granules, were more numerous and larger in synovial cells of rheumatoid joints (Barland et. al., 1964).

Fluorescent microscopic studies disclosed that the rheumatoid factors were primarily localized in the cytoplasm of plasma cells. Two different rheumatoid factors were isolated by special staining methods. Plasma cells contained either one or both factors (Mellors *et al.*, 1961).

III. Personal Studies

A. Purpose

In view of the differences in interpretation of the findings in synovial cells, further investigations are indicated to clarify details in the structure of the synovial membrane in rheumatoid arthritis. Correlation of the light microscopic findings and electron microscopic findings appears especially apt to enhance the understanding of such details. Furthermore, correlation of the morphologic findings to clinical data may assist in the interpretation of the observed histopathologic alterations.

B. Material and Methods

The studies were carried out with cooperation of the Institute of Pathology of the University of Düsseldorf and the Rheumatic Diseases Study Group of New York University School of Medicine. Twenty-one patients, aged 27 to 64 years, were incorporated in the studies. The patients suffered from joint disease for seven to twenty-two years, and presented permanent deformities of three to five major joints of the extremities; fourteen of the patients had also typical deformities of the fingers and ulnar deviations of the hands. The laboratory studies disclosed positive latex tests in 19 patients (positive tests for sheep cell agglutination in 16 patients) elevated sedimentation rate up to 74 mm in all patients, and positive tests for C-reactive protein in 14 patients. Analyses of synovial fluids of 13 patients disclosed a range of 3.6–6.4 g/l of total protein concentration with concentration of albumin ranging 1.9–3.0 g/l. All patients had clinically as well as microbiologically the signs of active joint disease. According to the criteria of the American Rheumatism Association seven of these patients were classified as having definite rheumatoid arthritis, and fourteen were classified as having classical rheumatoid arthritis. The patients underwent synovectomies or arthroplasties during which portions of the inner part of the joint capsule were removed.

The tissue specimens were fixed in buffered glutar aldehyde. Further fixation was done by 10% formaline for light microscopy, and by osmium tetroxyde for electron microscopy. Osmium fixed pieces of 1 mm thickness were embedded in Durcupan. Orthograde sections of synovial membrane were elected from methylen blue stained sections. Ultrathin sections were cut, and their contrast was enhanced by treatment with uranyl acetate and lead citrate. Paraffin sections were stained with hematoxylin-eosin, iron-hematoxylin-picrofuchsin (van Gieson) combined with resorcin, PAS method, Berlin blue, and Goldner's modification of Masson's trichrome. Sections from the inner layer of the joint capsule were cut perpendicularly to the surface to ensure comparison as to thickness of the synovial cell layer and extent of infiltrates. Also the degree of regressive changes, fibrinoid necrosis or hyalinization could thus be appropiately estimated.

C. Light Microscopic Findings

In accordance with the clinical data on the activity of the rheumatoid disease, the histological findings in the investigated 21 cases differed, and were grouped as follows:

In the first group (16 cases), florid inflammatory and old reactive alterations were present. No correlation between duration and phase of the disease could be established; florid inflammatory and old reactive changes were observed

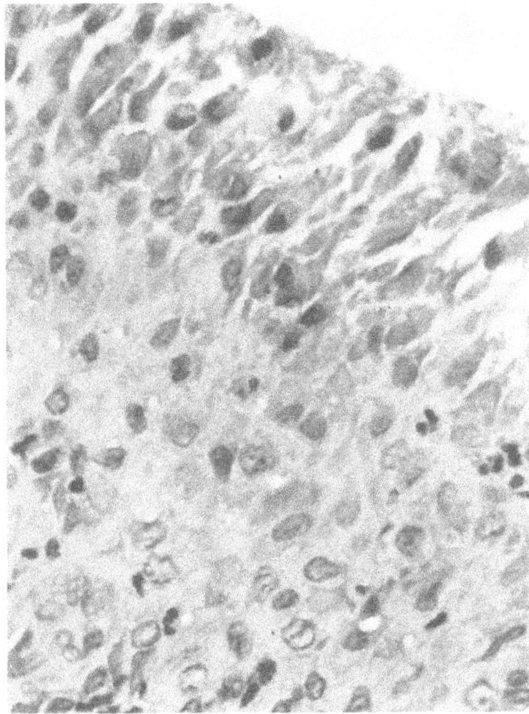

Fig. 1. Hypertrophic synovial membrane with polymorphic cells and nuclei in rheumatoid arthritis of 8 years. HE, 500 ×

after seven years as well as after 22 years of clinical manifestation of the rheumatoid joint disease. Proliferation of synovial cells to more than two or three layers was regarded as an indication for the degree of activity of the rheumatoid process. The augmented, closely apposed synovial cells displayed a distinct orientation toward the articular cavity (Figs. 1 and 2). More pronounced polymorphy of the cytoplasmic structures and nuclei of synovial cells was suggestive of a very active process. Sometimes mono- or multinuclear giant cells appeared among the polymorphic cells (Fig. 2). Predominantly, however, the giant cells were located in somewhat deeper zones. Usually, hyperplasia and polymorphy of synovial cells were combined with focal infiltrates of lymphocytes and plasma cells (Fig. 2). These infiltrates were mostly situated in deeper zones of the inner joint capsule, and had no immediate contact to the surface. In some cases, the lining cells were covered by fibrinoid material which contained fibrocytes and collagen fibrils. In other cases, the cover of lining cells was disrupted by fibrin or hyaline material (Fig. 3). These findings differed in intensity, but were rather constant. Alterations of the blood vessels in the subsynovial tissue varied greatly. Often, the capillaries and the pre- and postcapillary branches were hyperemic, but not sclerotic. Less often, blood vessels had walls thickened by concentric accumulation of fibrocytes and collagen fibers (Fig. 4). The fibrosis was limited to the outer layer of the

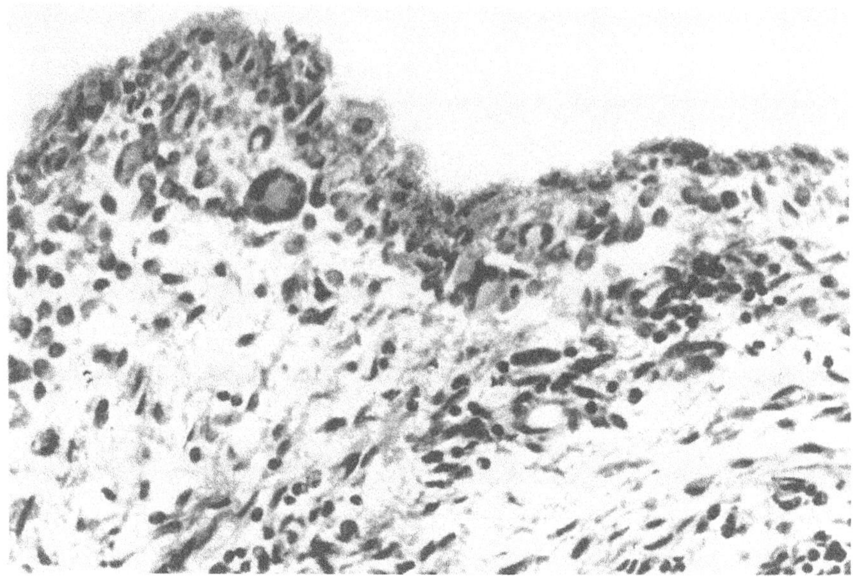

Fig. 2. Slightly hyperplastic synovial membrane with giant cells and round cell infiltrates in subsynovial tissue in rheumatoid arthritis of 16 years. HE, 310 ×

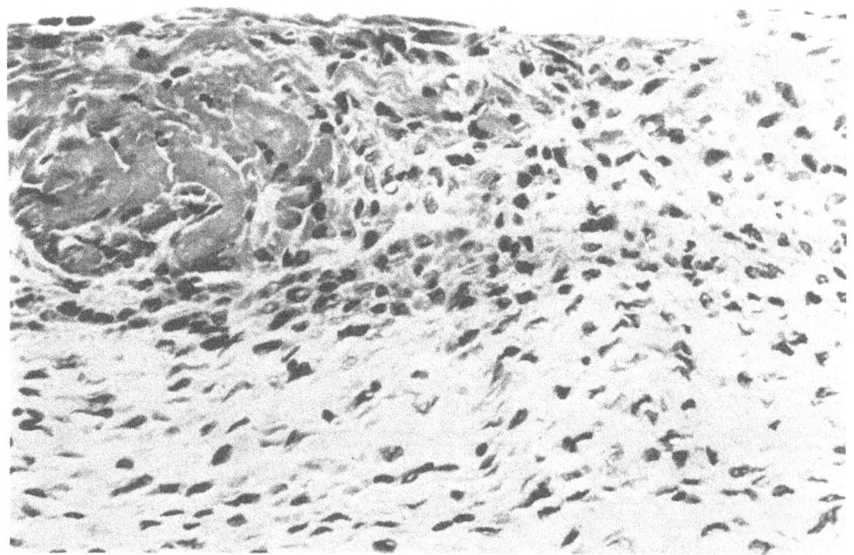

Fig. 3. Fibrinoid necrosis on synovial membrane in rheumatoid arthritis of 22 years. HE, 310 ×

vascular wall, and did not involve the intima or muscularis. The intensity of vascular sclerosis increased with distance between blood vessels and articular space. Fibrosis of the subsynovial tissue was as infrequent as the former fibrosis. Thrombotic obturation or hyalin obstruction of blood vessels was not observed.

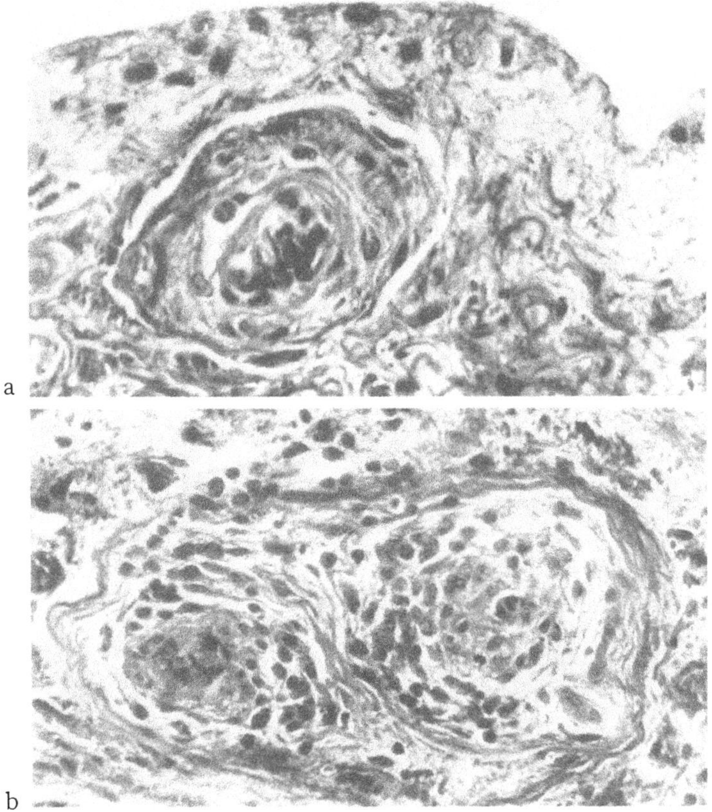

Fig. 4. Sclerosis of the outer vascular wall and adventitial infiltration by round cells in rheumatoid arthritis of 7 years. El. van Gieson, 500 ×

In the second group (4 cases), the arthritis was no longer florid. The alterations of the inner part of the joint capsule were associated with more or less diffuse fibrosis of the subsynovial tissue, vascular sclerosis, and villous thickening. Infiltrates of chronic inflammatory cells were mostly lacking. The synovial membrane was usually composed of one or two cell layers, and was often covered with cellular fibrin; in some places, the lining cells were replaced by fibrin precipitates. In one case, synovial membranes from an ankle joint and a knee joint were examined 7 and 10 years respectively after onset of the rheumatoid process, and displayed similar inflammatory reactions. The layer of lining cells was mostly thin. Fibrosis of the subsynovial tissue and subsynovial blood vessels had advanced with duration of the disease.

D. Electron Microscopic Findings

Degree of hyperplasia and other morphological changes of the synovial membrane in toto could only incompletely be determined by electron microscopy. Therefore, the changes of single synovial cells, of the interstitial tissue, and of blood and lymph vessels were chiefly studied.

1. Changes of Synovial Cells

In active synovitis, electron microscopy disclosed enlarged synovial cells which lay in a relatively loose network with rather wide spaces. The cells contained one or more polymorphic nuclei, and were in reciprocal connection by their filopodial cytoplasmic processes. The cell processes were broader than those of normal synovial cells. Cells with a vacuolated cytoplasm corresponding to type A of the differentiation of Hamerman *et al.* predominated; they often contained electron-dense cytosomes of various sizes (Fig. 5). The matrix of the lysosomal organelles was either homogeneous or sometimes loosened by small vesicles and fine granules. The type A cells with stronger lysosomal

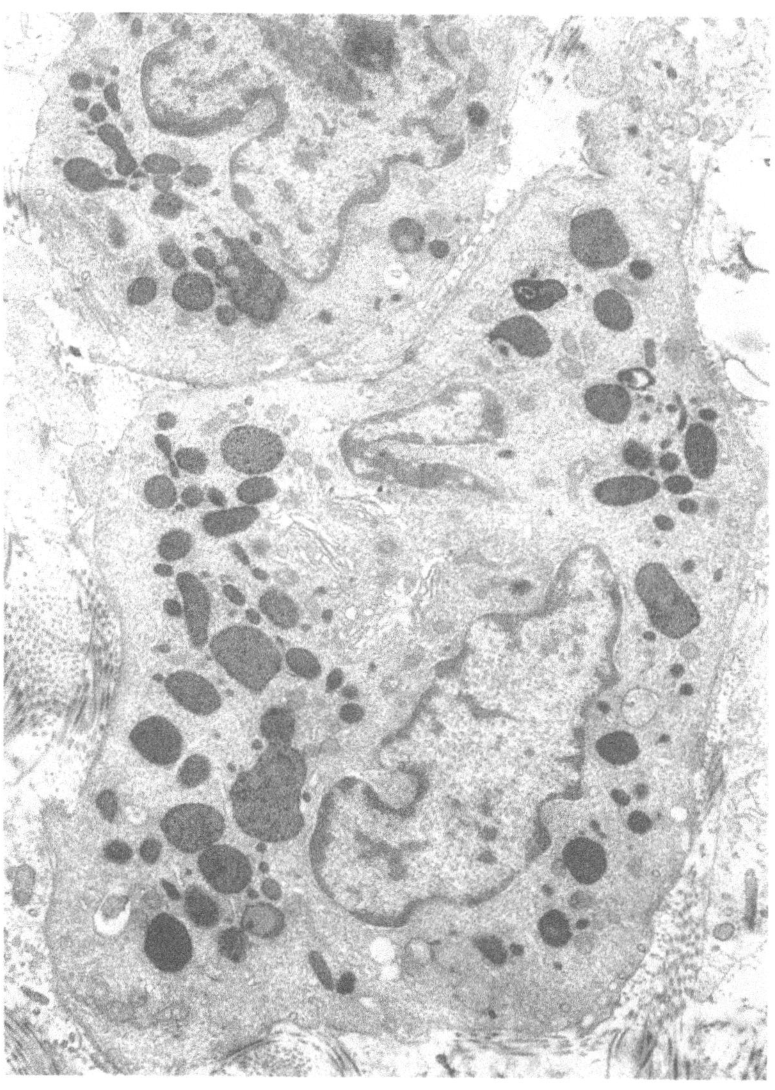

Fig. 5. Synovial cells of type A with strong lysosomal activity and well developed Golgi apparatus. Electr.-micr.: 1800; total magnific.: 7000

activity could often not be distinguished from the other type cells with enlarged ergastoplasm (Fig. 8). This indicated that cells existed with intermediate content of ergastoplasm and with simultaneous formation of granules (Fig. 6). In some cases, a great variation could be observed in the density of the cytoplasmic basic substance. In no case did significant swelling of the mitochondria occur. The number of mitochondria and the structure of their cristae did not

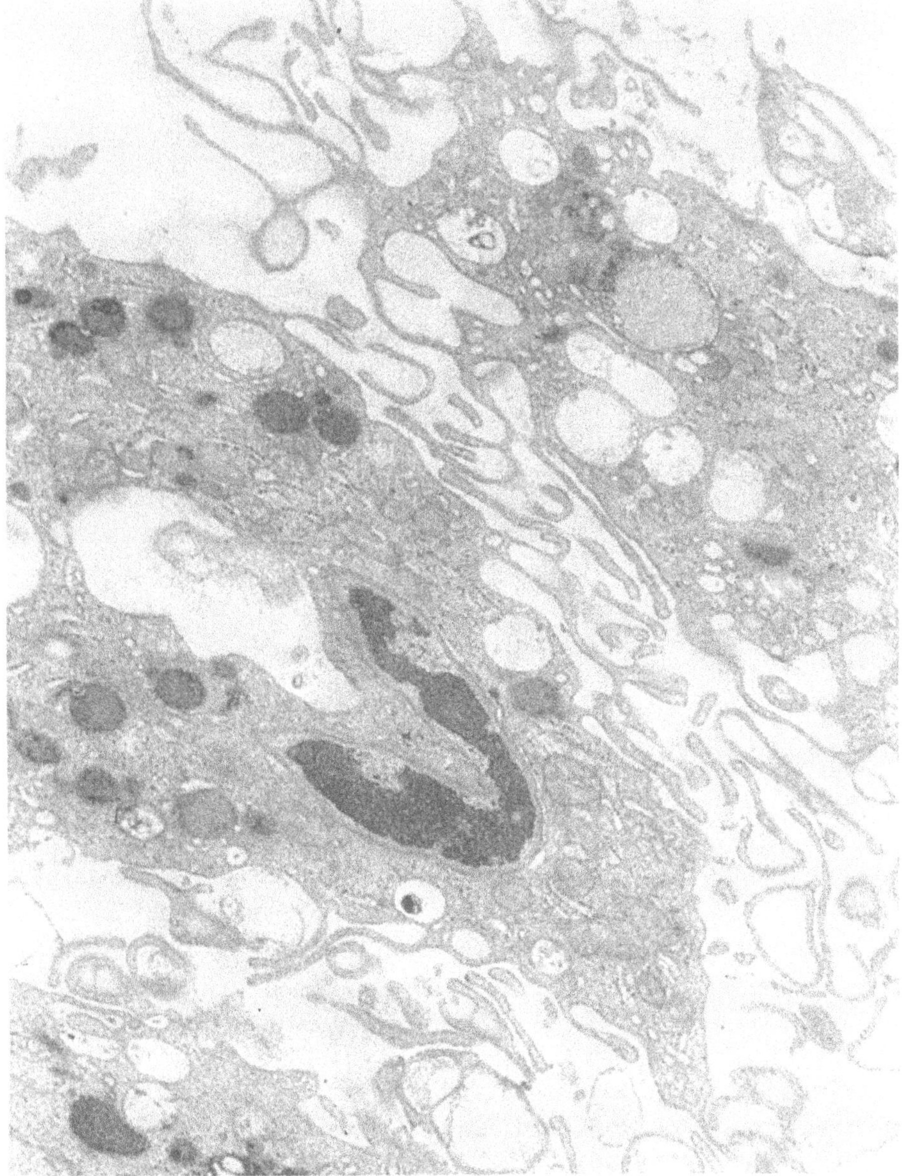

Fig. 6. Intermediate cell type with filopodial cell protrusions and a few lysosomes.
Electr.-micr.: 3400; total magnific.: 13000

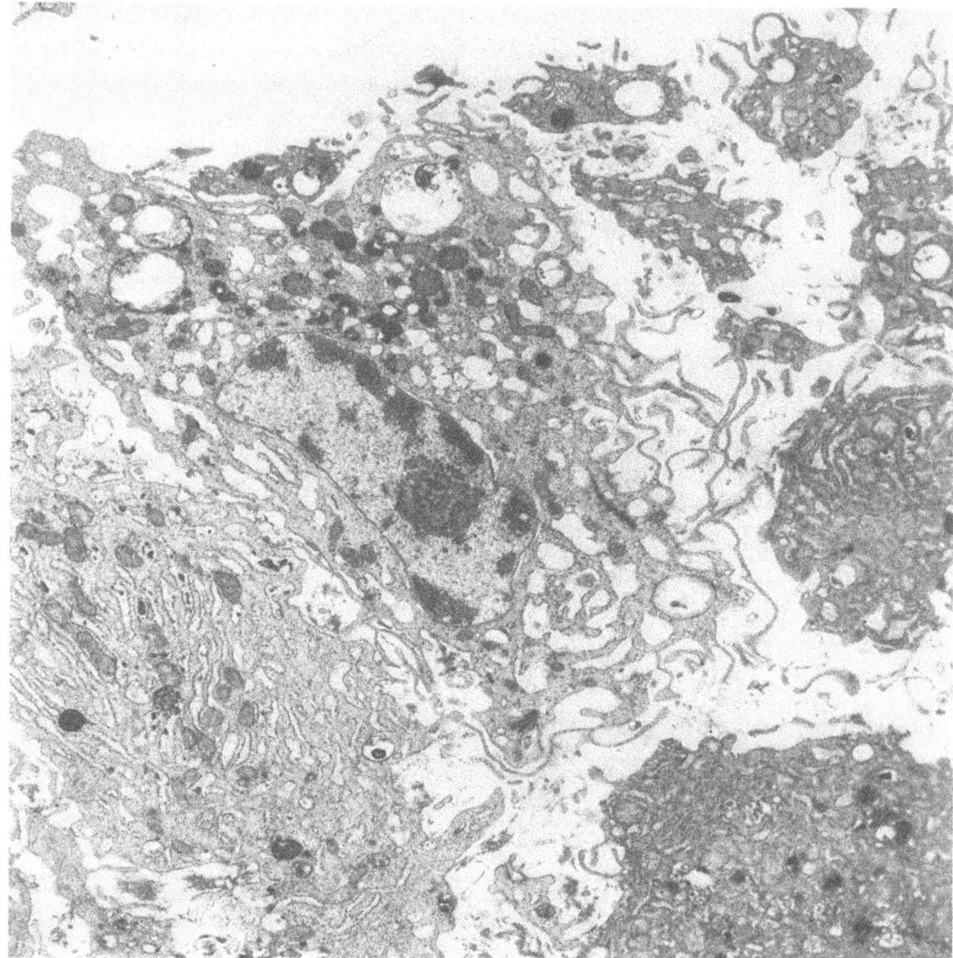

Fig. 7. Synovial cells of type B with dense ergastoplasm. Electr.-micr.: 1800; total
magnific.: 5800

differ from those of normal synovial cells. Now and then occurred clumpy
syncytial complexes with several nuclei and incomplete cytoplasmic infoldings.

2. Changes of Intercellular Spaces and on the Surfaces of Synovial Cells

In some cases, precipitates of fibrin were observed between synovial cells.
The fibrin lay often in contiguity with degenerating cells and cell debris
(Fig. 9). Other intercellular spaces contained small bundles of collagen fibrils,
and sometimes almost reached the surface of synovial membrane, or directly
conveyed the impression of open connections between joint space and subsynovial tissue. In some cases, a thick layer of fibrin and cell fragments
containing vacuoles and lipid droplets covered the lining cells (Fig. 9). The
synovial cells beneath the debris were mostly flattened and often lacked

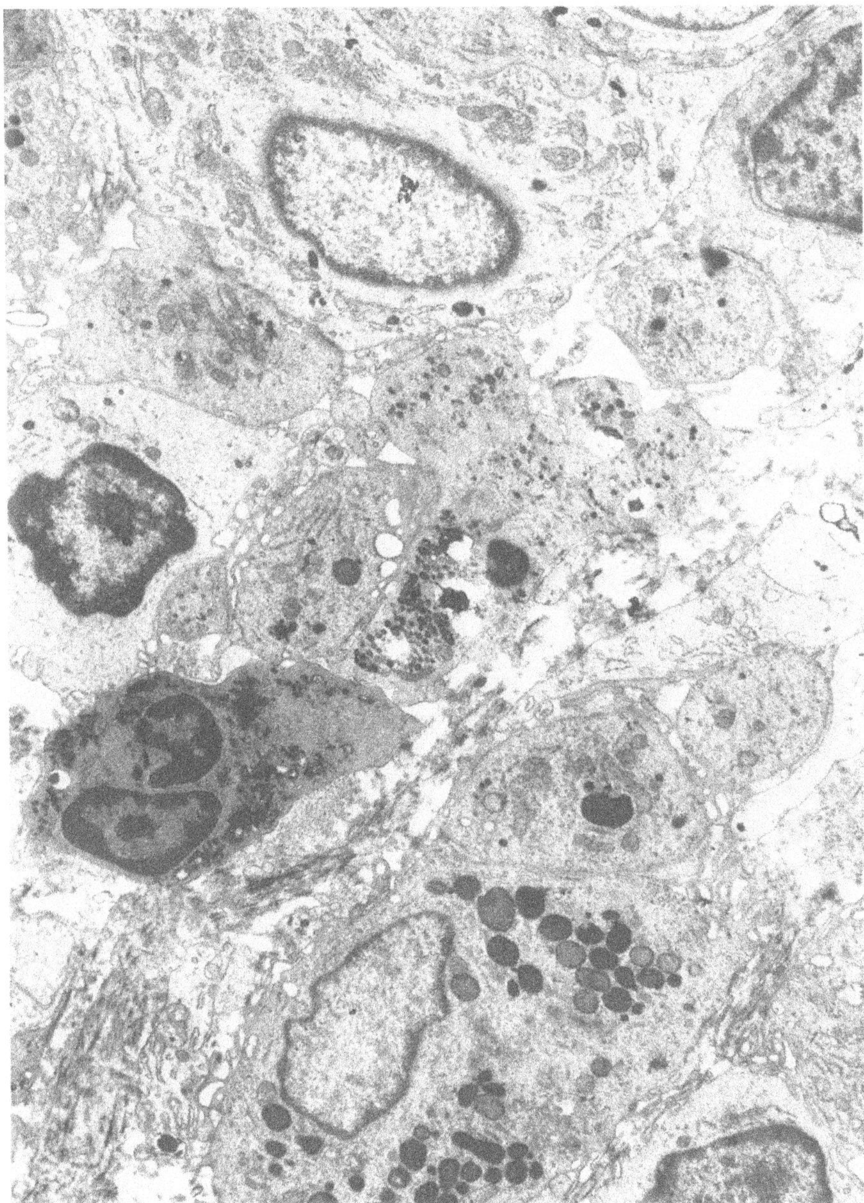

Fig. 8. Synovial cells with various lysosomes. Electr.-micr: 1800; total magnific.: 7000

protrusions or organelles (Fig. 10) In two cases, outgrowth of collagen fibrils into the debris was observed. No infiltrates of leukocytes, lymphocytes and plasma cells occurred between the lining cells.

3. Changes of Subsynovial Tissue

Below the synovial cells, lymphocytes and plasma cells occurred in diffuse infiltrates and often also accumulated around blood vessels (Fig. 15). Plasma

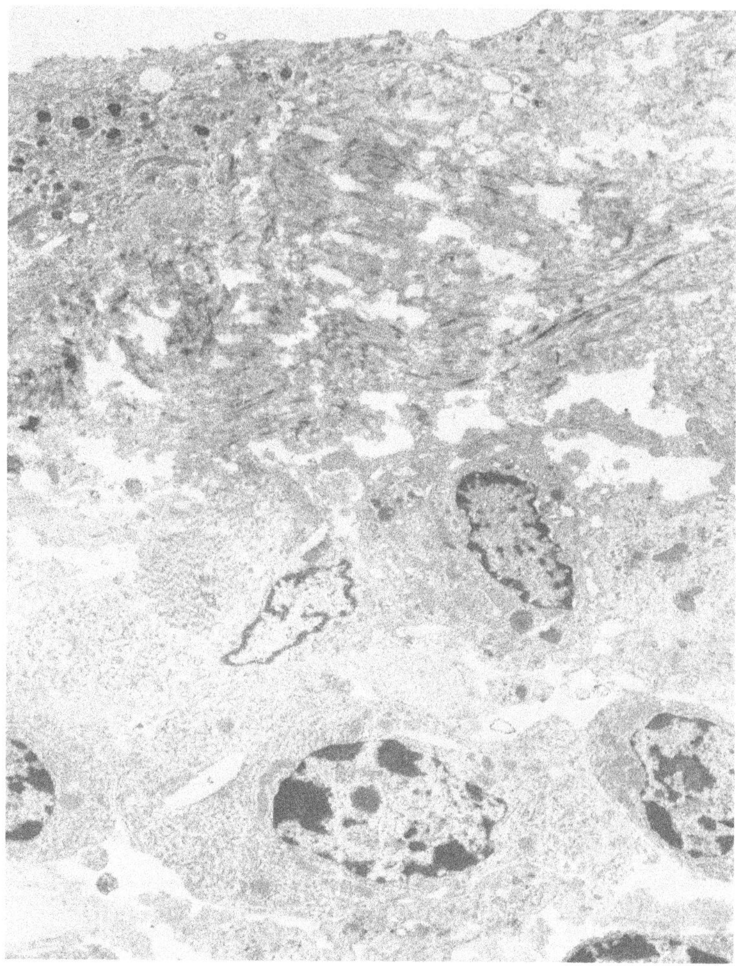

Fig. 9. Fibrinoid material and cell debris on the surface of synovial cells with collagen fibrils in the acellular layer. Electr.-micr.: 2 500; total magnific.: 5 000

cells with densely distributed ergastoplasma tubules predominated; they had characteristic nuclei with rough chromatin structure. Some plasma cells included cytosomes of different size with partly fine, partly rough granular matrix. Polymorphonuclear leukocytes were noticed in two cases only. The subsynovial connective tissue often displayed extraordinary density of collagen fibers.

4. Changes of Blood and Lymph Vessels

Alterations of the walls of blood vessels were inconstant. In some cases, capillaries and small blood vessels were hyperemic (Fig. 11), but not altered. In other cases, capillaries were surrounded by a thin network of fibril bundles. Arterioles had the basal membrane broadened to a layer of homogeneous or fine fibrillar tissue which was surrounded by atrophic smooth muscle cells

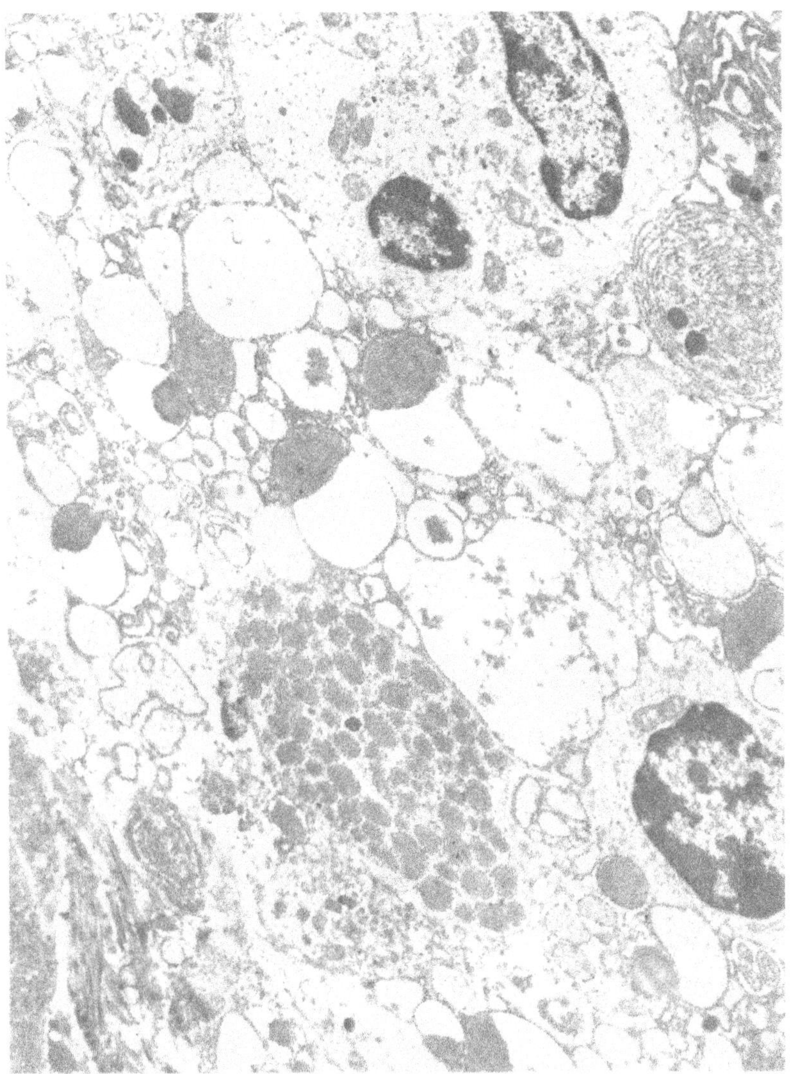

Fig. 10. Partly course vacuolar, partly granular debris in necrosis of synovial membrane in rheumatoid arthritis of 7 years. Electr.-micr.: 1800; total magnific.: 7000

(Fig. 13 and 14). Adventitial cells and pericytes were increased and enlarged up to formation of giant cells (Fig. 12). Essential alterations of the endothelial cells were absent as well as complete obliterations of blood vessels. Sometimes dilated lymph vessels could be observed; their endothelium often contained larger lipoprotein complexes (Fig. 16).

IV. Discussion

Morphological investigations of synovial membranes may contribute to understanding of rheumatoid arthritis, if the latter has been substantiated by

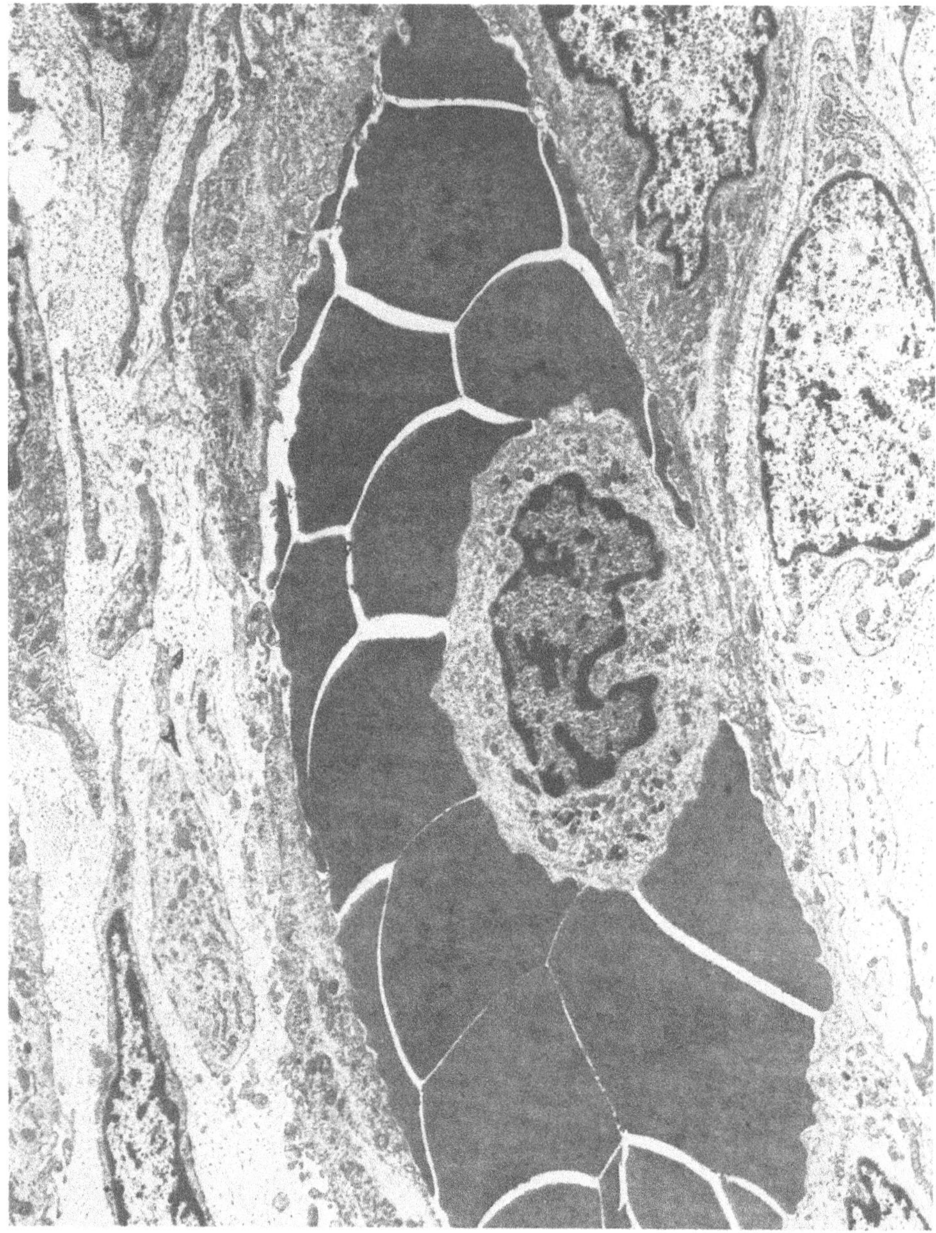

Fig. 11. Hyperemic subsynovial blood vessel in rheumatoid arthritis. Electr.-micr.: 1800; total magnific.: 7000

clinical observations and laboratory tests. The noticed alterations represented findings in arthritis often associated with recurrent exudation.

Although the findings varied individually, several morphological features were common. The layer of synovial cells was mostly broadened. The cells

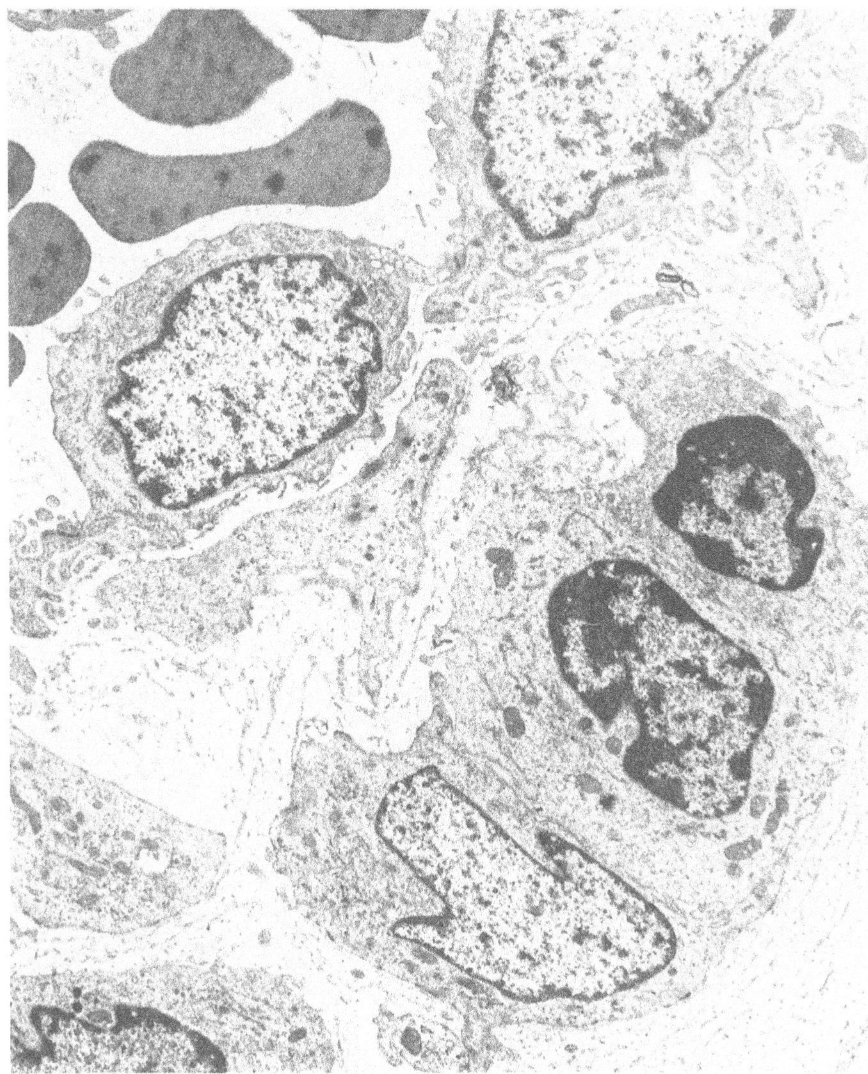

Fig. 12. Syncytial giant cell formation in the adventitia of a subsynovial blood vessel in rheumatoid arthritis of 8 years. Electr.-micr.: 1 800; total magnific.: 7 000

and their nuclei were polymorphic; a great number of cells were often strongly vacuolated. Their ergastoplasmic tubules were widened, the lysosomal cytosomes varied in number and size, and the filopodial cell processes were prominent. NORTON and ZIFF (1966) differentiated a cell type of an intermediate morphological position between the A- and B-cells of HAMERMAN *et al.* (1961). This cell type often occurred in our cases. Precipitations of fibrin and hyalin were lying between the lining cells and on their surface; the precipitated material consisted electron microscopically of fibrin with cell debris and collagen fibrils.

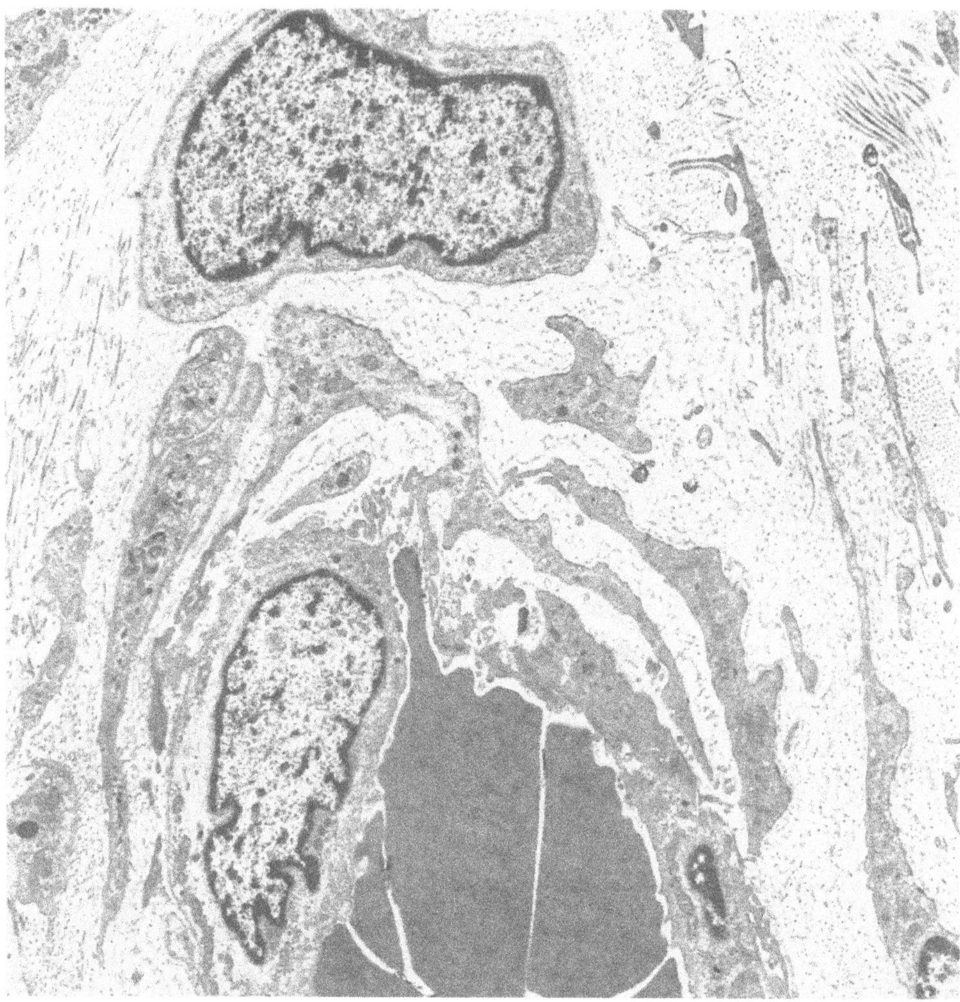

Fig. 13. Disruption of vascular wall by increased collagen fibers in rheumatoid arthritis of 8 years. Electr.-micr.: 1800; total magnific.: 7000

Interpretation of the alterations in shape and content of the synovial cells is difficult, because the cells of the normal synovial membrane are polygonal and contain varying cytoplasmic structures and organelles. Barland, Novikoff and Hamerman (1964) demonstrated by histochemical methods and fluorescent microscopy that the synovial cells have greater lysosomal activity than the other cells of the joint capsule. In some of our cases, the lysosomal activity was more pronounced than in normal synovial membrane. The lysosomal activity was even more intensive than the granule formation noticed under phagocytotic activity in synovial cells after injection of colloidal iron or colloidal carbon particles (Goldberg et al., 1962; Muirden, 1963; Ball et al., 1964; Huth and Langer, 1965; Adam, 1966). However, increased

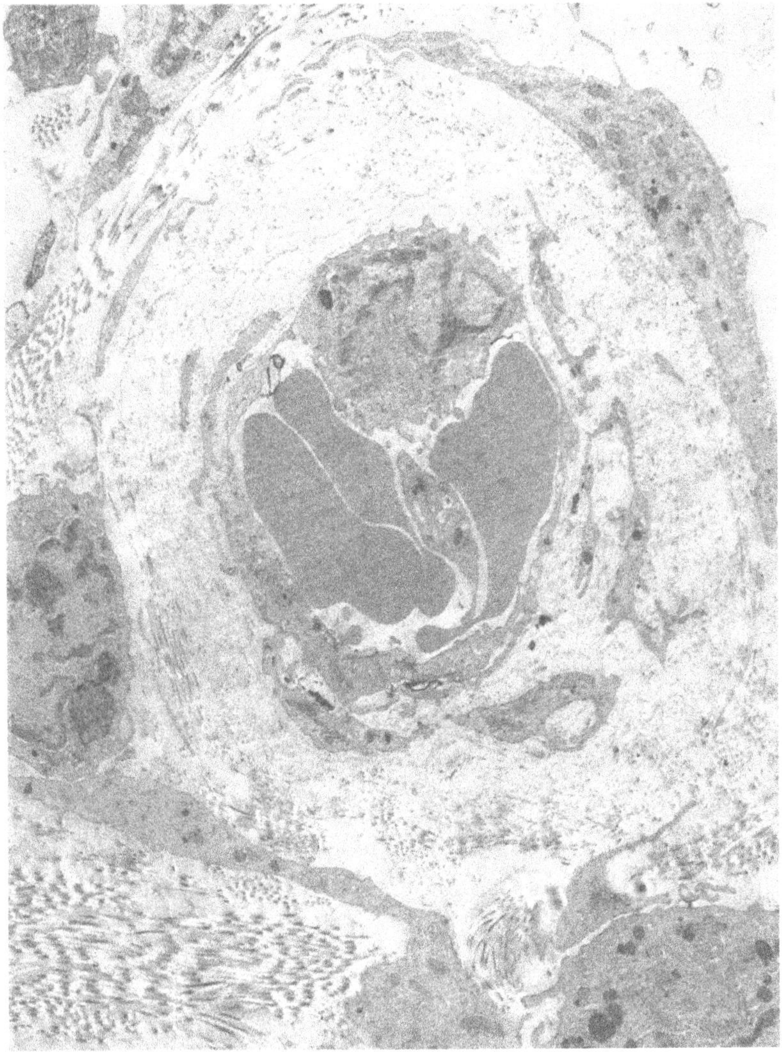

Fig. 14. Marked sclerosis of vessel wall with compression of smooth muscle cells. Electr.-micr.: 1 800; total magnific.: 7 000

lysosomal activity was not a constant finding. Mitochondrial alterations like swelling, as described by HAMERMAN *et al.* (1963), were not observed in our cases; also abnormalities of mitochondrial cristae were absent.

Polymorphism of cellular protrusions—observed by us as well as by other investigators—and nuclear polymorphism were probably an expression of enhanced cell degeneration and regeneration of hyperplastic synovial membrane. The rather frequent occurrence of giant cells in the synovial membrane was regarded as a characteristic finding in rheumatoid arthritis by DONALD and KERR (1968). Covering of the synovial cells with electron microscopically identifiable cell debris, fibrin, and outgrowing collagen fibers was even more

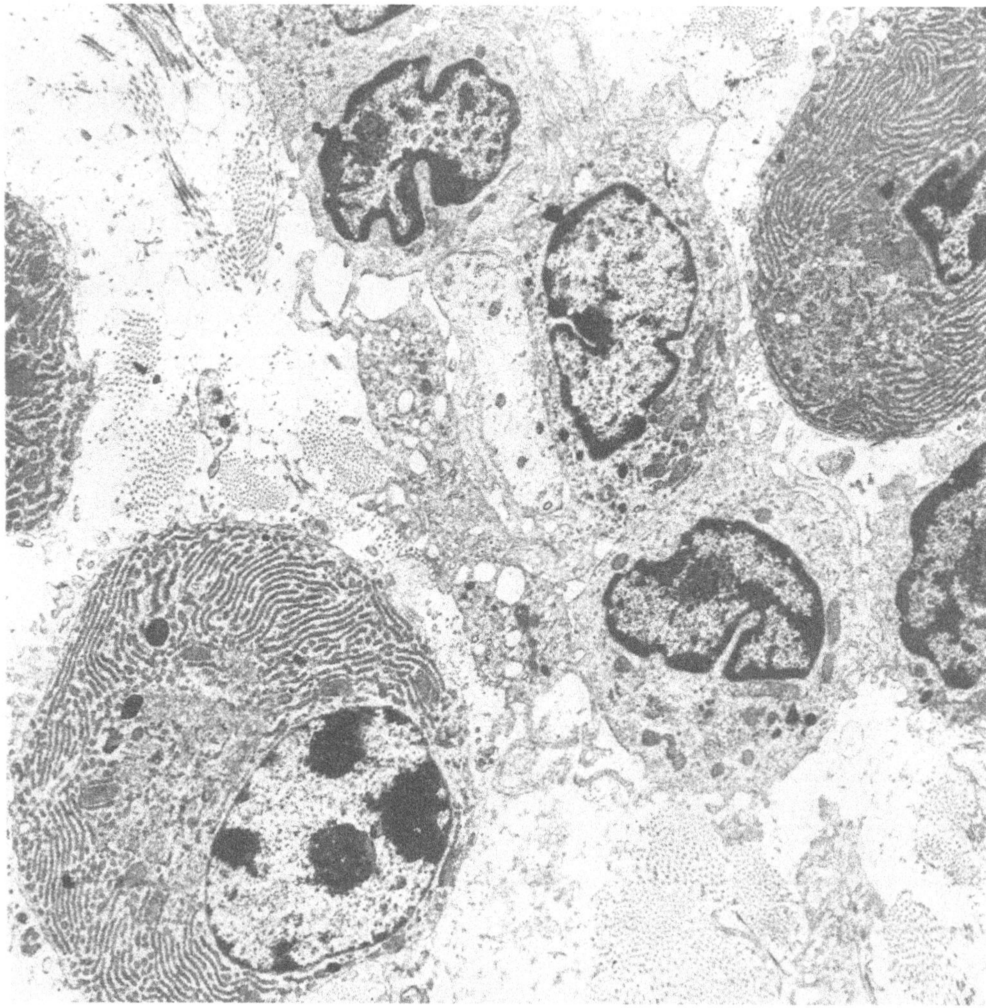

Fig. 15. Plasma cells in perivascular infiltrate in subsynovial tissue. Electr.-micr.: 1800; total magnific.: 5800

frequent. The increased cell regeneration and the more frequent necroses went along sometimes with very polygonal phagosomal inclusions in synovial cells. The presence of necroses in the synovial membrane was considered by Fass-bender (1970) as more typical for rheumatoid synovitis than the proliferation of synovial cells or the round cell infiltrates in the subsynovial tissue.

Fibrosis of the subsynovial tissue in rheumatoid arthritis caused a deeper position of the subsynovial vessels in relationship to the synovial surface than described by Ruckes et al. (1962) and Lang (1958) in arthrosis deformans. The increase of distance became more pronounced by marked hyperplasia of the lining cells. Additional increase of the distance between the vascular lumen and the synovial cavity was caused by proliferation of adventitial cells.

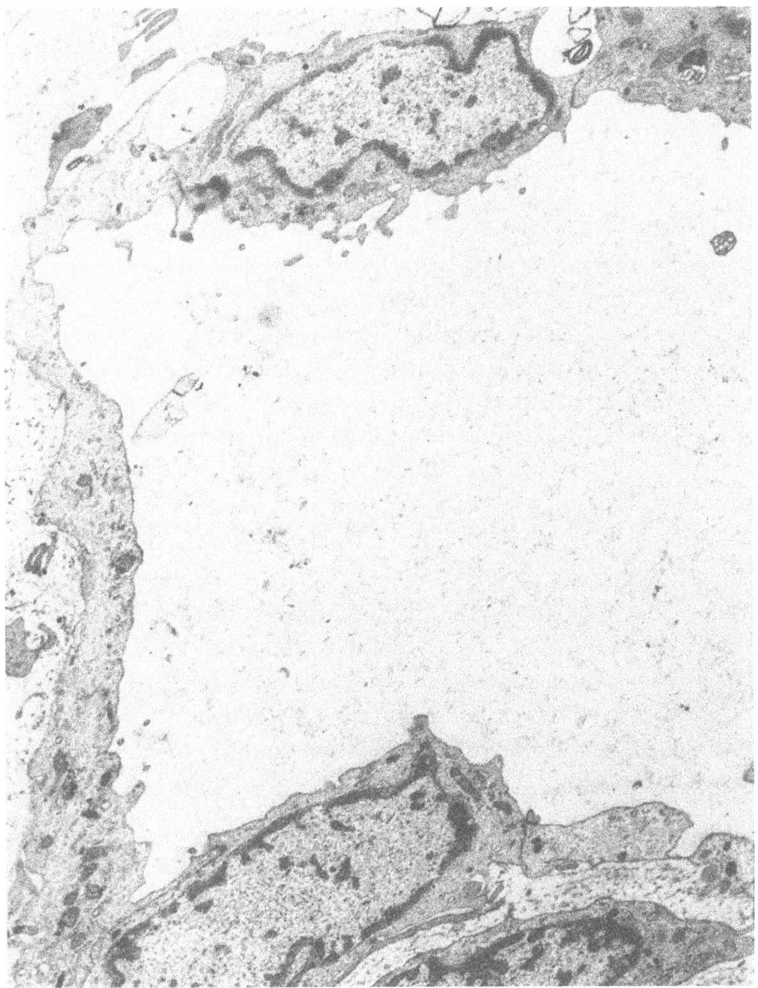

Fig. 16. Widely patent lymph vessel of subsynovial tissue in rheumatoid arthritis of 15 years. Electr.-micr.: 1 800; total magnific.: 5 800

Such proliferation seemed to occur sometimes in a precipitated way, and to be then associated with formation of multinuclear giant cells. Comparative examinations of synovial membranes in posttraumatic synovitis disclosed similar alterations of the vascular walls. Therefore, the sclerosing alterations of blood vessels appear to be uncharacteristic changes, and not to represent a specific feature of the rheumatoid process. Alterations of blood vessels in the vulnerable synovial membrane were also observed following arthrotic changes of the articular surface. A specific rheumatoid vasculitis as assumed by KULKA *et al.* (1959) could not be verified by our studies.

Similarly, the lymphocyte and plasma cell infiltrates were not a constant finding. Plasma cells predominated, having exceptionally dense ergastoplasmic tubules. MELLORS *et al.* (1961) differentiated two rheumatoid factors in plasma cells by fluorescent microscopy. The importance of these factors is subject to argument, because plasma cell infiltrates may be absent in phases of hyperplastic reaction of synovial lining cells in rheumatoid arthritis. This question might be clarified by further investigations of experimental arthritis which Rawson *et al.* (1968) induced in rabbits.

Finally, alterations of the subsynovial lymph vessels in rheumatoid arthritis were often noted. The density of lymphatic vascular nets in the synovial membrane—demonstrated especially by Lang (1958)—indicates important function in the normal synovial membrane. These lymph vessels of the subsynovial tissue were often exceptionally dilated. Their endothelial cells were blown up by larger lipoprotein inclusions which may be regarded as signs of increased drainage of lymphatic fluid. The high content of protein in rheumatoid synovial exudates possibly may induce further unfolding of lymphatic vessels.

V. Summary and Conclusion

The morphologic appearance of synovitis in rheumatoid arthritis varies. The characteristic hyperplasia and hypertrophy of synovial cells may regress; changes of blood vessels may be absent. Nevertheless, both comparative light and electron microscopic studies and the correlation of the morphological to clinical observations do allow a certain histopathologic definition of diagnosed rheumatoid synovitis. The finding permitting such definition are:

1. Clinically, progressive disease over many years with persistent thickening of joints and effusions in some joints.
2. Serologically, positive laboratory tests for rheumatoid factor in more than 90% of cases.
3. Light microscopically:
   a) Hyperplasia and hypertrophy of synovial cells in 80% of the cases;
   b) Polymorphism of synovial cells and their nuclei;
   c) Fibrosis of the subsynovial tissue with increase of the distance between synovial surface and subsynovial blood vessels;
   d) Fibrinoid necrosis of synovial membrane (not constant);
   e) Sclerosis of subsynovial blood vessels (not constant).
4. Electron microscopically:
   a) Relative increase of B-cells in synovial membrane
   b) Occurrence of an intermediate cell type (not constant);
   c) Increase in lysosomal activity of synovial cells (not constant);
   d) Increase of ergastoplasmic tubules in synovial cells (not constant);
   e) Greater vacuolization of synovial cells (not constant).

Hyperplasia of synovial lining cells, their degeneration and desquamation, and the frequent augmentation of their ergastoplasmic tubules may be reactions to the noxious agent as well as the cause of the relatively high content of protein, cells, and cell debris in synovial fluid. The formation of intraarticular exudates, however, cannot be ascribed exclusively to the hyperplastic elements of the synovial membrane, especially if one considers how fast exudates recur after aspiration. Occurrence of exudates in cases with atrophic or fibrosed synovial membrane suggests the production of exudates not only by synovial cells.

An important pathogenetic factor in the symptom "hydrarthrosis" appears to be increased permeability of the subsynovial blood vessels. The broad perivascular infiltrates very likely stem from this permeability. The sclerosing alterations of the outer vascular wall and of the perivascular tissue may possible be a sequel of long time increased permeability. The inconstancy of vascular alterations does not imply necessarily that the sclerosing changes are not akin to the picture of the primary disease.

References

ADAM, W. S.: Fine structure of synovial membrane: Phagocytosis of colloidal carbon from the joint cavity. Lab. Invest. **15**, 680–691 (1966).

ASCHOFF, L.: Spezielle Pathologische Anatomie 4. Aufl., S. 263. Leipzig: Breitkopf und Härtel 1919.

BALL, J., CHAPMAN, J. A., MUIRDEN, K. D.: The uptake of iron in rabbit synovial tissue following intraarticular injection of iron dextran. J. Cell Biol. **22**, 351–364 (1964).

BARLAND, P., NOVIKOFF, A. B., HAMERMAN, D.: Electron microscopy of the human synovial membrane. J. Cell Biol. **14**, 207–320 (1962).

— — — Fine structure and cytochemistry of the rheumatoid synovial membrane with special reference to lysosomes. Amer. J. Path. **44**, 853–866 (1964).

BAUMECKER, H.: Untersuchungen über die Veränderungen an der Gelenkkapsel und ihre Beziehung zu den Ergüssen des Kniegelenkes. Langenbecks Arch. klin. Chir. **170**, 511–569 (1932).

BICHAT, X.: Anatomie générale. Paris 1806.

BLAU, S., JANIS, R., HAMERMAN, D., SANDSON, J.: Cellular origin of hyaluronate protein in the human synovial membrane. Science **150**, 353–355 (1965).

BRÅNEMARK, P. I., EKHOLM, R., GOLDIE, I.: To the question of angiopathy in rheumatoid arthritis. Acta orthop. scand. **40**, 153–175 (1969).

CAMPBELL, W. G.: Localization of adenosine 5-triphosphate in vascular and cellular synovium of rabbits. Lab. Invest. **18**, 304–316 (1968).

CHAPMAN, J. A., MUIRDEN, K. D., BALL, J., HYDE, P. A.: Synovial tissue and uptake of iron following intraarticular injection. Electron microscopy. SS 12. New York and London: Acad. Press 1962.

COOPER, N. S.: Pathology of rheumatoid arthritis. Med. Clin. N. Amer. **52**, 607–621 (1968).

COTTA, H.: Elektronenmikroskopische Untersuchungen an der Gelenkkapsel und ihre Bedeutung für die morphologisch-funktionelle Einheit des Gelenkes. Arch. orthop. Unfall-Chir. **53**, 443–494 (1962).

COULTER, W. H.: The characteristics of human synovial tissue as seen with the electron microscope. Arthr. and Rheum. **5**, 70–87 (1962).

CRUICKSHANK, B.: Interpretation of multiple biopsies of synovial tissue in rheumatic diseases. Ann. rheum. Dis. **11**, 137–145 (1952).

DONALD, K. J., KERR, J. F. R.: Giant cells in the synovium in rheumatoid arthritis. Med. J. Aust. **55** (I), 761–762 (1968).

Efskind, L.: Experimentelle Untersuchungen über die Anatomie und Physiologie der Gelenkkapsel. Acta orthop. scand. **12**, 214–266 (1941).

Fassbender, H. G.: Spezifische und unspezifische Strukturen entzündlich-rheumatischer Erkrankungen. Med. Klin. **49**, 2152–2157 (1970).

— Morphologische Kriterien für die Beurteilung und Klassifikation von Synovialisgewebe. Therapiewoche **20**, 720–724 (1970).

— Die primär nekrotisierende Form der primär chronischen Polyarthritis. Therapiewoche **20**, 3191–3194 (1970).

Franceschini, P.: La formatione reticuloistiocitaria della membrana sinoviale. Monit. zool. ital. **40**, 411–412 (1930).

Ghadially, F. N. A., Roy, S.: Ultrastructure of synovial membrane in rheumatoid arthritis. Ann. rheum. Dis. **26**, 426–443 (1967).

Goldberg, B., Kantor, F., Benacerraf, B.: An electron microscopic study of delayed sensivity to ferritin in guinea pigs. Brit. J. exp. Path. **43**, 621–626 (1962).

Grimley, P. M.: Rheumatoid arthritis: Ultrastructure of the synovium. Ann. intern. Med. **66**, 623–624 (1967).

Gross, D.: Die sogenannten Kollagenosen. In: Documenta Geigy: Folia rheumat. **16**, 1–16 (1967).

Gugelberger, M.: Zur Differenzierung der Gelenkpunktate. Sandoz Z. med. Wiss. Triangel **9**, Nr 4 (1970).

Hagen-Torn, O.: Entwicklung und Bau der Synovialmembran. Arch. mikr. Anat. **21**, 591–663 (1882).

Hamerman, D., Sandson, J., Schubert, M.: Biochemical events in joint disease. J. chron. Dis. **16**, 835–852 (1963).

— Stephens, M., Barland, P.: Comparative histology and metabolism of synovial tissue in normal and arthritic joints. In: Inflammation and disease of connective tissue, p. 158–168. Philadelphia: W. B. Saunders 1961.

Hammar, J. A.: Über den feineren Bau der Gelenke. Arch. mikr. Anat. **43**, 266–325 (1894).

Hidvegi, E.: On the finer structure and blood supply of the synovial membrane with special regard to its physiological circulation. Acta morph. Acad. Sci. hung. **4**, 319–331 (1954).

Hirohata, K.: Studies on ultra thin sections of synovial tissue with the phase contrast microscope and the electron microscope. Kobe J. med. Sci. **4**, 241–257 (1958).

— Kobayashi, J.: Fine structures of the synovial tissues in rheumatoid arthritis. Kobe J. med. Sci. **10**, 195–203 (1964).

Hollander, J. L., McCarty, D. J., Astorga, G., Castro-Murillo, E.: Studies on the pathogenesis of rheumatoid joint inflammation. Ann. intern. Med. **62**, 281–291 (1956).

Huth, F., Langer, E.: Elektronenmikroskopische Untersuchungen der Aufnahme von Myofer durch die Synovialmembran. Beitr. path. Anat. **131**, 435–449 (1965).

Jordan, P.: Synovial membrane and fluid in rheumatoid arthritis. Arch. Path. **26**, 275–288 (1938).

Kulka, J. P.: The vascular lesions associated with rheumatoid arthritis. Bull. rheum. Dis. **19**, 201–219 (1957).

Lang, L.: Die Gelenkinnenhaut, ihre Aufbau- und Abbauvorgänge. Jb. Morph. mikr. Anat. **98**, 387–482 (1958).

Langer, E., Huth, F.: Untersuchungen über den submikroskopischen Bau der Synovialmembran. Z. Zellforsch. **51**, 545–559 (1960).

Lever, J. D., Ford, E. H. R.: Histological, histochemical and electron microscopic observations on synovial membrane. Anat. Rev. **132** 525–540 (1958).

LINDNER, J.: Der rheumatische Bindegewebsstoffwechsel und die pathologische Struktur des Bindegewebes bei rheumatoider Arthritis. Verh. dtsch. Ges. inn. Med. **73**, 1315–1349 (1968).

MARIN, D., NEGOESCU, M., STOIA, J., PIERRETTE, A., PETRESCU, A. L., CONSTANTINESCU, S. P.: The morphology of the synovial tissue and articular fluid cells in rheumatoid polyarthritis — studied with the optical and elctron microscope. Acta rheum. scand. **15**, 126–134 (1969).

MARQUART, W.: Zur Histologie der Synovialmembran. Z. Zellforsch. **12**, 34–52 (1931).

McFARLAND, G. B. et al.: Rheumatoid nodules in synovial membranes and tendons. Clin. Orthop. **58**, 165–170 (1968).

MELLORS, R. C., NOWOSLAWSKI, A., KORNGOLD, L.: Rheumatoid arthritis and the cellular origin of rheumatoid factors. Amer. J. Path. **39**, 533–546 (1961).

MUIRDEN, K. D.: An electron microscopic study of the uptake of ferritin by the synovial membrane. Arthr. and Rheum. **6**, 289–302 (1963).

NORTON, L. W., ZIFF, M.: Electron microscopic observations on the rheumatoid synovial membrane. Arthr. and Rheum. **9**, 589–610 (1966).

NOWOSLAWSKY, A., BRZOSKO, W. J.: Imunpathology of rheumatoid arthritis. I. The rheumatoid synovitis. Path. europ. **2**, 198–219 (1966).

PERLMANN, G. E., ROPES, M. W., KAUFMANN, D., BAUER, W.: The electrophoretic pattern of proteins in synovial fluid and serum in rheumatoid arthritis. J. clin. Invest. **33**, 319–322 (1954).

RAWSON, A. J., QUISMORIO, E. P., ABELSON, N. M.: The induction of synovitis in the normal rabbit with Fab.: A possible experimental model of rheumatoid arthritis. Amer. J. Path. **52**, 9a Abstract (1968).

RESTIFO, R. A., LUSSIER, A. J., RAWSON, A. J., ROCKEY, H. J., HOLLANDER, J. I.: Studies on the pathogenesis of rheumatoid joint inflammation. III. The experimental production of arthritis by the intraarticular injection of purified S-gamma globulin. Ann. intern. Med. **62**, 281–285 (1965).

RIDDLE, J. M., BLUHM, G. B., BARNHART, M. J.: Interrelationships between fibrin, neutrophils and rheumatoid synovitis. J. reticuloend. ath. Soc. **2**, 420–436 (1965).

ROBERTS, E. D., RAMSEY, F. K., SWITZER, W. P., LAYTON, J. M.: Electron microscopy of porcine synovial cell layer. J. comp. Path. **79**, 41–45 (1960).

ROPES, M. W., MULLER, A., BAUER, W.: The entrance of glucose and other sugars into joints. Arthr. and Rheum. **3**, 496–502 (1960).

ROY, S., GHADIALLY, F. N.: Ultrastructure of normal rat synovial membrane. Ann. rheum. Dis. **25**, 26–38 (1966).

RUCKES, J.: Experimentelle Untersuchungen über die Resorptionsfähigkeit des Stratum synoviale. Z. Zellforsch. **55**, 313–369 (1961).

— SCHUCKMANN, F.: Über die Topic der Kapillaren im Stratum synoviale des Kniegelenkes in Abhängigkeit vom Lebensalter unter besonderer Berücksichtigung der Arthrosis deformans. Frankfurt: Z. Path. **72**, 243–255 (1962).

SIGURDSON, A.: The structure and function of articular synovial membranes. J. Bone Jt Surg. **12**, 603–639 (1930).

SOKOLOFF, L., BUNIM, J.: Vascular lesions in rheumatoid arthritis. J. chron. Dis. **5**, 668–687 (1957).

STANFIELD, A. B., STEPHENS, C. A. L., JR.: Studies of cells cultured from 188 rheumatoid and non rheumatoid synovial tissues. Tex. Rep. Biol. Med. **21**, 400–411 (1963).

SUTER, E. R., MAJNO, G.: Ultrastructure of the joint capsule in the rat: presence to two kinds of capillaries. Nature (Lond.) **202**, 920–921 (1964).

Thomas, D. P. P., Dingle, J. T.: Studies on human synovial membrane in vitro. The metabolism of normal and rheumatoid synovial and the effect of hydrocortisone. Biochem. J. **68**, 231–238 (1958).

Tillmann, H.: Die Lymphgefäße der Gelenke. Arch. mikr. Anat. **12**, 649–664 (1878).

Wilkinson, M., Jones, B. S.: Serum and synovial fluid proteins in arthritis. Ann. rheum. Dis. **21**, 51–63 (1961).

Wyllie, J. C., Haust, M. D., More, R. H.: The fine structure of synovial lining cells in rheumatoid arthritis. Lab. Invest. **15**, 519–529 (1966).

— More, R. H. Haust, M. D.; The fine structure of normal guinea pig synovium. Lab. Invest. **13**, 1254–1263 (1964).

Cancer Research Institute, Department of Pathology and Carcinogenesis,
Sofia, Bulgaria

Experimental Thyroid Carcinogenesis

KONSTANTIN CHRISTOV and RAIKO RAICHEV

With 2 Figures

Contents

Introduction

Thyroid carcinomas have recently become one of the main problems in theoretical, experimental and clinical oncology. This is due, on the one hand, to their specific biological properties with regard to growth, metastasis, functional activity, hormonal control, radiobiological changes after treatment with ^{131}I and resistance to antitumour agents, and, on the other hand, to the possibility of studying them by means of radioactive iodine. There is no other type of tumour in the human body presenting a more favourable target for functional investigations than thyroid tumours. The wide use of radioactive iodine in the diagnosis and treatment of thyroid diseases inevitably brought up the problem of its carcinogenic effect. Experimental data and some clinical observations show that radioactive iodine (^{131}I) is able to cause thyroid tumours both in animals and in man. The increased incidence of thyroid cancer among patients irradiated in childhood for thymic enlargement is indicative of the significant participation of X-ray irradiation in thyroid carcinogenesis.

Experimental models of thyroid tumours in mice, rats and hamsters have elucidated the causes and mechanisms determining tumour growth. Moreover, they have shown that most factors supposed to have a carcinogenic effect on man have caused the appearance of thyroid carcinomas and adenomas under experimental conditions. Because there are differences in the biological properties and the morphological structure of thyroid tumours in man and in animals it is necessary to make comparisons.

I. Methods of Thyroid Tumour Induction

1. Spontaneous Thyroid Tumours

In comparing the carcinogenic effect of the various agents, it es particularly important to know the incidence of spontaneous tumours in the thyroid gland. In mice they are comparatively infrequent. Among 51700 mice Slye et al. (1926) found only twelve with thyroid carcinomas. The existence of thyroid tumours in adult mice is also reported by Jacobs (1963), Roe (1965). Jones et al. (1966) published nine thyroid tumours in C3H mice and in hybrids of C3H and C3Hf. Zaidela et al. have discovere a high percentage (about ten) in several subsequent generations of XVIInc/ZE mice.

Spontaneous thyroid tumours are most frequent in rats. This is true of adenomas predominantly. Van Dike (1953) reported ten thyroid adenomas among sixteen adult albino rats aged between 801 and 906 days. The author relates the histogenesis of these tumours with the epithelium of the ultimo-bronchial bodies. The percentage of these naturally occuring thyroid tumours varies a great deal in inbred animals (see Table 1).

In publications by Lindsay et al. (1968a), naturally occurring tumours of the thyroid gland are attributed to the group of carcinomas, owing to their infiltrative growth and metastatic capacity. Their small size and the character-

Table 1. *Incidence of naturally occurring thyroid carcinomas in rats.*
(Lindsay *et al.*, 1968b)

Rat strain	No. of rats	Age of incidence		
		6 months	12 months	24 months and over
Long-Evans	40	1 (2%)	—	16 (40%)
Sprague	160	—	—	36 (22%)
Fischer	90	—	—	20 (22%)
Wistar	61	—	—	12 (19%)
Buffalo	47	—	—	12 (25%)
Ostborne-Mendel	30	—	—	10 (33%)
Lewis	4	—	—	0 (0%)
Rattus norvegicus (wild)	6	—	—	1 (16%)
Rattus rattus (wild)	24	—	—	0 (0%)

istic histological structure differentiate them very well from induced follicular and papillary tumours. The authors relate their histogenesis predominantly to the "light cells".

2. Induction of Thyroid Tumours by Goitrogens

Intensive investigations in the field of thyroid carcinogenesis started only after the goitrogenic effect of sulphonamides and thiourates was established (MACKENZIE and MACKENZIE, 1943; ASTWOOD et al., 1943). It has been clarified that these compounds inhibit thyroid hormone synthesis and cause hyperplasia of the thyroid cells (BIELSCHOWSKY et al., 1949; KABAK, 1949; BEID et al., 1955). For the first time BIELSCHOWSKY (1945) combined the thyroidblocking effect of alylthiourea with the blastomogenic effect of acetylaminofluorene (AAF) and obtained numerous benign tumours of the thyroid gland within a short period of time (197 days). For the same period of time AAF and alylthiouresa, separately applied, did not cause thyroid tumours. Subsequently it was established that thiouracil can also induce thyroid adenomas and carcinomas, provided that the period of treatment is extended to two years (GRIESBACH et al., 1945; PASCHKIS et al., 1948; MORRIS and GREEN, 1951; MORRIS and DALTON, 1951; MONEY and ROWSON, 1950). A number of other thiouracil compounds have a similar carcinogenic effect. Most commonly applied among them are methylthiouracil (MTU) and propylthiouracil (PTU) (DONIACH, 1950; VOITKEVIC, 1957; LEATHEM, 1958; WILLIS, 1961; GREER et al., 1964). Iodinization of thiouracil in fifth position eliminates its goitrogenic and carcinogenic effects (MONEY et al., 1957).

Thyroid carcinogenesis in animals treated with thiourates passes three morphological stages: (SEIFTER et al., 1949; BIELSCHOWSKY, 1955; NAPALKOV, 1958; WOLLMAN, 1961; CHRISTOV, 1968a).

1. Diffuse hyperplasia of the thyroid epithelium. This stage normally lasts until about the 6th or the 8th month after the beginning of the experiment.

2. Nodular proliferation of the follicular and parafollicular cells (light cells) with formation of benign tumours. This stage starts from the 8th month and continues until the 16th or 18th month approximately.

3. Malignant tumour growth later than 18 months after the beginning of the experiment.

The latent period given for thyroid adenoma varies in publications by different authors, but it is never shorter than six months (BIELSCHOWSKY, 1955; MORRIS, 1955; NAPALKOV, 1958). Upon extension of the treatment period, there is an increase both in the percentage of animals with thyroid tumours and in the incidence of tumours in one and the same gland. After the 16th to 18th month the size of individual adenomas grows rapidly and the cells in separate regions show signs of malignant growth (PURVES and GRIESBACH, 1947; PURVES et al., 1951; SELLERS et al., 1953; PETREA, 1961).

Upon comparing the goitrogenic effect of the different derivatives of thiourea, it was established that the degree of hyperplasia caused by them is different in the individual experimental animals (Morris, 1955). Thus, for example PTU has about eleven times stronger effect on the thyroid tissue of rats than MTU, whereas in man their effect is almost identical (Greer et al., 1964). Although hyperplastic changes in the thyroid gland of rats are most clearly expressed in the case of PTU treatment, the latent period for thyroid tumours is the same as with MTU treatment. Obviously the degree of thyroid hyperplasia is not the most important factor in the neoplastic transformation of the thyroid cells. There are a number of other factors which modify the goitrogenic effect of the different thioureates and influence the appearance and growth of thyroid tumours (Isler, 1962).

Dose of the goitrogenic agent. The significance of the goitrogenic effect is discussed in the works of many authors. Applying doses of 2,5, 10, 20, and 50 mg of PTU, Willis (1961) came to the conclusion that large doses not only farled to stimulate hyperplastic and tumour growth of the thyroid cells, but they even inhibited them. Napalkov (1958, 1959a) maintained a similar opinion. The Rumanian authors Milcu and Petrea (1959) preferred MTU doses of 25 mg. The quantities of goitrogenic substance which block thyroid hormone synthesis entirely without damage to the parenchyma organs and the haemopoietic apparatus should be considered optimum. This is achieved by daily doses of 5 to 10 mg of PTU and 10 to 20 mg of MTU.

The age, sex and genetic characteristics of the experimental animals also have an effect on the process of thyroid carcinogenesis. According to Money and Rowson (1950), the age of the animals does not play a significant role since the incidence of thyroid tumours and their latent period are almost identical in the different age groups. Particularly interesting in this respect are Napalkov's (1969) investigations of the appearance of thyroid tumours in animals treated with MTU in utero and after birth for several subsequent generations. In control animals (not treated with MTU during their embryogenesis) the percentage of thyroid tumours is lower than that established between the 1st and the 4th, the 8th and the 9th generations of the experimental group (MTU was applied during embryonic and post-embryonic development up to the 17th generation). This twophase curve of the frequency of thyroid tumours is also observed in the brother-sister crossing of animals, only the peaks of the curves are shifted two or three generations backward. The author does not give a satisfactory explanation of these phenomena, but it es obvious that both age and genetic factors interfere. The relation of genetic factors to the latent period and the frequency of thyroid tumours has also been discussed in publications by Wollman (1961). He has established that, among rats of the Fischer-344, AC-9935 black and Marshall-520 strains, thyroid adenomas appeared earliest in rats of the Fischer-344 strain. Zajdela (1967) reported a high frequency of thyroid tumours in XVII nc/ZE mice. A rather interesting fact is that under conditions of increased TSH (after MTU treatment), predominantly parafollicular cells show hyperplastic growth (Petrea, 1996). These cells from mainly solid tumour variants in the thyroid gland. MTU causes the appearance of thyroid adenomas and carcinomas not only in rats but also in mice (MORRIS *et al.*, 1951) and hamsters (FORTNER *et al.*, 1960; AKIMOVA and KULIK, 1966; SICHUK *et al.*, 1968; AKIMOVA *et al.*, 1969; RAICHEV and CHRISTOV, 1971). The latent period of these tumours and their frequency are close to those of the rats and therefore we are not going to dwell on them in detail.

In the case of MTU treatment it seems that the sex of the animals does not have much effect on the latent period and the incidence of thyroid adenomas and carcinomas (MONEY, 1969), as the data of most authors are rather contradictory and inconvincing. In hamsters the goitrogenesis in females is more intensive compared with rats (SICHUK *et al.*, 1968). When thyroid tumours are means of ionizing radiation, however, the sex of the experimental animals is of considerable importance (POTTER *et al.*, 1960; LINDSAY *et al.*, 1963; LINDSAY, 1969).

In animals treated with ionizing radiations, the incidence of thyroid adenomas and carcinomas was higher for males. DONIACH (1969a) tried to explain these differences as due to the greater height of the follicular cells in male rats which is indicative of an inborn state of increased thyrotrophic stimulation. The differences disappear when the effect of ^{131}I or of X-rays is combined with subsequent treatment with goitrogens, most probably due to the greater increase in TSH in both female and male animals. No differences in the frequency of thyroid adenomas and carcinomas were established in males and females in the course of our experiments with hamsters (RAICHEV and CHRISTOV, 1971). However, certain authors (SICHUK *et al.*, 1968 have found that goitrogenesis in hamsters was more marked in females.

Depriving the organism of thyroid hormones for a longer period of time has an unfavourable effect on growth and metabolism (BIELSCHOWSKY, 1955). This condition of the body adversely affects the experiments themselves. Therefore SELLERS and SCHÖNBAUM (1957, 1962a, 1965) added minimum quantities of desiccated thyroid powder (DTP) to the food or injected thyroxine animals. The administration of small quantities of thyroid hormones improved the experimental conditions without inhibiting TTS. In animals so treated hyperplasia of the thyroid cells is more clearly expressed and the latent period of the tumours is shorter (LINDSAY *et al.*, 1966).

Mechanism of action of the thioureates. According to most authors, hyperplastic and tumour growth in the thyroid gland after treatment with thioureates is due, not to their direct carcinogenic effect on thyroid cells, but to their increase of TSH (BIELSCHOWSKY and HORNING, 1958; D'ANGELO and TRAUM, 1958; NAGASAKA, 1961/1962; PURVES, 1964; BROWN-GRANT, 1967; FURTH, 1969). When thyroid hormonesynthesis is inhibited with thioureates, the lack of thyroid hormones in the body and the existing feedback correlations between the thyroid gland and the adenohypophysis bring about a compensatory increase in TSH production. TSH is a physical stimulator of thyroid epithelia, and a definite quantity of thyroid hormones is necessary to inhibit its effect. Dissenting from this generally accepted view, NAPALKOV (1962, 1965) assumes that the thyrostatics are in a position to upset, perhaps directly, certain enzyme systems in the thyroid cells and to lead to their neoplastic transformation (Gucha, 1964; Chu Chick-Mei and Chen Hann-Yuan, 1965). In favour of this view, Napalkov (1965) adduced numerous examples of the blastomogenic effect of thioureates on other organs, such as liver, kidneys, and lymphoreticular apparatus. We can accept the arguments of Napalkov (1965) as perfectly valid without ignoring the leading part played by increased TSH in thyroid carcinogenesis (Raichev and Christov, 1971). The same mechanism of tumour induction is also found in animals treated with a low-iodine diet, or by transplantation into the host of adenopituitary tumours producing TSH, or by intrasplenic transplantation of thyroid tissue.

3. Induction of Thyroid Tumours by Low-Iodine Diet

Many years ago the higher frequency of thyroid adenomas and carcinomas in regions with endemic goitre raised the problem of the etiological role of iodine insufficiency in thyroid cancer (Wegelin, 1928). Considerably later it was established that continuons feeding of a low-iodine diet to mice and rats leads to the appearance of malignant and benign epithelial tumours of the thyroid gland (Bielschowsky, 1953). Exhaustive investigations in this field have been carried out by Axelrad and Leblond (1955). Depending on the cytological features of the tumours induced, the authors divided them into three groups: thyroid tumours of α, β and γ cellular types, respectively. The tumours of γ cellular type show the most considerable cytological atypism and susceptibility to infiltrative growth. Thyroid adenomas and carcinomas were also obtained in mice of C3H/Hey strain by means of a low-iodine diet (Schaller and Stevenson, 1966) and in hamsters (Fortner et al., 1959). The malignant tumour variants showed infiltrative growth and metastatic susceptibility. In these experiments, too, the appearance of thyroid tumours was preceded by diffuse hyperplasia of the thyroid epithelium. The first malignant tumour variants of this strain were observed among 11 out of 78 mice (14 per cent) in the 12th month after the beginning of the experiment. Thyroid carcinomas developed in 8 out of the 30 remaining mice (27 per cent) when the period of thyroid insufficiency was extended. The number and size of the adenomas also increased.

Combined treatment of the animals with low-iodine diet and AAF (Axelrad and Leblond, 1955) or with low-iodine diet and X-rays (Nadler et al., 1969), considereably shortens the latent period for the appearance of thyroid tumours and increases their frequency (Table 2). After this combined treatment there is an increase in the percentage of malignant tumours in the thyroid gland, the structural and cytological atypism in the tumours also being strongly expressed. In most animals adenomas and carcinomas of a follicular type predominated, papillary and solid tumour variants occurring less frequently.

The mechanism of inducing thyroid tumours by means of a low-iodine diet is similar to that of MTU treatment. Here hormone synthesis is disturbed by the absence of inorganic iodine, necessary for the iodization of the thyrosines.

Table 2. *Quantitative assessment of follicular cell tumours.* (NADLER *et al.*, 1969)

Treatment	No. of rats surviving	Proportion of thyroids[a] with tumours %	Average	
			No. of tumours per thyroid[a]	volume of tumours per thyroid $\times 10^9$ cu[a]
300 R X-ray + low iodine diet	115	98.3	2.97	5.5
No. radiation + low-iodine diet	125	62.4	0.90	2.2

[a] All three parameters were statistically different ($p < 0.05$) between the two groups receiving different treatments.

4. Induction of Thyroid Tumours by Chemical Carcinogens

In the first experiments aimed at inducing thyroid tumours the carcinogenic agents were injected directly into the parenchyma of the thyroid gland. However, in these experiments mainly sarcomas and spinocellular carcinomas were obtained (BIELSCHOWSKY, 1955 and MORRIS, 1955). MONEY and ROWSON (1950, 1965) applied DMBA subcutaneously and directly in the thyroid of rats and established that this substance not only did not have any carcinogenic effect on the thyroid cells, but that when its effect was combined with the effect of MTU the number of thyroid tumours was smaller than in groups treated with MTU only. Consequently the carcinogen had an inhibiting effect on MTU induction of thyroid tumours. The results obtained by GNATISHAK (1956) are also unconvincing. He injected benzopyrene, scarlet dye and quinine into the thyroid gland of rats which had had hyperplasia and discovered individual spinocellular carcinomas and sarcomas after different periods of time. MILCU and PETREA (1959) kept thyroid tissue in immediate contact with methylholanthrene crystals and afterwards implanted this tissue in the animals. Only one adenoma and one angiosarcoma were obtained in this experiment. Obviously the direct introduction of various carcinogenic agents into the thyroid gland causes the appearance chiefly of mesenchymatous tumours and spinocellular carcinomas, greatly differing from the functioning thyroid tumours in man.

Unlike the carcinogenic agents mentioned above, acetylaminofluorene (AAF) proved much more promising for the induction of thyroid tumours. By means of this agent and in combination with alylthiourea, BIELSCHOWSKY (1945) succeeded in inducing thyroid adenomas in a short period of time (197 days). Large doses were used in the first experiments with this carcinogenic agent: BIELSCHOWSKY (1966) gave a dose of 600 mg over a period of 20 weeks, PASCHKIS *et al.* (1948)—400 mg over 15 weeks, NAPALKOV (1959b)—1 000 mg over a year, and LAPIS and VEBERDI (1962)—120 mg over 12 weeks. HALL

(1948) worked with comparatively smaller doses. Applied independently in large doses and over a long period of time, AAF causes mainly the appearance of tumours in the liver, stomach, kidneys, the external aural duct, and comparatively rarely in the thyroid gland (Bielschowsky, 1946, 1955). When the effect of AAF was combined with that of the thioureates (Doniach, 1950) or with a low-iodine diet (Axelrad and Leblond, 1955), its carcinogenic effect on the visceral organs was reduced, while at the same time an increase in the incidence of thyroid tumours and a shortening of their latent period was observed. All efforts by Napalkov (1959) to induce mainly malignant thyroid tumours through the combined treatment with large doses of AAF and MTU were unsuccessful. It was found (Hall, 1948; Doniach, 1950, and Napalkov, 1959; Christov, 1967b) that even small doses of AAF (in the range of 12 to 40 mg) were capable of shortening the latent period of thyroid tumours and of increasing their incidence. However, a state of thyroid insufficiency is evoked in the body after their administration. The percentage of animals with thyroid carcinoms and the period of their appearance are almost identical in groups treated with MTU only and in those treated with AAF and MTU in combination. The capacity for malignant growth is consequently determined not by the doses and duration of AAF treatment but mainly by the degree and duration of TSH (Morris, 1955). The latent period for thyroid tumours in combined AAF and MTU treatment is about 4 to 5 months. Hall (1948) observed isolated adenomas in similar experimental conditions as early as the 12th week after beginning the experiment. Thyroid carcinomas appeared 15 to 18 months after the beginning of the experiment in a comparatively small percentage of the animals, and their frequency increased progressively with the extension of the period of MTU treatment.

Particularly interesting are the problems related to the mechanism of action of AAF on thyroid cells under conditions of normal and increased TSH. Hall (1948) considers that AAF initiates neoplastic changes in the thyroid cells, changes which appear as a result of the increased TSH acting as a promoter. This theory of Hall (1948) is in agreement with the concept of the two-stage character of carcinogenesis. In support of this theory Hall (1948) pointed to the fact that the initiating effect of the carcinogenic agent on thyroid epithelia is not eliminated even if MTU treatment begins 18 weeks after the administration of the carcinogenic agent. The induction of thyroid tumours by means of low-iodine diet and after transplants into the host of pituitary tumours producing TSH, shows that the existence of initiating effects is not inevitably necessary for the tumour transformation of the thyroid epithelium, i. e. that the appearance of thyroid tumours in experimental animals does not conform to the principles of the two-stage character of carcinogenesis. Although contemporary methods of study are not yet able to show what particular cellular systems are affected by AAF, it is obvious that this carcinogenic agent leaves a "trace" on the metabolism of certain thyroid epithelia. This is also confirmed by the observations of Paschkis et al. (1948) who discovered that a double quantity of thyroxine is needed to inhibit thyroid hyperplasia caused by combined treatment with AAF and MTU, compared with treatment with MTU alone.

5. Induction of Thyroid Tumours by Radioactive Iodine and X-Rays

Ionizing radiation has an important place in experimental studies of thyroid carcinogenesis. DONIACH (1950) was the first to succeed in inducing thyroid adenomas in rats injected with 32 µGI [131]I. The incidence of tumours was considerably higher in the animals subjected to combined treatment with ^{131}I and MTU and with AAF and MTU. Thyroid carcinomas were found in these groups together with the adenomas. Two years later, GOLDBERG and CHAIKOFF (1952) treated rats of the Long-Evans strain with 400 µCI ^{131}I and, 18 months later, found that 9 out of the 25 animals had thyroid tumours, 7 of which were carcinomas. These results obtained by GOLDBERG and CHAIKOFF were criticized by many authors, such as DONIACH (1958, 1963), MALOOF et al. (1952), FRANTZ et al. (1957), MOLE (1958), FIELD et al. (1959), and CHRISTOV (1968a). This prompted LINDSAY et al (1957) to undertake a revision of the material used by GOLDBERG and CHAIKOFF in 1952. The revision established that three of the tumours originally described as carcinomas were actually adenomas. Besides that, the changes in the remaining parenchyma of the gland were very similar to those obtained from appreciably lower activities of [131]I. The studies undertaken by FELLER et al. (1949), MALOOF et al. (1952), DONIACH (1953), LINDSAY and CHAIKOFF (1964), and HINDAWI and WILSON (1965) showed that activities at the rate of 700–800 µCi ^{131}I cause radiation ablation of the thyroid inrats, while amounts of over 100 µCi ^{131}I considerably damage the hyperplastic capacities of the thyroid cells. The teams working under the guidance of DONIACH in London and of LINDSAY in San Francisco (Table 3) have offered the most significant contributions in the field of thyroid carcinogenesis in the last 20 years. Table 3 shows that the activities most suitable for inducing thyroid adenomas and carcinomas are those of the order of 25–40 µCi [131]I. DONIACH (1950, 1953) administered single injections of 5, 30, 32 and 100 µCi ^{131}I in a group of animals, while to another group of animals he applied the same quantities in two injections at an interval of 4 to 6 months from one another without ascertaining any significant difference in the incidence and latent period of the tumours. In the course of similar experiments, POTTER et al. (1960) injected 25 µCi ^{131}I in a single dose, while to another group of animals they administered four successive doses of 10 µCi [131]I. The results of their observations were a larger number of thyroid tumours observations were a larger number of thyroid tumours in the case of a single dose of 25 µCi [131]I. It is therefore obvious that the division of the total amount of ^{131}I into two or more doses has no essential effect on neoplastic changes in the thyroid cells.

The existence of clinical data about the carcinogenic effect of X-rays when the thyroid is irradiated led to the question whether X-rays could be used in obtaining experimental tumours. A number of experiments were carried out

Table 3. *Carcinogenic action of various doses of* ^{131}I

Author	Treatment µCi ^{131}I	No. of ♀+♂ animals	Adenomas %	Carci- nomas %
Doniach (1953) 13–15 months	Controls	9 ♀+♂	7 (77)	0
	5	6 ♀+♂	3 (50)	0
	30	14 ♀+♂	7 (50)	0
	100	7 ♀+♂	0 (0)	0
Lindsay et al. (1957) 18–29 months	Controls	156 ♀+♂	1 (06)	0
	10	6 ♀+♂	3 (50)	1 (16)
	25	20 ♀+♂	9 (45)	3 (15)
	100	10 ♀+♂	2 (20)	1 (10)
	200	16 ♀+♂	4 (25)	0
	400	146 ♀+♂	2 (1.3)	0
Lindsay et al. (1968a) 6 months to 2 years	Controls	140	♂	0
	1–6 months	100 ♂	0	1 (1)
	12 months	100 ♂	1 (1)	0
	24 months	55 ♂	1 (2)	0
	1–6 months	100 ♂	0	0
	12 months	100 ♂	9 (9)	0
	24 months	59 ♂	7 (12)	0
Lindsay et al. (1963) 2 years	Controls	31 ♀	1 (3)	0
	40	49 ♀	19 (39)	3 (6)
Potter et al. (1960) 2 years	Controls	56 ♂	1 (0.6)	0
	25	23 ♂	22 (95)	6 (26)
	40	28 ♂	28 (100)	6 (21)

to this end by Doniach (1956, 1958) and by Lindsay et al. (1961); these showed that the highest percentage of thyroid tumours is obtained in animals treated with 1000–1100 rads of X-rays. The efficiency of these doses in inducing thyroid tumours is equal to 30 µCi ^{131}I (Table 4). However, there are considerable differences in the radiobiological effects of ^{131}I and of X-rays, since 30 µ ^{131}I provide the thyroid with a dose of about 10000 to 15000 rads (beta rays in the first place) within several days (Feller et al., 1949), whereas X-rays induce changes in the thyroid cells in 1 or 2 minutes, i. e. during the exposure time.

The combined administration of ^{131}I and MTU auf of X-rays and PTU, respectively, considerably shortens the latent period of the thyroid tumours and increases their incidence. Gross et al. (1968) compared the carcinogenic effect of 25 µCi ^{131}I and 25 µCi ^{125}I and found 2 thyroid tumours among 23 rats treated with ^{125}I. During our experiments (Christov, 1970) the injection of 30 µCi ^{131}I led to thyroid adenomas after the 9th month. The combined treatment of the animals with ^{131}I and MTU shortened the latent period of tumour appearance to 5–6 months (Stoll and Marand, 1963; Garner, 1963; Georgadze et al., 1966). A similar pattern is to be found in hamsters, where

Table 4. *Carcinogenic action of X-rays*

Author	Treatment	No. of male or female rats	Adenomas	Carcinomas papillary and folliculary
DONIACH (1958)	Controls	41	0	0
13—15 months	MTU	50	39 (77 %)	0
male +	30 μCi [131]I	52	21 (40 %)	0
female	30 μCi [131]I + MTU	48	47 (98 %)	11 (23 %)
	1 100 rads X-rays	13	4 (30 %)	1 (7 %)
	1 100 rads X-rays + MTU	22	21 (95 %)	7 (32 %)
LINDSAY *et al.* (1961)	Controls	33	1 (3 %)	0
2 years male	500 r X-rays both lobes	22	4 (18 %)	1 (4 %)
	100 r X-rays both lobes	22	12 (54 %)	5 (22 %)
	1000 e X-rays right lobes	26	10 (38 %)	2 (7 %)
	2000 r X-rays both lobes	4	3 (75 %)	1 (25 %)

the combined treatment of the animals with 10 μCi ^{131}I and MTU leads to thyroid adenomas as early as the 5th month, and thyroid carcinomas in the 8th to 9th months after the beginning of the experiment (RAICHEV and CHRISTOV, 1971). LINDSAY *et al.* (1966) followed up the carcinogenic effect of ^{131}I in treatment with propylthiouracil (PTU) and desiccated thyroid powder (DTP) (Table 5). Obviously, DTP applied in small quantities potentiates goitrogenesis and the appearance of thyroid adenomas and carcinoms. Attempts to induce predominantly malignant tumours through the combined effect of ^{131}I, AAF and MTU proved unsuccessful, as the incidence rate of the carcinomas is almost identical in the groups treated with ^{131}I and MTU and with ^{131}I, AAF and MTU (DONIACH, 1950; CHRISTOV, 1968b).

It was established in recent years that a number of carcinogenic agents have a considerably more marked blastomogenic effect when applied in small quantities in newborn animals than in adult animals (DELLA-PORTA and

Table 5. *Thyroid tumours in animals treated with* [131]I, *PTU and DTP.*
(LINDSAY *et al.*, 1966)

Treatment	No. of male rats	Adenomas	Carcinomas papillary and follicular
Controls	68	0	0
25 μCi [131]I	65	7 (10 %)	2 (3 %)
25 μCi [131]I + DTP	69	0	0
PTU	35	16 (48 %)	0
25 μCi [131]I + PTU	35	23 (65 %)	0
25 μCi [131]I + PTU + DTP	65	51 (78 %)	13 (20 %)
PTU + DTP	60	39 (65 %)	4 (6 %)

DTP = desiccated thyroid powder; PTU = propylthiouracil.

Terracini, 1969; Toth, 1968; Chernozemski and Warwick, 1970). In order to trace this phenomenon in the thyroid gland, Doniach (1969b) injected small amounts of ^{131}I in newborn rats (on the 4th day after their birth). In determining the dose the author took into consideration the weight of the thyroid gland of the newborn and the most active carcinogenic ^{131}I dose in adult animals. The incidence of thyroid adenomas at the end of the first year is almost identical in animals treated with ^{131}I immediately after birth and 10 weeks later. The lack of difference in the course of thyroid carcinogenesis in newborn and older animals may be due to the low mitotic level of the thyroid cells in newborn rats.

The adenomas of the thyroid gland induced by irradiation are mainly of the follicular type, with predominance of the macrofollicular variants (Doniach, 1950). This pattern is similar to the tumours obtained with goitrogens or with low-iodine diet. The thyroid carcinomas are mainly of the papillarly type (incidence about twice that of the follicular type), with a markedly infiltrative growth and metastatic potential (Lindsay, 1969). There are also mixed variants composed simultaneously of papillary and follicular structures. The histogenesis of both follicular and papillary adenomas and carcinomas is related to the follicular cells, while the spontaneous thyroid blastomas start from the parafollicular cells (Lindsay et al., 1968b). Most of the thyroid carcinomas originate from adenomas whose neoplastic cells undergo malignant transformation in certain sections.

The carcinogenic effect of irradiation (^{131}I and X-rays) is a result of both the direct changes that have taken place in the thyroid cells, probably mutations (Doniach, 1950; Lindsay et al., 1966, 1969) and of the intensified TSH. However, it seems that the leading role is that of direct radiation changes in the thyroid cells, since the degree of TSH is less marked due to the capacity preserved by the follicular cells of synthesizing thyroid hormones—thyroxine and tri-iodothyronine (Christov, 1968a).

The concept expressed about the two-stage character of thyroid carcinogenesis (Hall, 1948) in animals subjected to the combined treatment of ^{131}I and MTU or with X-rays and MTU it not acceptable, since thyroid tumours are also obtained in animals with transplanted pituitary tumours producing TSH, or fed on a low-iodine diet or on goitrogens. This concept might become acceptable only if we assume that (1) there is an unknown initiator in the environment or in the food of the animal, (2), that since birth its thyroid gland contains cells with initiated neoplastic changes, and (3) that TSH acts simultaneously both as promoter and initiator (Doniach, 1958; Lindsay, 1968 and Christov, 1967a and b).

6. Induction of Thyroid Tumours after Subtotal Thyroidectomy

In the case of subtotal thyroidectomy, the level of TSH also increase, since the thyroid tissue that remains after the operation is not capable of meeting the body's need for thyroid hormones (Dent et al., 1956; Israel and

ELLIS, 1960). The percentage of animals with thyroid tumours is considerably lower in these experiments than after treatment with thioureates or with a low-iodine diet. Thus, for example, two years after thyroidectomy DONIACH and WILLIAMS (1962) found two adenomas and a carcinoma of the thyroid gland in three out of 26 rats of the Lister strain. The authors removed about 85 per cent of the thyroid gland together with the isthmus. In similar experiments GOLDBERG et al. (1964) combined subtotal thyroidectomy with subsequent treatment with 1 μCi of ^{131}I and with desiccated thyroid powder (DTP) and discovered a higher percentage of thyroid adenomas in the groups which had undergone subtotal thyroidectomy and had subsequently been injected with 1 μCi of ^{131}I. In two out of 68 animals with thyroidectomy only, and in one animal subjected to combined ^{131}I treatment and subtotal thyroidectomy, papillary carcinomas were found in the region of the isthmus. MILCU and PETREA (1959) described thyroid carcinosarcomas in three out of ten rats treated with MTU for eight months, after which unilateral thyroidectomy was carried out, the administration of MTU being restarted thirty days after the operation. The animals were also subjected to painful electric stimuli. The authors believe that these conditions, as well as previous and subsequent MTU treatment of the animals, stimulate tumour growth in the thyroid gland. IRD (1968) combined subtotal thyroidectomy, removing 3/4 to 5/6 of the gland, with subsequent MTU treatment and succeeded in raising the percentage of animals with thyroid tumours to 24. The low percentage of thyroid tumours after subtotal thyroidectomy is probably due to low thyrotrophic stimulation, owing to the partial supply of the organism with thyroid hormones from the remaining thyroid tissue. The absence of sufficient quantities of thyroid tissue (IRD, 1968) or the exhaustion of the hyperplastic capacity of the thyroid cells (VOITKEVIC, 1964) may be factors conducive to the low tumour incidence in these experiments.

7. Induction of Thyroid Tumours by Means of Intrasplenic Transplants

Transplantation of thyroid tissue in the spleen after complete removal of the recipient's thyroid gland leads to hyperplasia of the transplanted tissue and, 15 to 16 months later, to the appearance of thyroid adenomas (BRACHETTO-BRIAN and GRINBERG, 1951). In analogous experiments with ovaries, BISKIND and BISKIND (1944) found a higher percentage of tumour growths in the transplants. These differences are due either to incomplete thyroxine breakdown in the liver or to the more strongly marked hyperplastic capacities of the mesenchymal cells in the ovary. In these experiments, too, hyperplastic and tumoral growths in the transplanted thyroid tissue are due to increased thyrotrophic stimulation resulting from inhibition of the thyroid hormone produced by the transplant in the spleen. The changes in the adenopituitary cells producing TSH also indicate this mechanism of thyroid hyperplasia and neoplasia under conditions of intrasplenic transplantation.

8. Induction of Thyroid Tumours after Transplantation of Adenohypophyseal Tumours Producing Thyrotrophic Hormone (TSH)

Dent et al. (1956), Haran-Shera et al. (1960) and Sincha et al. (1965) induced thyrotrophin-producing tumours of the adenohypophysis after thyroidectomy of mice of LAF_1 strains. At first these tumours could be transplanted only in hosts with thyroid insufficiency. In subsequent transplants the tumours acquired autonomous growth, preserving their capacity to produce TSH. The authors Haran-Shera et al., 1960) traced the effect of these thyrotrophin-producing transplants on the host's thyroid gland and on parallel-transplanted thyroid tissue. It was established that hyperplastic and neoplastic growths (adenomas) are to be discovered in the thyroid gland of the same time the tissue transplanted changed from differentiated to undifferentiated under the influence of increased TSH. Although it underwent considerable morphological changes, the thyroid transplant did not acquire functional independence. It is rather interesting to note that the rate of growth of the thyroid tissue transplant was considerably higher when transplants of the thyrotrophin- producing tumour preceded those of the thyroid tissue by two to four months. The induction of hyperplastic and neoplastic growths in the host's thyroid gland after transplantation of thyrotrophin-producing pituitary tumours is one of the most convincing proofs of the idea of the causative role of increased TSH in the genesis of thyroid tumours.

II. Functional Changes of the Thyroid Gland in Carcinogenesis

In the last twenty years, using the labelled isotopes of iodine, as well as scintigraphic, autoradiographic and chromatographic methods of investigation, the basic stages of thyroid hormone synthesis have been studied under normal and pathological conditions. The correlations between the thyroid gland and the remanining endocrine glands have been elucidated and it was established that the adenohypophysis with its thyrotrophic hormone (TSH) play a major part in thyroid regulation.

In view of the mechanism of action of thioureates in animals treated with MTU, the ^{131}I uptake per mg of thyroid tissue is many times smaller than that of the controls (Mackenzie and Mackenzie, 1943; Money et al., 1953; Lapis and Veberdi, 1962; Calvert, 1963, and Brodhead et al., 1965). The cumulative capacity per mg of thyroid tissue changes, depending on the duration of MTU treatment (Money et al., 1953; Wolff, et al. 1959; Christov and Kristeva, 1971; Table 6). The accumulation of ^{131}I was traced in rats with diffuse hyperplasia of the thyroid epithelium (animals killed on the 120th day after the beginning of the experiment), with focal hyperplasia (animals killed on the 250th day), and with wellformed epithelial tumours (animals killed on the 450th day). The higher value of ^{131}I per mg for the 250th day is due to the inorganic ^{131}I, and to some unseparated organically bound ^{131}I ingredients which are probably retained in the gland for a longer period of time. In the

Table 6. [131]I *Metabolism in conditions of hyperplasia and tumour growth.* (CHRISTOV and KRISTEVA, 1971)

	Animals treated with methylthioruacil (MTU) — days							Tumours		[131]I
	Controls	120	250	450	120[a]	250[a]	450[a]	I	II	uptake
Thyroid gland (mg)	18.4 ± 3.7	118 ± 33	189 ± 65	219 ± 65	98.6 ± 12.5	173 ± 14.5	19.8 ± 37.6	126	94	114 ± 5
[131]I (%)	9.1	0.82	9.2	1.31	33.6	47.3	39.3	1.20	2.36	—
[131]I (mg)	0.5	0.007	0.05	0.006	0.34	0.27	0.20	0.01	0.025	—
Thyr. tss.										
Start	4.1 ± 0.50		8.0 ± 3.1		9.2 ± 2.3	8.1 ± 2.2	10.4 ± 3.3	10.8	9.3	—
MIT	33.2 ± 4.20				35.5 ± 8.3	28.7 ± 5.4	34.2 ± 6.6	61.2	52	—
DIT	38.3 ± 7.33				19.4 ± 4.8	21.3×7.1	24.6 ± 8.2	22	24.2	—
I	3.6 ± 0.62	100	92 ± 7.9	100	5.2 ± 1.9	10.9 ± 2.3	4.3 ± 0.82	6	14.5	—
T_3	5.5 ± 0.48				15.0 ± 3.8	24.1 ± 6.3	11.2 ± 3.7	—	—	—
T_4	15.8 ± 0.67				17.3 ± 6.4	16.0 ± 3.7	13.8 ± 4.3	—	—	—

[a] Without MTU 14 days before killing.

MIT = Monoiodothyrosine, DIT = Diiodothyrosine, T_3 = Triiodothyronine, T_4 = Thyroxine.

same period, colloid was found in the gland (Morris and Dalton, 1951; Napalkov, 1959a and Christov, 1967a). This colloid accumulation in the lumen of the follicles at a high level of TSH shows that the hyperplastic thyroid cells have acquired a relative functional independence and do not react adequately to increased thyrotrophic stimulation. The low ^{131}I values recorded on the 120th day are due to the complete blocking of thyroid hormone-synthesis by MTU and to the total absence of colloid in the thyroid gland where ^{131}I is to be deposited. In the case of animals treated for more than 450 days with MTU, neoplastic nodules were found, together with hyperplastic changes in the thyroid gland. In these glands the ^{131}I quantity per mg of thyroid tissue decreases, most probably because the tumour cells lose their capacity for accumulating [131]I.

In the thyroid hyperplasia induced by a low-iodine diet, the ^{131}I uptake per mg thyroid tissue many times exceeds the values for control animals. The data of the different authors vary a great deal owing to the application of diets with different iodine content and to the different experimental conditions (Hatway and Lipscomb, 1962).

In thyroid gland tumours induced by different methods, the ^{131}I values per mg of thyroid tissue were most frequently smaller than in the case of thyroid hyperplasia because of the functional dedifferentiation of the neoplastic cells (Fitzgerald et al., 1950; Doniach, 1950; Money et al., 1953; Wollman et al., 1953 a and b; and Wollman, 1963). In animals treated with MTU for more than 450 days, organically bound ^{131}I in the form of MIT and DIT was demonstrated in some well-differentiated tumours. The neoplastic cells consequently skip the thiouracil block, though only to the level of the iodotyrosines (Christov and Kristeva, 1971). Fourteen days after discontinuation of the MTU treatment, the thyroid hyperplastic cells resume their hormone-synthesis. In a number of neoplastic nodules separated from the adjacent parenchyma, ^{131}I metabolism also reaches the levels of T_3 and T_4. In other cases MIT and DIT or organic iodine only are discovered in the tumours. This absence of individual links of the thyroid hormone-synthesis in the process of tumorigenesis is particularly apparent in the transplantable tumour variants of the thyroid gland (Tata, 1958; Pittman et al., 1963; Boat and Halmi, 1965; Robbins, 1968; and Matovinovic et al., 1968) (Table 7). Table 7 clearly shows how the more differentiated variant of one and the same transplantable tumour strain synthesizes thyroid hormones, while the cells of the undifferentiated tumours synthesize MIT and DIT only. In a later generation, the cells of the same tumour variant lose their capacity to combine iodine in a organic form. These changes in the values of the individual iodine-containing components show how in the process of carcinogenesis important links of the thyroid function disappear. In the more differentiated epithelial tumours, the neoplastic cells metabolize ^{131}I to the thyroxine and triiodothyronine, in the less differentiated ones only precursors of the thyroid hormones MIT and DIT are synthesized, and in the anaplastic thyroid tumours the cells lose their capacity to bind radioactive iodine in an organic form.

Table 7. *Rat thyroid transplant tumours-follicular and sarcomatous variants* (Matovinovic *et al.*, 1968)

	Generation	Body weight	Tumour pair [131]I	Tumour pair weigth	Tumour pair PB[131]I	Thyroid 12 hour [131]I	Tumour 131-iodide compounds						Serum PB [127]I
		g	uptake % dose	g	% of 12 hour uptake	uptake % dose	[131]I	MIT	DIT	T_3	T_4	$U_{\hat{t}}$	
Follicular	6	267.8	43.8	2.4	59.0	9.6	40.2	33.2	8.8	5.1	12.5	0	3.2
		7.5	3.7	0.5	5.4	0.8	3.0	4.0	0.9	0.7	1.7	—	0.1
Sarcomatous	5	221.2	56.6	26.1	0.9	8.5	52.8	2.0	1.5	0.0	0.0	42.9	1.7
		4.0	3.3	2.7	0.9	1.2	5.8	0.2	0.1	0.0	0.0	5.8	0.1
Sarcomatous	13	221	69.8	14.1	47.3	12.7	82.5	0.0	0.0	0.0	0.0	12.7	0.0
		3.9	4.1	3.8	5.9	1.7	7.6	0.0	0.0	0.0	0.0	1.7	0.0

$U_{\hat{t}}$ = unknown total, MIT = Monoiodothyrosine, DIT = Diiodothyrosine, T_3 = Triiodothyronine, T_4 = Thyroxine.

In the transformation of the normal thyroid cell into a neoplastic cell, protein synthesis is adversely affected, as a result of which a number of atypical thyroproteins are discovered in the thyroid gland and in the circulation (Lissitzky, 1969; Valenta et al., 1969). The existence of thyroproteins is not always indicative of carcinoma of the thyroid gland, since they can be observed in insignificant quantities in the normal thyroid gland, too, as well as in a number of other thyroid diseases (Robbins et al., 1959; Tata and Pochin, 1964).

As the tumour progresses, not only do the separate links of hormone-synthesis disappear, but there is also a change in the relationship between the tumour and the host. From being hormonally dependent in the first generation, the tumours become hormonally independent in later generations (Wollman, 1963; Matovinovic et al., 1968).

The autoradiographic method gives much more precise information about the functional capacities of the thyroid epithelium. This method makes it possible to trace the distribution of the organically bound and inorganic iodine among the individual thyroid structures (Dobins and Lenan, 1948; Doniach and Pelc, 1949; Pitt-Rivers and Trotter, 1953; Andros and Wollman, 1967). By neams of this method, as early as 1950 Fitzgerald et al. (1950) and Doniach (1950) established that tumours differing in morphological structure accumulate different quantities of ^{131}I. These data have been obtained in animals treated with MTU to which the administration of a goitrogenic agent discontinued twelve days before they were killed. The 12-day interval is necessary for the disappearance of the MTU-inhibiting effect on thyroid hormone-synthesis and for the normalization of the hormonal balance between the thyroid and the pituitary glands. In similar experiments, we (Christov, 1969; 1971) tried to find a dependence between the morphological structure of the pre-neoplastic and neoplastic changes in the thyroid gland on one hand and the accumulation and organic binding of ^{131}I on the other (Table 8). Table 8 shows that about 50 per cent of thyroid adenomas and carcinomas do not bind ^{131}I in an organic form. The quantity of ^{131}I in the tumours with functional activity is smaller than that in the surrounding parenchyma. Adenomas with a cumulative capacity exceeding that of the adjacent hyperplastic follicles were observed in individual animals only, and, with regard to this particular behavioural pattern, these adenomas resemble the "hot nodes" of the thyroid gland in man. Among the different tumour variants, follicular adenomas show predominantly functional activity, though among them, too, it is possible to find types that do not accumulate ^{131}I. The opinion maintained by certain authors (Fitzgerald and Foote, 1949; Doniach, 1950) that the tumour follicles which are small in size accumulate a greater quantity of ^{131}I has not been confirmed by our studies (Christov, 1969). No dependence was established between the height of the follicular neoplastic cells and the quantity of the isotope accumulated. It is obvious that the diameter of the follicles and the height of the follicular cells, i. e. the morphological parameters deter-

Table 8. *Experimental groups, histological structure and functional activity of induced thyroid tumors*[a] (CHRISTOV to be published)

Experimental groups groups	No. of animals	Histological structure	Functional activity		
			none[b]	scanty	considerable
Controls	4 ♀	—	—	—	—
	4 ♀	—	—	—	—
^{131}I-*treated*	12 ♀	10 f.	4	6	—
		2 p.	2	—	—
	8 ♂	6 f.	2	4	—
MTU-treated	12 ♀	15 f.	10	5	—
		3 p.	2	1	—
	14 ♀	10 f.	3	6	1
		5 p.	3	2	—
		1 s.	1	—	—
$^{131}I + MTU$ *treated*	16 ♀	20 f. (2 Ca)	4 (2 Ca)	14	—
		7 p.	6	1	—
		3 s.	2	1	—
	10 ♂	18 f. (2 Ca)	6 (1 Ca)	10 (1 Ca)	2
		5 p. (2 Ca)	2 (1 Ca)	3 (1 Ca)	—
		2 s.	2	—	—
Total	44 ♀	79 f. (4 Ca)	29 (3 Ca)	45 (1 Ca)	5
		22 p. (2 Ca)	15 (1 Ca)	7 (1 Ca)	—
	36 ♀	6 s.	5	1	—

[a] STUDENT-FISCHER criterion ($P < 0.01$) for reliability
[b] Functional activity according to the surrounding follicles. f. = Follicular adenomas, p. = Papilliferous adenomas, s. = Solid adenomas, Ca = Carcinomas.

mining the functional condition of the follicle and of the thyroid gland, respectively, lose their significance in the process of tumorigenesis.

Positive theoretical interest was aroused by the experiments of MONEY *et al.* (1953) who treated the animals with MTU until the last day of the experiment. Under these conditions, in view of the inhibiting effect of MTU on thyroid hormone-synthesis, there should have been no organically bound ^{131}I. It has been proved, however, that the majority of pathologically changed thyroid follicles and certain tumour nodules accumulate ^{131}I. This capacity of the thyroid epithelia to metabolize ^{131}I, even in the presence of MTU in the circulation, shows that they overcome the thiouracil block. This partial deblocking of thyroid hormone-synthesis may be explained by assuming (MORRIS, 1955; CHRISTOV, 1968a) that a greater quantity of MTU is necessary to inhibit ^{131}I metabolism in the preneoplastic and neoplastic thyroid tissues, or that the mechanism of ^{131}I binding has changed. It is hardly probable that the large size of the tumours prevents MTU from reaching the all neoplastic cells in order to inhibit the organic combination of ^{131}I, since both the thyroid gland and the thyroid tumours are very well vasculated (Sellers and Schönbaum, 1962b). Contrary to our data (Christov and Kristeva, 1971) and those of Money et al. (1953), Lapis and Veberdi (1962) could not discover organically bound ^{131}I on the autograms, most probably owing to the shorter period for which the animals were treated with MTU (400 days), a period insufficient for the thyroid epithelia to aquire functional independence.

In recent years the functional condition of the "C" cells in the thyroid gland has been the subject of intense experimental studies because of the thyroid calcitonin they produce (Young and Leblond, 1963; Sarkar and Isler, 1963; Kiyama et al., 1968). Most authors believe that medullary carcinomas of the thyroid gland have their origin in a particular type of cells (Taylor, 1960; Lindsay et al., 1968b; Silverberg and Vidone, 1966). In order to establish whether the "C" cells lose their capacity for producing thyrocalcitonin during neoplastic transformation, certain medullary carcinomas have been examined by immunofluorescent methods. It was proved by Cunliffe et al. (1968), Bussolati et al. (1969) and Milhaud et al. (1969) that a large part of the cells of the blastomas investigated produce calcitonin, its quantity in the tumour being many times greater than in the remaining parenchyma. There is still no convincing evidence in the literature about the existence of calcitonin in experimentally induced thyroid tumours, although we have every reason to believe that their cells, too, preserve their functional capacities to a considerable degree during the process of tumorigenesis.

In the present paper we have deliberately refrained from discussing the functional activity of thyroid tumours in man and the factors relevant to this activity (see publications by Fitzgerald, 1955; Tata, 1958; Tata and Pochin, 1964; Nunez et al., 1965; Papazov, 1967; Lemarchand-Berand et al., 1969; Lissitzky, 1969; Pochin and Thompson, 1969; Valenta et al., 1969; Stanbury, 1969), owing to the particular task that we have set ourselves.

In conclusion, we may point out that in the process of neoplastic transformation the thyroid cells, follicular and parafollicular, show both morphological and functional changes. Moreover, regardless of the fact that they acquire new biological properties, namely the capacity for infiltrative and metastatic growth, in a considerable percentage of cases they retain the property of accumulating ^{131}I and of metabolizing it to the level of iodothyrosines and iodothyronines. There exists no close dependence between structure and function in the thyroid tumours, although follicular variants have the most clearly expressed functional activity. In the process of tumorigenesis, protein synthesis in the thyroid cells is adversely affected a number of non-specific thyroproteins appearing, some of which pass into the circulation. The complete cycle of thyroid hormone-synthesis with formation of thyroxine and triiodothyronine is effected in the hyperplastic thyroid tissue. This is how hormonogenesis takes place in some induced and transplantable thyroid tumours. In only a small proportion of thyroid adenomas and carcinomas is there disturbance of the hormone-synthesizing function of the gland: ^{131}I metabolism reaching the level of the precursors MIT and DIT of the thyroid hormones, or the tumour cells not being in a position to accumulate ^{131}I. The changes in the functional activity of the thyroid tumours are nonspecific and can also be observed in a number of non-neoplastic diseases of the thyroid gland.

III. Radiation Thyroid Carcinogenesis in Man

Interest in thyroid tumours has grown considerably in recent years, owing to the high incidence of carcinomas among people who have been irradiated in the cervical region for some reason (GOOLDEN, 1957 and 1958; HANFORD et al., 1962; DE WITT et al., 1963; SAENGER et al., 1963; SOCOLOV et al., 1963; CARROLL et al., 1964; PIEFER, 1964; McGROW and MACKENZIE, 1965; DOLPHIN, 1968; HEMPELMANN, 1968a and b, 1969; HARPER and PAVOYAN, 1969; CONARD et al., 1970a and b). The data are particularly convincing when irradiation has taken place in early childhood (SIMPSON et al., 1955 and 1957; SAENGER et al., 1960; PIEFER and HEMPELMANN, 1964; PINCUS et al., 1967, and HEMPEL-MANN, 1969). In the 'thirties and 'forties, and in some countries even in the early 'fifties, a number of diseases in the cervical and head regions were treated mainly by means of X-rays. This "vogue" was particularly popular in the United States, where almost one per cent of the babies born between 1935 and 1945 (in Rochester) underwent such treatment for thymic enlargement. The thyroid gland was also irradiated during treatment of chronic cervical lymphadenitis and tonsilitis, as well as in the case of certain skin diseases in the same region. Later in the 'fifties, when X-ray treatment was no longer used as a therapeutical method for these diseases, the incidence of thyroid cancer began to show a gradual decline (WINSHIP and ROSVOLL, 1969). These authors studied the percentage of thyroid cancer in childhood and adolescence and established that, while in the early years of the present century this type of tumour was a very rare phenomenon, its frequency showed a rapid increase after 1930 (Fig. 1). The values were particularly high between 1950 and 1960, when more than ten years had elapsed after the irradiation of the first children. In a group of 286 children with thyroid cancer aged under 15, 80 per cent had been irradiated in early childhood for thymic enlargement (WINSHIP and ROSVOLL, 1961). The epidemiological investigations of CARROLL et al. (1964, FERBER et al. (1962) deal with the same problem. The authors have traced the incidence of thyroid cancer in upstate New York over a period of twenty years between 1941 and 1962 and have established that the number of thyroid carcinomas had almost doubled. Comparing the data for the different age groups, CARROLL et al. (1964) found that the incidence of thyroid carcinomas rose chiefly among adolescents and young people, while the values relating to the age group over 55 years remained unchanged. The authors ascribe this increase to irradiation in the cervical region for thymic enlargement and other chronic diseases. Higher incidence of thyroid carcinomas has also been reported by PIEFER et al. (1968), who studied a group of 958 patients from

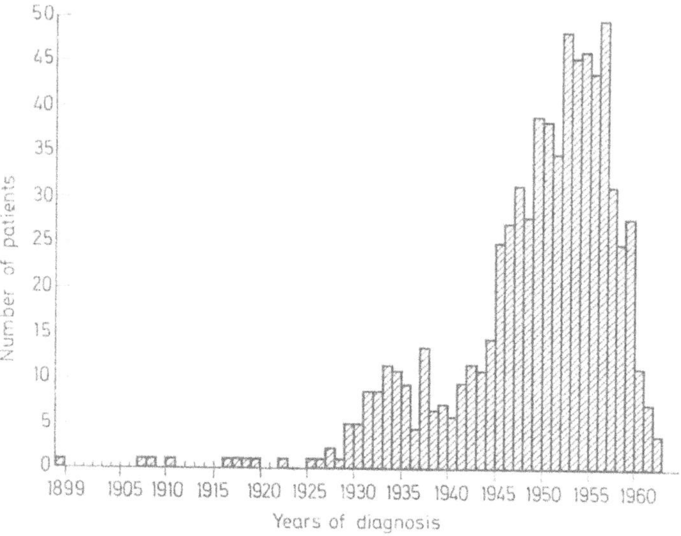

Fig. 1. Incidence of childhood thyroid carcinom. (WINSHIP and ROSVOLL, 1969)

Ann Arbor, Michigan, irradiated for thymic enlargement. Approximately one-half of the children were treated with X-rays before the age of two months and nearly 90 per cent were irradiated before the age of one year. In 1965, when all subjects were over 15 years of age, thyroid adenomas were found in seven of them and thyroid carcinoma in one. The fact that X-irradiation increases the incidence of thyroid tumours has brought to the fore a number of problems for further discussion, as follows:

1. The most effective X-ray dose for inducing thyroid tumours (adenomas and carcinomas) in man.

2. The significance of the patient's age in the production of the carcinogenic effect.

3. Latent period between irradiation and tumour appearance.

4. Factors modifying the carcinogenic effect of X-rays.

The dose received by the thyroid gland during X-irradiation of the neck region shows big differences, for instance, between 100 and 600 rads during treatment for thymic enlargement (Fig. 2). It is obvious that there is no close connection between the dose of X-rays and the incidence of thyroid tumours. The authors show, moreover, that both bigger and smaller doses are able to induce thyroid adenomas and carcinomas. Obviously, tumour incidence is determined not only by the cumulative thyroid dose (rads) but also by other biological factors modifying its carcinogenic effect. Judging by the experiments of PIEFER et al. 1968) and of CONARD et al. (1970a and b), doses in the range 200–300 rads have the most clearly expressed carcinogenic effect on the thyroid gland.

The age of the patients is of considerable significance for the appearance of thyroid tumours after irradiation. Most of the cases studied by WINSHIP

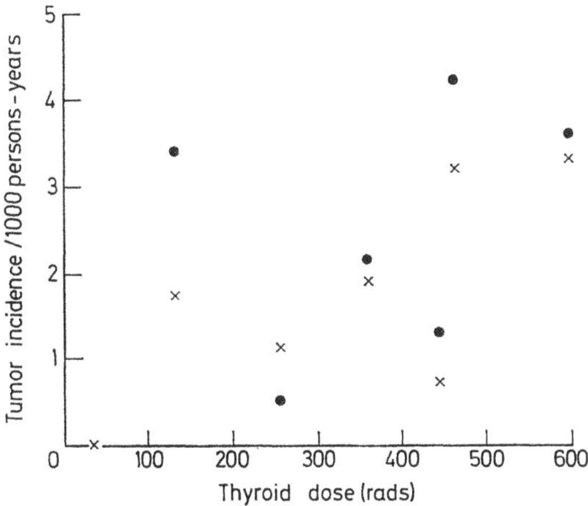

Fig. 2. Incidence of pooled thyroid neoplasms plotted against cumulative thyroid dose (rads). The circles refer to incidence in the oldest cohort of the Rochester thymus-irradiated population (born 1926–1939) and the crosses to the two oldest cohorts (born 1926–1949). The incidence is given in terms of 100 person-years-at-risk. (HEMPELMANN *et al.*, 1967)

and ROSVOLL (1961), PIEFER *et al.* (1968), HEMPELMANN *et al.* (1967) were treated for thymic enlargement below the age of one year. The significance of dose and age has been very well studied by CONARD *et al.* (1969 and 1970a and b). CONRAD, helped by a small team, traced the incidence of thyroid abnormalities among the population of the Rongelap and Utirik islands which belong to the group of the Marshall Islands. In 1954, the population of the above two islands received considerable Falloutradiation.

In addition to gamma irradiation, the thyroid gland accumulated ^{131}I, ^{132}I, ^{133}I, ^{135}I released during the thermonuclear reaction on Bikini Island (Table 9). Table 9 clearly shows, the high incidence of thyroid tumours among patients irradiated below the age of ten years. SOCOLOV *et al.* (1960) reached similar conclusions after examining 19. 962 patients exposed to irradiation from the atomic explosions over Hiroshima and Nagasaki in 1945. In the period between 1958 and 1961 they found among them 168 cases of thyroid adenomas and 18 carcinomas. About 71 per cent of the cases were under thirty years of age at the time of the explosions.

The latent period for the appearance of thyroid tumours in patients irradiated for thymic enlargement is more than five yeats, the percentage of thyroid adenomas being higher between 20 and 24 years of age and that of thyroid carcinomas between 15 and 19 years of age. RAVENTOS and WINSHIP (1964), and WINSHIP and ROSVOLL (1969) give similar data.

Calculation of risks of developing radiation induced malignancies, based on the assumption of linear dose response, are usually expressed as cases developing per year per million people into have been irradiated with one rad of radiation. HEMPELMANN *et al.* (1967) calculated a higher risk value of thyroid

Table 9. *Thyroid lesions in Marshallese, March 1969* (Conard, 1970)

Island group radiation dose (γ)	Age at exposure (year)	Estimates thyroid dose (rad, radioactive iodines)[a]	Thyroid lesions %	Malignant lesions %
Rongelap	<10	500–1 400	89.5 (17 of 19)	5.3 (1 of 19)
(175 Rad)	>10	160[b]	8.8 (3 of 34)	5.9 (2 of 34)
	all	—	39.6 (21 of 35)	5.7 (3 of 53)
Rongelap	<10	275–550	0.0 (0 of 6)	—
(69 Rad)	>10	55	12.5 (1 of 8)	—
	all	—	7.1 (1 of 14)	—
Utirik	<10	55–100	0.0 (0 of 40)	—
(74 Rad)	>10	14	5.1 (3 of 59)	1.7 (1 of 59)
	all	—	3.0 (3 of 99)	1.0 (1 of 99)
Rongelap	<10	—	0.0 (0 of 61)	—
(unexposed)	>10	—	2.3 (3 of 133)	—
	all	—	1.5 (3 of 194)	—

a ^{131}I, ^{132}I, ^{133}I, ^{135}I.

b Children 10 to 20 years of age at exposure received doses between 160 and 500 Rad.

cancer, namely 2,5 cases year (10^6) rad, based on data from the Rochester study. The relatively long latent period between irradiation and the appearance of thyroid tumours on one hand, and the absence of a direct dependence between the dose applied, the frequency and the biological properties of the tumours induced on the other, are facts indicating that there are other factors modifying the blastomogenic effect of X-rays. The hormonal changes at puberty seem to play an important role in this respect since thyroid tumours are most frequent at that time. The higher incidence of thyroid tumours in females is probably due to the influence of fluctuations in the level of oestrogens, which are known to stimulate hyperplasia of the thyroid cells (Fortner et al., 1960; Money, 1969).

While the evidence concerning the carcinogenic effect of X-rays on the thyroid gland in man is absolutely convincing, the epidemiological investigations of the tumorigenic effect of ^{131}I cannot as yet provide a conclusive answer as to whether ^{131}I is carcinogenic in man or not (Pochin, 1965; 1969). Publications about the appearance of thyroid gland cancer in patients treated with ^{131}I for hyperthyroidism are insufficient to allow as to assume that ^{131}I has a carcinogenic effect in the doses used for the treatment of thyrotoxicosis (Sheline et al., 1959). It is necessary to examine a sufficiently large group of patients treated with ^{131}I for a longer period of time in order to accept or reject such an assumption. Observations on patients treated with ^{131}I for thyrotoxicosis over twenty years ago do not offer grounds for the belief that the incidence of thyroid gland cancer has increaseed among them (Pochin, 1969). Radioactive iodine represents a danger mainly for young people who have been irradiated in childhood or adolescence (HEMPELMANN, 1969; LIND-SAY, 1969). The thyroid epithelium of young people seems to be more sensitive to the carcinogenic effect of X-rays, probably owing to the higher mitotic activity of the cells and their higher hyperplastic capacities.

The following should be pointed out in conclusion. X-rays in doses between 100 and 600 rads administered in childhood in the neck region have a carcinogenic effect on the thyroid gland. The latent period between irradiation and the appearance of the tumours is normally longer than ten years. Tumour incidence is highest between 15 and 30 years of age. Radioactive iodine ^{131}I accumulated by the gland in childhood raises the incidence of thyroid tumours. The combination of the effects of X-rays and radioactive isotopes of iodine shortens the latency period for the development of thyroid tumours and increases their frequency.

IV. Similarities and Differences between Thyroid Tumours in Man and in Experimental Animals

Thyroid tumours in man show great structural variety, and this leads to certain difficulties in classifying them. A considerable number of differentiated thyroid carcinomas posses functional activity. The capacity of ^{131}I accumulation does not always correspond to their morphological structure. Together with these functional and structural features, thyroid tumours differ a great deal from other tumours in man with regard to their biological behaviour. For instance, there are tumour variants whose growth takes dozens of years, while on the other hand there are certain undifferentiated carcinomas which lead to an early death. Some thyroid carcinomas lead to early metastasis, while others are very late in doing so (LINDSAY et al., 1954; LINDSAY, 1964; BOWENS and VANDER, 1962; GUINET, 1966; PAGES, 1966; MONEY and ROWSON, 1968). The radiobiological changes in thyroid carcinomas after ^{131}I treatment also show great differences, due to their morphological structure and their capacity for accumulating ^{131}I. All this justifies the great interest shown in this type of tumour from the both clinical and experimental point of view.

Quite logically, the question arises: Is there a close parallel between the morphological structure and the biological properties of thyroid tumours in man and those induced in experimental animals, and to what extent do experimental models resemble tumours in man? Spontaneous thyroid tumours in man are chiefly of a differentiated type, predominantly papillary and follicular. About 90 per cent of all malignant thyroid tumours in man belong to these two groups. Papillary and the socalled intermediary carcinomas are more frequent than follicular ones. Naturally occuring thyroid adenomas and carcinomas in mice and rats have a follicular or solid histological structure. The histological structure of those thyroid adenomas and carcinomas in man which are supposed to be due to radiation effects, or to low-iodine diet for the inhabitants of endemic regions, is particularly interesting. In such cases

Table 10

	Man	Experimental animals (rats)
Spontaneous tumours:		
Adenomas	Frequent in the endemic regions	Frequent (Table 1)
Carcinomas	Below 1 % ; in endemic regions— 1—2 %	Frequent[a]
Histogenesis	From follicular and parafollicular cells	Parafollicular
Induces thyroid tumours:		
Causes	Iodine-deficient diet, natural Goitrogens, X-rays, ^{131}I, unknown factors	Thioureates, low-iodine diet, X-rays, ^{131}I, AAF, transplantation of thyroid tissue in the spleen
Pathogenic mechanism	Increases thyrotrophic stimution (TTH), direct carcinogenic effect, unknown endogenous and exogenous factors	Increased TTH, direct carcinogenic effect and a combination of the two
Latent period	Adenomas 10 to 15 years Carcinomas 16 to 25 years	Adenomas 6 to 8 mths. Carcinomas 15 to 18 months
Frequency	Reaching 70–80 % in patients irradiated for thymic enlargement and in the children of Rongelap Island	At the end of the second year adenomas in 80*100 % of the animals treated with MTU, independently or in combination with ^{131}I, AAF, low-iodine diet, X-rays. Carcinomas 20–40 %
Morphological structure:		
	Papillary, follicular, anaplastic carcinomas	Papillary, follicular, solid
	Predominantly mixed variants	Predominantly pure variants
Follicular carcinomas	Scanty colloid formation	Considerable colloid formation
Cytological atypism	Considerable	Scanty
Number of tumours per gland	Single	Multiple
Mesenchymatous changes	Considerable	Scanty
Biological properties:		
Growth	Slow—in differentiated variants. Rapid—in anaplastic variants	Slow, after elimination of TSH tendency towards reverse development
Infiltration	Strongly expressed in adjacent parenchyma and the soft tissues	Poorly expressed predominantly within the limits of the tumour and in adjacent soft tissues

Table 10 (Continued)

	Man	Experimental animals (rats)
Invasion:		
Follicular variants	Blood vessels	Blood vessels
Papillary variants	Lymphatic vessels	Lymphatic vessels
Metastases:		
Follicular variants	Lungs, bones, early metastases	Lungs
Papillary variants	Cervical lymph nodes Late metastases, slow evolution	Cervical lymph nodes, lungs
Anaplastic carcinomas	Early metastases in the lungs and other organs	Seldom in the lungs
Death rate	Generally lethal	Seldom cause the death of the animal
Functional activity:		
Follicular variants	Well marked	Well marked
Papillary variants	Scanty	Scanty
Anaplastic variants	Deficient	Deficient
Transplantibility	Hetero- seldom successful	Isotransplantation successful tumour strains

[a] Naturally occurring thyroid carcinomas.

experimental thyroid tumours in animals may be compared with "induced" thyroid tumours in man.

The following Table 10 sets out the differences and the similarities between thyroid adenomas and carcinomas in man and in experimental animals.

The above brief parallel between the morphological and biological behaviour of thyroid epithelial tumours in man and in experimental animals shows that they differ in a number of features. Certain animal species, owing to their specific biological features, show variants mostly as regards the latent period for the appearance of the tumours and their malignancy. In hamsters, for instance, the latent period for the appearance of thyroid tumours is shorter compared with that in mice and rats and the frequency of malignant variants is very high. In mice, however, diffuse thyroid hyperplasia creates conditions for metastatic growth of thyroid epithelia into the lungs. If increased thyrotrophic stimulation is suppressed, this metastatic thyroid tissue undergoes reverse development.

Although existing experimental models of thyroid tumours in mice, rats and hamsters cannot explain certain permanent trends in the development of thyroid tumours in man, they provide very extensive information about the basic stages in the transformation of normal thyroid tissue into tumour tissue. By applying different experimental conditions aimed at the induction of thyroid tumours, experimental methods can elucidate some of the relations between the endocrine glands.

References

Akimova, P., Gonina, R., Zotikov, L. A., Kulik, G. I.: Results of a biochemical, histochemical and ultrastructural study of the thyroid gland in the process of experimental carcinogenesis. In: Thyroid cancer. UICC monog., p. 149–154. Berlin-Heidelberg-New York: Springer 1969.

— Kulik, G. I.: Some biochemical and functional peculiarities of thyroid carcinogenesis in hamsters after treatment with 6-methylthiouracil. In: Problems of experimental Oncology, p. 133–141. Kiev: Health 1966.

Andros, G., Wollman, S. H.: Autoradiographic localisation of radioiodine in the thyroid gland of the mouse. Amer. J. Physiol. **213**, 198–208 (1967).

Astwood, E. B., Sullivan, I., Bissell, A., Tyslowitz, R.: Action of certain sulfonamides and of thiourea of the function of the thyroid gland of the rat. Endocrinology **32**, 214–226 (1943).

Axelrad, A. A., Leblond, C. D.: Induction of thyroid tumours in rats by a low iodine diet. Cancer (Philad.) **8**, 339–367 (1955).

Beid, L. C., Davis, D. A., Ainton, J. V.: The mechanism of action of some antithyroid drugs. Trans. Amer. Goitre Ass. 158–166 (1955).

Bielschowsky, F.: Experimental nodular goitre. Brit. J. exp. Path. **26**, 270–276 (1945).

— Comparison of the tumours production by 2-acetylaminofluorene in Piebold and Wistar rats. Brit. J. exp. Path. **27**, 135–140 (1946).

— Chronic iodine deficiency as cause of neoplasia in thyroid and pituitary of aged rats. Brit. J. Cancer **7**, 203–213 (1953).

— Neoplasia and internal enviromnent. Brit. J. Cancer **9**, 80–116 (1955).

— Griesbach, W. E., Hall, W. H., Kennedy, T. H., Purves, H. D.: Studies on experimental goitre: The transplantability of experimental thyroid tumours of the rat. Brit. J. Cancer **3**, 541–546 (1949).

— Horning, E. S.: Aspects of endocrine carcinogenesis. Brit. med. Bull. **14**, 106–115 (1958).

Biskind, M. S., Biskind, G. S.: Development of tumours in the rat ovary after transplantation into the spleen. Proc. Soc. exp. Biol. (N.Y.) **55**, 176–179 (1944).

Boat, T. F., Halmi, N. S.: Perticulate iodoproteins of the rat thyroid. In: Current topics in thyroid research, p. 122–128. New York: Academic Press Inc. 1965.

Bowens, O. M., Vander, J. D.: Thyroid nodules and thyroid malignancy. Ann. intern. Med. **2**, 245–253 (1962).

Brachetto-Brian, D., Grinberg, R.: Histological development of intraplenic thyroid autografts in thyroidectomized rats. Rev. Soc. argent. Biol. **27**, 199–204 (1951).

Broadhead, G. D., Wilson, I. B., Pearson, G. M.: The effect of prolonged feeding of goitrogens on thyroid function in rats. J. Endocr. **32**, 341–351 (1966).

Brown-Grant, K.: The control of thyroid secretion. J. clin. Path. **20**, 527–532 (1967).

BUSSOLATTI, G., FOSTER, G. V., CLARK, M. B., PEARSE, A. G. E.: Immunofluorescent localisation of calcitonin in medullary (C cell) thyroid carcinoma, using antibody to the pure porcine hormone. Virchows Arch. Abt. B 2, 234–238 (1969).

CALVERT, D.: Antithyroid drugs. Wis. med. J. 62, 440–441 (1963).

CARROLL, R. E., HADDON, R. E., HANDY, V. H., WIEBEN, E. E.: Thyroid cancer: Cochot analysis of increasing incidence in New York state 1941–1962. J. nat. Cancer Inst. 33, 277–283 (1964).

CHERNOZEMSKI, I. N., WARWICK, G. P.: Production of hepatomas in suckling mice after single application of β-propiolactone. J. nat. Cancer Inst. 45, 709–717 (1970).

CHRISTOV, K.: Dynamic changes in the thyroid gland of rats after treatment with acetylaminofluorene and methylthiouracil. Oncologia (Sofia) 4, 157–163 (1967a).

— Early morphological changes in the thyroid gland of rats after treatment with 4-methylthiouracil and 2-acetylaminofluorene. Abstr. 3rd Natl. Conf. Path. Sofia, 61–62 (1967b).

— Early morphological changes in the thyroid gland of rats after treatment with ^{131}I and methylthiouracil. Proc. nat. Cancer Inst. Sofia, 12 19–27 (1968a).

— Experimental tumours of the thyroid gland in rats treated with 2-acetylamino-fluorene and methylthiouracil. Oncologia (Sofia) 5, 49–60 (1968b).

— Autoradiographic investigation on thyroid carcinogenesis in rats after treatment with 131-iodine and methylthiouracil Oncologia (Sofia) 6, 53–58 (1969).

— Thyroid carcinogenesis in rats after treatment with ^{131}I and methylthiouracil. C. R. Acad. Bulg. Sci. 23, 891–894 (1970).

— Autoradiographic characteristics of experimental thyroid tumours in rats. Endocrinologie (to be published).

— KRISTEVA, M.: Funktionelle Charakteristik der Schilddrüsenkanzerogenese bei den Ratten. Arch. Geschwulstforsch. 37, 257–265 (1971).

CHU CHICK-MEI, CHEN HANN-YUAN: Studies on experimental thyroid tumours in rats: Histochemical demonstration of the changes in peroxidase activity during tumorigenesis. Acta Biol. exp. sin. 10, 41–51 (1965).

CONARD, R. A., DOBINS, B. M., SUTOV, W. W.: Thyroid neoplasia as late effect of exposure to radioactive iodine in fallout. J. Amer. med. Ass. 214, 316–324 (1970b).

— SUTOV, W. W., BATEMAN, J. L., DOBINS, B. M., RIKLON, E., DEMOISE, C. F.: Medical survey of the people of Rongelap and Utirik Islands, 13, 14 and 15 years after exposure to fallout radiation. March 1967–March 1969. Brookhaven Natl. Lab. Upton, N.Y. 50226, 1–127 (1970a).

— — COLCOCK, B. P., DOBINS, B. M., PAGIA, D. E.: Thyroid nodules as a la teeffect of exposure to fallout. In: Radiation induced cancer. Intern. Atomic Energy Agency, Wienna, 325–336 (1969).

CUNLIFFE, W. J., HALL, R., HUDSON, P., GUDMUNDSSON, T. W., WILLIAMS, E. D., GALANTE, L., MACINTIRE, I.: A calcitonin-secreting thyroid carcinoma. Lancet 1968I, 63–66.

D'ANGELO, S. A., TRAUM, R. E.: An experimental analysis of the hypothalamic-hypophyseal-thyroid relationship in rat. Ann. N.Y. Acad. Sci. 72, 239–270 (1958).

DELLA-PORTA, G., TERRACINI, B.: Chemical carcinogenesis in infant animals. In: Progress in exp. tumour res., vol. 2, p. 334–369. New York-Basel: Karger 1969.

DENT, I. N., GADSDEN, E. L., FURTH, I.: Futher studies on induction and growth of thyrotropic pituitary tumours in mice. Cancer Res. 16, 171–174 (1956).

DIKE, J. H. VAN: Experimental thyroid tumorigenesis in rats: predominance of neoplasms type and influence of age. Arch. Path. 56, 613–628 (1953).

DOBINS, B. M., LENAN, B. A.: Study of the histopathology and function of thyroid tumours using radioactive iodine and radioautography. J. clin. Endocr. 8, 732–748 (1948).

DOLPHIN, G. W.: The risk of thyroid cancer following irradiation Hlth Phys. **15**, 219–221 (1968).

DONIACH, I.: The effect of radioactive iodine alone and in combination with methylthiouracil and acetylaminofluorene upon tumour production in rats thyroid gland. Brit. J. Cancer **4**, 223–234 (1950).

— The effect of radioactive iodine alone and in combination with methylthiouracil upon tumour production in rats thyroid gland. Brit. J. Cancer **7**, 181–202 (1953).

— Comparison of the carcinogenic effect of X-irradiation with radioactive iodine in rats thyroid. Brit. J. Cancer **11**, 67–76 (1956).

— Experimental induction of tumours of the thyroid by irradiation. Brit. med. Bull. **14**, 181–183 (1958).

— Effect including carcinogenesis of ^{131}I and X-rays on the thyroid of experimental animals: A review. Hlth Phys. **9**, 1357–1362 (1963).

— Correlation of thyroid cells height with sex difference in tumour induction. Discussion on carcinogeneic role of TSH. In: Thyroid cancer, UICC monog. Ed. by E. Hedinger, vol. 12, p. 131–154. Berlin-Heidelberg-New York: Springer 1969a).

— Tumour production in thyroids of rats given varying doses of radioactive iodine at birth. In: Thyroid cancer. Ed. by Chr. E. Hedinger. UICC monog., vol. 12, p. 174–183. Berlin-Heidelberg-New York: Springer 1969b.

— PELC, S. R.: Autoradiographs with radioactive iodine. Proc. roy. Soc. Med. **42**, 957–959 (1949).

— WILLIAMS, E. D.: Development of thyroid and pituitary tumours in rats two years after partial thyroidectomy. Brit. J. Cancer **16**, 222–321 (1962).

FELLER, D. D., CHAIKOFF, I. L., TAUROG, A., JONES, H. B.: The changes induced in iodine metabolism of the rat by internal radiation of the thyroid with ^{131}I. Endocrinology **45**, 464–479 (1949).

FERBER, B., HANDY, V. H., GERHARDT, P. R., SOLOMON, M.: Cancer in New York state exclusive of New York City 1941–1960. Bureau of Cancer Control, New York State Department of Health (1962).

FIELD, I. B., McCOMMAN, C. I., VALENTINE, R. I., BERNICK, S., ORR, C., STARR, P.: Failure of radioiodine to induce thyroid cancer in the rat. Cancer Res. **19**, 870–873 (1959).

FITZGERALD, P. J.: ^{131}I concentration and thyroid morphology. In: Thyroid gland, p. 220. Upton-New York: Brookhaven Natl. Lab. 1955.

— FOOTE, F. W.: The function of various types of thyroid carcinoma as revealed by the radioautographic demonstration of radioactive iodine. J. clin. Endocr. **9**, 1153–1157 (1947).

— — HILL, R. F.: Concentration of ^{131}I in thyroid cancer shown by radioautography. Cancer (Philad.) **3**, 86–105 (1950).

FORTNER, J. G., GEORGE, P. A., STERNBERG, S. S.: The development of thyroid cancer and other abnormalities in Syrian hamsters maintained on an iodine deficient diet. Surg. Forum **9**, 646–650 (1959).

— — — Induced and spontaneous thyroid cancer in the Syrian (golden) hamster. Endocrinology **66**, 364–376 (1960).

FRANTZ, V. K., KLIGERMAN, M. M., HARLAND, W. A., PHILLIPS, M. E., QUIMBY, E. H.: A comparison of the carcinogenic effect of internal irradiation on the thyroid gland of the male Long-Evans rats. Endocrinology **61**, 574–581 (1957).

FURTH, J.: Concepts of thyroid carcinogenesis. Interpretation and events. Needed research. In: Thyroid cancer. Ed. by Chr. Hedinger. UICC monog., vol. 12, p. 171–174. Berlin-Heidelberg-New York: Springer 1969.

GARNER, R. J.: Comparative early and late effects of single and prolonged exposure to radioiodine in young and adults of various animal speties. A review. Helth Phys. **9**, 1333–1339 (1963).

GEORGADZE, O. E., BARAMDZE, T. G., CHECHELOSHWILY, G. L.: Thyroid tumours induced with 131-iodine and chemical carcinogens. 9th Intern. Cancer Congr., Tokyo, 144 (1966).

GNATISHAK, A. I.: Thyroid tumours in experiments and changes in some endocrine glands. Vop. Onkol. 3, 659–666 (1957).

GOLDBERG, R. C., CHAIKOFF, I. L.: Induction of thyroid cancer in the rat by radioactive iodine. Arch. Path. 53, 22–28 (1952).

— LINDSAY, S., NICHOLS, C. V., CHAIKOFF, I. L.: Induction of neoplasms in the thyroid gland of rats by subtotal thyroidectomy and by the injection of 1 μCi ^{131}I. Cancer Res. 24, 35–48 (1964).

GOOLDEN, A. W. G.: Radiation cancer. Review with spetial references to radiation tumours in the pharynx, larynx and thyroid. Brit. J. Radiol. 30, 626–640 (1957).

GREER, M. A., KENDALL, J. W., SMITH, M.: Antithyroid compounds. In: The Thyroid Gland. Ed. by R. PITT-RIVERS and W. TROTTTER, Vol. 2, pp. 357–390. London: Butterworth 1964.

GRIESBACH, W. E., KENNEDY, T. H., PURVES, H. D.: Studies on experimental goitre. Thyroid adenomata in rats on Brassica seed diet. Brit. J. exp. Path. 26, 18–24 (1945).

GROSS, J., BEN-PORATH, M., ROSIN, A., BLOCH, M.: A comparison of radiobiologic effects of ^{131}I and ^{125}I respectively on the rat thyroid. In: Thyroid neoplasia. Ed. by S. Young and D. R. Inman, p. 291–306. London-New York: Academic Press 1968.

GUCHA, S.: Studies of oxidative enzymes in rat thyroid epithelium under normal and experimental conditions. Ann. Histochem. 9, 107–113. (1964)

GUINET, P.: Histological and histochemical criteria of malignancy in thyroid epitheliomas. In: Tumours of the thyroid gland. Ed. by H. Appaix, p. 106–109. Basel-New York: Karger 1966.

HALL, W. H.: The rolr of initiation and promoting factors in the pathogenesis of tumours of the thyroid. Brit. J. Cancer 2, 273–280 (1948).

HANFORD, J. M., QUIMBY, E. H., FRANTZ, V. K.: Cancer arising many years after radiation therapy; incidence after irradiation of benign lesions in the neck. J. Amer. med. Ass. 181, 404–410 (1962).

HARAN-CHERA, N., PULLAR, P., FURTH, J.: Induction of thyrotropin dependent thyroid tumours by thyrotropes. Endocrinology 66, 694–701 (1960).

HARPER, P. V., PAVOYAN, D.: Thyroid carcinoma associated with radiation therapy. Surg. Clin. N. Amer. 49, 57–60 (1968).

HATWAY, D. S., LIPSCOMB, H. S.: Chemical, Chromatographic and radioisotopic technique in an experimental study of thyroid function. Tex. Rep. Biol. Med. 20, 204–213 (1962).

HEMPELMANN, L. H.: Radiation induced thyroid neoplasms in man. Science 160, 1959–1963 (1968a).

— Radiation induced thyroid neoplasms in man. In: Thyroid neoplasia. Ed. by S. Young and A. D. Inman, p. 267–277. London-New York: Academic Press 1968b.

— Radiation exposure and thyroid cancer in man. In: Thyroid cancer. Ed. by Chr. Hedinger, UICC monog., vol. 12, p. 103–111. Berlin-Heidelberg-New York: Springer 1969.

— PIEFER, J. F., BURKE, G. J., TERRY, R., AMES, W. R.: Neoplasms in persons treated in infancy with X-rays for thymic enlargement. Report of the 3rd follow-up survey. J. nat. Cancer Inst. 38, 317–341 (1967).

HINDAWI, A. I., WILSON, C. M.: The effect of irradiation on the function and survival of rat thyroid. Clin. Sci. 28, 555–571 (1965).

IRD, E. A.: Effect of subtotal thyroidectomy on the development of thyroid tumours in rats treated with methylthiouracil. Probl. Endocrinology 14, 87–94 (1968).

Isler, H.: Effect of iodine intake, prophyltiouracil and environmental temperature on the induction of thyroid tumours in the rat. Sci. Proc. Amer. Ass. Cancer Res. 3, 331 (1962).

Israel, M. S., Ellis, I. R.: The neoplastic potencialities of mouse thyroid under extreme stimulation. Brit. J. Cancer 14, 206–212 (1960).

Jones, E. E., Barker, J., Dietrich, S.: Spontaneous tumours of the thyroid gland in rats. J. nat. Cancer Inst. 36, 1–14 (1966).

Kabak, I. M.: Drugs blocking thyroid function. Usp. sovrem. Biol. 28, 187–196 (1949).

Kiyama, H., Totsuka, S., Yoshimura, F.: Chronic changes of the parafollicular cells in the rats fed diets of high or low calcium contant. Endocr. jap. 15, 439–455 (1968).

Lapis, K., Veberdi, L.: Simultaneous histological, autoradiographic and biochemical examination of experimental induced thyroid tumours. Acta morph. Acad. Sci. hung. 11, 2–14 (1962).

Leathem, J. H.: Goitrogen induced thyroid tumours. Ciba Found. coll. Endocr. 12, 50–58 (1958).

Lemarchand-Berand, T., Valenta, L., Vannotti, A.: In: Thyroid cancer. Ed. by Chr. Hedinger. UICC monog., vol. 12, p. 205217. Berlin-Heidelberg-New York: Springer 1969.

Lindsay, S.: Pathology of the thyroid gland. In: The thyroid gland, ed. by R. Pitt-Rivers and W. Trotter, vol. 2, p. 223–271. London: Butterworhs 1964.

— Ionising radiation and experimental thyroid neoplasmas: A review. In: Thyroid cancer. Ed. by Chr. Hedinger. UICC monog., vol. 12, p. 161–171. Berlin-Heidelberg-New York: Springer 1969.

— Chaikoff, L.: The effects of irradiation on the thyroid gland with particular reference to the induction of thyroid neoplasmas. Cancer Res. 24, 1099–1107 (1964).

— Daivy, M. E., Jones, M. D.: Histologic effects of various types of ionising radiation on normal and hyperplastic human thyroid glands. J. clin. Endocr. 14, 1179–1186 (1954).

— Nichols, C. W., Chaikoff, I. L., Jr.: Induction of benign and malignant thyroid neoplasms in the rat. Arch. Path. 81, 308–317 (1966).

— — — Induction of thyroid neoplasms in the rat by injection of 1 or 5 Ci ^{131}I. Arch. Path. 85, 487–492 (1968a).

— — — Naturally occurring thyroid carcinoma. Arch. Path. 86, 353–365 (1968b).

— Potter C. D., Chaikoff, I. L.: Thyroid neoplasms in the rat. A comparison of naturally occurring and ^{131}I induced tumours. Cancer Res. 17, 183–189 (1957).

— — — Radioiodine induced thyroid carcinoma in female rats. Arch. Path. 75, 8–12 (1963).

— Sheline, G. E., Potter, G. D., Chaikoff, I. L.: Induction of neoplasms in the thyroid gland of the rat by X-irradiation of the gland. Cancer Res. 21, 9–16 (1961).

Lissitzky, S.: Thyroglobulin and other iodinated proteins in relation to cancerous thyroid tissue. In: Thyroid cancer. Ed. by Chr. Hedinger. UICC monog., vol. 12, p. 217–224. Berlin-Heidelberg-New York: Springer 1968.

Mackenzie, J. B., Mackenzie, C. G.: Effect of sulfonamides and tioureas on the thyroid gland and basal metabolism. Endocrinology 32, 185–209 (1943).

Maloof, F., Dobyns, B M., Vickery, A. D.: The effect of various doses of radioactive iodine on the function and structure of the thyroid of the rat. Endocrinology 50, 612–619 (1952).

MATOVINOVIC, J., LEAHY, M. S., ARMSTRONG, W. F., HILL, H. C.: The effect of environment on the growth and function of rat thyroid transplant tumours. In: Thyroid neoplasia. Ed. by S. Young and D. R. Inman, p. 211–248. London-New York: Academic Press 1968.

McGROW, R. W., MACKENZIE, A. D.: Carcinoma of the thyroid and laryngopharings following irradiation. Cancer (Philad.) 18, 692–679 (1965).

MILHAUD, G., TUBIANA, M., PARMENTIER, C., COUTRIS, G., LACOUR, J.: Thyrocalcitonin-secreting thyroid carcinoma. In: Thyroid cancer. Ed. by Chr. Hedinger. UICC monog., vol. 12, p. 237–242. Berlin-Heidelberg-New York: Springer 1969.

MILCU, ST., PETREA, I.: Experimental cancer of the thyroid. Probl. Morfopat. (Buc.) 1, 9–49 (1959).

MOLE R. H.: The dose-response relationship in radiation carcinogenesis. A Review. Brit. med. Bull. 14, 184–189 (1958).

MONEY, W. L.: Chemical carcinogenesis and sex hormones in experimental thyroid tumours. In: Thyroid cancer. Ed. by Chr. Hedinger. UICC monog., vol. 12, p. 140–149. Berlin-Heidelberg-New York: Springer 1969.

— FITZGERALD, P. J., GODWIN, T. I., ROWSON, R. W.: The effect of thiouracil on the colletcion of radioactive iodine in experimental induced thyroid tumours. Cancer (Philad.) 6, 111–120 (1953).

— GODWIN, J. T., ROWSON, R.: The experimental production of thyroid tumours in the rat by the administration of sodium-5-iodo-2-thiouracil. Cancer (Philad.) 10, 690–697 (1957).

— ROWSON, R. W.: The experimental production of thyroid tumours in the rat exposed to prolonged treatment with thyrouracil. Cancer (Philad.) 3, 321–335 (1950).

— — Intrathyroid implantation of chemical carcinogens in the rat. Arch. Path. 79, 470–474 (1965).

— — Factors influencing malignancy versus benignancy of thyroid neoplasms in man and experimental animals. 2-Experimental animals. In: Thyroid neoplasia. Ed. by S. Young and D. R. Inman, p. 179–199. London: Academic Press 1968.

MORRIS, H. P.: The experimental development and metabolism of thyroid gland tumours. In: Advances in cancer research. Ed. by J. Greenstein and A. Haddow, vol. 3, p. 51–115. London-New York: Academic Press 1955.

— DALTON, A. I.: Malignant thyroid tumours occurring in the mouse after prolonged hormonal imbalance during the ingestion of thiouracil. J. clin. Endocr. 11, 1281–1295 (1951).

— GREEN, C. D.: The role of thiouracil in induction, growth and transplantability of mouse thyroid tumours. Science 114, 44–46 (1951).

NADLER, N. J., MANDAVIA, M. G., LEBLOND, C. P.: Influence of preirradiation of thyroid tumorogenesis by low iodine diet in the rat. In: Thyroid cancer. Ed by. Chr. Hedinger. UICC monog., vol. 12, p. 125–131. Berlin-Heidelberg-New York: Springer 1969.

NAGASAKA, T.: The experimental studies of the hormonal regulation of the thyroid gland. Abstr. J. Jap. Soc. Inter. Med. 49, 44–48 (1961/62).

NAPALKOV, N. P.: Experimental tumours of the thyroid gland. Vop. Onkol. 4, 138–150 (1958).

— Morphological properties of the experimental thyroid tumours induced in rats by treatment with 6-methylthiouracil. Vop. Onkol. 5, 578–592 (1959a).

— Experimental tumours of the thyroid gland in rats after treatment with acethylaminofluorene and methylthiouracil. Vop. Onkol. 5, 23–33 (1959b).

— New aspects of thyroid carcinogenesis. 8th Intern. Cancer Congr., Moscow, 1962, 5, 502–506 (1962).

— Tumorigenic action of antithyroid drugs. In: Sovr. Probl. Oncologii, p. 34–42. Leningrad: Medgisdat 1965.

Napalkov, N. P.: Thyroid carcinogenesis in rats treated with 6-methylthiouracil for several successive generations. In: Thyroid Cancer. Ed. by Chr. Hedinger. UICC monog., vol. 12, p. 134–140. Berlin-Heidelberg-New York: Springer 1969.

Nunez, J. J., Brun, D., Roche, J.: Solubilisation of thyroid particulate iodoproteins. Current topics in thyroid research, p. 129–138. London-New York: Academic Press 1965.

Pages, A.: Diagnostic elements of malignant tumours of the thyroid gland. In: Tumours of the thyroid gland, p. 117–135. Basel-New York: Karger 1966.

Papazov, G.: Thyroid iodoproteins. In: Sovr. Probl. Endocrin. 2, 175–179 (1967).

Paschkis, K. E., Cantarow, A., Stasney, I.: Influence of thyrouracil on carcinoma induced by 2-acetylaminofluorene. Cancer Res. 8, 257–263 (1948).

Petrea, I.: Recherches sur la tumorigenesis de certaines glandes endocrines (thyroide, hypophyse et surrenale). Neoplasma (Bratisl.) 8, 145–156 (1961).

— Experimental thyro-oncogenesis in XVII nc/ZE mice. In: Thyroid cancer. Ed. by Chr. Hedinger. UICC monog., vol. 12, p. 154–160. Berlin-Heidelberg-New York Springer 1969.

Piefer, I. W., Hempelmann, L. H.: Radiation induced thyroid carcinoma. Ann. N.Y. Acad. Sci. 114, 838–848 (1964).

— — Dodges, H., Hodges, F. J.: Neoplasmas in Ann Arbor series of thymus irradiation children: Rereat Survey. Amer. J. Roentgenol. 103, 13–18 (1968).

Pincus, R. A., Reichlin, S., Hempelmann, L. H.: Thyroid abnormalities after radiation exposure in infancy. Ann. intern. Med. 66, 1154–1164 (1967).

Pittman, S. S., Lin, A., Jones, E. E.: Hormone synthesis by a transplantable thyroid tumour in mice. Endocrinology 73, 403–409 (1963).

Pitt-Rivers, R., Trotter, W. R.: The site of accumulation of iodide in the thyroid of rats treated with thiouracil. Lancet 265, 918–919 (1953).

Pochin, E. E.: Questions involved in defining dose limits for occupational exposure of thyroid and other organs. Proc. 2nd Int. Congr. Radiol. Rome 1965, 1352–1355 (1965).

— Carcinogenic effects of a radiation in man: The importance of estimates for protection purposes. In: Radiation induced cancer. IAEA monog., Viena 1969, 3–13 (1969).

— Thompson, B.: Metabolic activity of tumour tissue. In: Thyroid Cancer. Ed. by Chr. Hedinger. UICC monog., vol. 12, p. 194–205. Berlin-Heidelberg-New York: Springer 1969.

Potter, C. D., Lindsay, S., Chaikoff, I. L.: Induction of neoplasms in rat thyroid gland by low doses of radioiodine. Arch. Path. 69, 257–269 (1960).

Purves, H. D.: Control of thyroid function. In: The thyroid gland. Ed. by R. Pitt-Rivers and W. Trotter, vol. 2, p. 1–39. London: Butterworths 1964.

— Griesbach, W. E.: Studies on experimental goitre. Thyroid carcinoma in rat treated with thiouracil. Brit. J. exp. Path. 28, 46–53 (1947).

— — Kennedy, T.: Studies in experimental goitre: Malignant changes in a transplantable rat thyroid tumour. Brit. J. Cancer 5, 301–310 (1951).

Raichev, R., Christov, K.: Thyroid carcinogenesis in hamsters after treatment with ^{131}I and methylthiouracil. (Submitted to Endocrinology.)

Raventos, A., Winship, T.: The latent interval for thyroid cancer following irradiation. Radiology 83, 501–505 (1964).

Robbins, J.: Abnormal thyroglobulin in experimental thyroid tumours. In: Thyroid neoplasia. Ed. by S. Young and D. C. Inman, p. 405–411. London-New York: Academic Press 1968.

— Wolff, J., Rall, J. I.: Iodoprotein in normal and abnormal human thyroid tissue and in normal sheep thyroid. Endocrinology 64, 37–52 (1959).

Roe, E. I. C.: Spontaneous tumours in rats and mice. Fol. Cosmetic Toxicol. 3, 97–114 (1965).

SAENGER, E. L., SELTZER, R. A., STARLING, T. D., KEREIAKES, I. G.: Carcinogenic effect of ^{131}I compared with X-irradiation. Studies on the association of irradiation and thyroid cancer in human. Hlth Phys. 9, 1371–1384 (1963).
SAENGER, E. L., SILVERMAN, E. M., STARLING, T. D., TURNER, M. E.: Neoplasia following therapeutic irradiation for benign conditions in childhood. Radiology 74, 889–904 (1960).
SARKAR, S. K., ISLER, H.: Origin of the "Light cells" of the thyroid gland. Endocrinology 73, 199–204 (1963).
SCHALLER, R. T., STEVENSON, J. K.: Development of carcinoma of the thyroid in iodine-deficient mice. Cancer (Philad.) 19, 1063–1080 (1966).
SEIFTER, I., EHRICH, W. E., HUDJAMA, G. M.: Effects of prolonged administration of antithyroid compounds on the thyroid gland and other endocrine glands of the rat. Arch. Path. 48, 536–549 (1949).
SELLERS, E. A., HILL, J. H., LEE, R. B.: Effect of iodine and thyroid on the production of tumours of the thyroid and pituitary by propylthiouracil. Arch. Path. 52, 118–203 (1953).
— SCHÖNBAUM, E.: Enhancement of goitrogenic action of propylthiouracil by thyroxine. Science 126, 1342–1345 (1957).
— — Goitrogenic action of thyroxine administered with propylthiouracil. Acta endocr. (Kbh.) 40, 39–50 (1962a).
— — Blood vessels of experimental thyroid tumours. Acta endocrin. (Kbh.) 40, 51–59 (1962b).
— — Further studies on the goitrogenic action of thyroxine, administered with propylthiouracil, methimazol or perchlorate. Acta endocr. (Kbh.) 49, 319–330 (1965).
SHELINE, G. E., LINDSAY, S., BELL, H. G.: Occurrence of thyroid nodules in children following therapy with radioiodine for hyperthyroidism. J. clin. Endocr. 19, 127–133 (1959).
SICHUK, G., MONEY, W. L., FORTNER, J. G.: Cancer of the thyroid. Goitrogenesis and thyroid function in Syrian (golden) hamster. Cancer (Philad.) 21, 952–963 (1968).
SILVERBERG, S. G., VIDONE, R. A.: Adenoma and carcinoma of the thyroid. Cancer (Philad.) 19, 1053–1062 (1966).
SIMPSON, C. L., HEMPELMANN, L. H., FULLER, L. M.: Neoplasms in children treated with X-rays in infancy for thymic enlargement. Radiology 64, 840–845 (1955).
— — The association of tumours and roentgen ray treatment of the thorax in infancy. Cancer (Philad.) 10, 42–56 (1957).
SINCHA, D., PASCAL, R., FURTH, J.: Transplantable thyroid carcinoma induced by thyrotropin. Arch. Path. 79, 192–198 (1965).
SLYE, M., HOLMES, H. F., WELLS, H. G.: Studies in the incidence and inheritability of spontaneous tumours in mice. XXII. The comparative pathology of cancer of the thyroid, with report of premary spontaneous tumours of the thyroid in mice and in a rat. J. Cancer Res. 10, 175–194 (1926).
SOCOLOV, E. L., HASHIZUMA, A., NERISHI, S., NITANI, N.: Thyroid cancer in man after exposure to ionising radiation. New Engl. J. Med. 268, 406–407 (1963).
STANBURY, J. B.: Thyroid-specific metabolic incopentence and tumour development. In: Thyroid cancer. Ed. by Chr. Hedinger. UICC monog., vol. 12, p. 183–191. Berlin-Heidelberg-New York: Springer 1969.
STOLL, R., MARAND, R.: Sur l'induction de tumeurs thyridiennes chez le rat treite par le ^{131}I et propylthiouracil. Bull. du Cancer. 50, 359–398 (1963).
TATA, J. R.: Normal and abnormal iodinated compound in the serum of subjects with carcinoma of the thyroid. Ciba Found. Coll. Endocrin. 12, 33–41 (1958).
— POCHIN, E. E.: Thyroid cancer. In: The thyroid gland. Ed. by R. Pitt-Rivers and W. Trotter, vol. 2, p. 208–223. London: Butterworth 1964.

Taylor, S.: Genesis of thyroid nodule. Brit. med. Bull. **16**, 102–111 (1960).

Toth, B.: A critical review of experiments in chemical carcinogenesis usings newborn animals. Cancer Res. **28**, 727–738 (1968).

Valenta, L., Lissitzky, S., Roques, M., Rolland, M.: A comparison of thyroglobulines from normal and carcinomatous thyroid tissue. In: Thyroid cancer. Ed. by Chr. Hedinger. UICC monog., vol. 12, p. 334–337. Berlin-Heidelberg-New York: Springer 1969.

Voitkevich, A. A.: Antithyroid action of sulfonamides and thioureates, Monog. 213. Moscow: Medgis 1957.

— Structural changes of the thyroid gland according to its repairing properties. Probl. Endocrinol. Hormonother. **10**, 89–98 (1964).

Wegelin, C.: Malignant disease of the thyroid gland and its relation to goitre in man and animals. Cancer Res. **3**, 297–313 (1928).

Willis, I.: The induction of malignant neoplasms in the thyroid gland of the rat. J. Path. Bact. **82**, 23–27 (1961).

Winship, T., Rosvoll, R. V.: A study of thyroid cancer in children. Amer. J. Surg. **102**, 747–752 (1961).

— — Cancer of the thyroid in children. In: Thyroid cancer. Ed. by Chr. Hedinger. UICC monog., vol. 12, p. 75–78. Berlin-Heidelberg-New York: Springer 1969.

Witt, S. de, Delamter, M. D., Winship, T.: Follow-up study of adults treated with roentgen rays for thyroid disease. Cancer (Philad.) **16**, 1028–1033 (1963).

Wolff, J., Robbins, J., Rall, J. E.: Iodide trapping without organification in a transplantable rat thyroid tumour. Endocrinology **64**, 1–19 (1959).

Wollman, S. H.: Effects of feeding thiouracil on thyroid glands of rats. J. nat. Cancer Inst. **26**, 473–487 (1961).

— Production and properties of transplantable tumours of the thyroid gland in Fischer rats. Recent Progr. Hormone Res. **19**, 579–585 (1963).

— Scow, R. O., Wagner, B., Morris, H. P.: Radioiodine uptake by transplantable tumours of the thyroid gland in C3H mice. Experimental results. J. nat. Cancer Inst. **13**, 785–805 (1953a).

— — — — Radioiodide concentrating ability of transplantable tumours of the thyroid gland in C3H mice. J. nat. Cancer Inst. **14**, 593–603 (1953b).

Yacobs, B. B.: Transplantability and function of a thyroid and pituitary tumours arising spontaneously in an Ha/ICR Swiss mouse. Proc. Amer. Ass. Cancer Res. **4**, 1 (1963).

Young, B. A., Leblond, C. P.: The "light cells" as compared to the follicular cells in the thyroid gland of the rat. Endocrinology **73**, 669–686 (1963).

Zajdela, F., Vignal, A., Triantaphyllidis, E.: Etude du fonctionement thyroidien de trois souches differents de souris. Rep. de l'Institut de Radium Paris, 99 (1967).

Division of Experimental Pathology, Walter Reed Army Institute of Research,
Walter Reed Army Medical Center, Washington, D. C.

Current Aspects of Bacterial Enterotoxins

DANIEL G. SHEAHAN

Contents

Introduction

It is a curious fact of medical history that entero (exo)toxin production by a wide variety of enteric pathogens has been appreciated only within the past decade while the pathogens themselves have been recognized since the beginning of bacteriology. Recent investigations have implicated toxins produced by *Staphylococcus aureus*, *Vibrio cholerae*, certain strains of "non-pathogenic" *Escherichia coli*, as well as *Shigella dysenteriae*, *C. perfringens* and possibly *Pseudomonas aeruginosa* as being responsible for diarrheal disease.

The purpose of this communication is to outline the recent advances in the knowledge and understanding of diarrheal disease mediated by these toxin-producing organisms. Particular emphasis will be placed on pathogenetic mechanisms as well as various facets of pathological and immunological relationships which exist between the organism and the host. Insights into the pathophysiological aspects of intestinal secretory and absorptive functions derived from investigations utilizing such toxins in experimental models as well as in human volunteers, will be discussed.

For the sake of simplicity and clarity, each specific toxin shall be dealt with separately. In this discussion it is the bacterial entero(exo)toxin which is being considered and no attempt is made to discuss endotoxin in this communication. The greatest emphasis shall be placed on cholera enterotoxin which is the most intensively studied.

Vibrio Cholerae Enterotoxin

Introduction

ROBERT KOCH (1884), who first described the comma bacillus in Alexandria, Egypt, in 1883, asserted the etiological relationship between the *Vibrio cholerae* organism and the disease. He noted that the vibrio was confined to the wall and contents of the intestine and suggested that the organism produced soluble, absorbable toxins. Subsequent laboratory investigations initiated by PFEIFFER (1892) demonstrated the existence of a toxic moiety. However, because the intraperitoneal route of challenge was used, only the effects of endotoxin and not those of entero(exo)toxin were recognized. VIRCHOW (1879) observed from post-mortem studies of cholera patients a denudation of the small intestinal epithelium which he ascribed to the effect of the vibrio and as the cause of the diarrhea.

COHNHEIM (1882) indicated that the choleraic stool had such a low protein content that it should not be considered an exudate but was the result of intestinal hypersecretion. Though GOODPASTURE (1923), studying cholera in the Phillipines, found evidence which supported COHNHEIM's view, the earlier views held sway and were cited in text books even as late as 10 years ago.

In 1894, METCHNIKOFF described the classic experiment whereby infant rabbits developed diarrhea following suckling on maternal tits previously smeared with vibrio organisms. Because of poor reproducibility, this approach received little support. DUTTA and HABBU (1955) demonstrated the consistent production of diarrhea in this experimental model following intraintestinal inoculation of viable organisms. DE and CHATTERJEE (1953) rediscovered the model of VIOLLE and CRENDIROPOULO (1915) and demonstrated that the adult rabbit produced fluid in ligated ileal loops in response to intraluminal inoculation of viable organisms.

Epithelial denudation was convincingly shown not to be a response to cholera by the observations of GANGAROSA et al. (1960) on biopsy material showing an intact intestinal epithelium in cholera. This has been repeatedly confirmed in the rabbit experimental model (NORRIS and MAJNO, 1968; FRESH et al., 1964; FORMAL et al., 1961). In the canine model the intestinal morphology remained unaltered from first mucosal contact with cholera enterotoxin through recovery as evaluated by both light and electron microscopy (ELLIOTT et al., 1970).

Products of Vibrio Cholerae and Their Terminology

The *vibrio cholerae* produces a number of toxic moieties which can be separated on the basis of heat stability, dialyzability, location in the bacterial cell and toxic effects in different assay systems. BURROWS (1968) has grouped cholera "toxins" into three types. Type I which is heat stable and nondialyzable, is only seen in liquid culture supernatants as a consequence of autolysis of vibrios. It includes the mouse lethal factor and is most probably endotoxin. Type II which is heat labile and non-dialyzable, occurs in the intracellular substance and diffuses into the liquid culture medium but is not a component of the cell wall. It includes the factors responsible for the net flux of ion and water from the tissues to the lumen of the small bowel, for increased skin capillary permeability and for the cytotoxic effects on cultured cells. Type III toxin includes the dialyzable, heat stable factors which inhibit active sodium transport in anuren epithelium and para-aminohippurate uptake by kidney tissues *in vitro*. Some evidence exists that the presence of ammonia may contribute to these latter activities.

The toxic moieties obtained from *V. cholerae* culture filtrates are also detectable in cholera stools. Filtrates of stools from bacteriologically proven cases of cholera when fed to infant rabbits caused a lethal disease similar to experimental cholera in such animals (PANSE and DUTTA, 1961). HUBER and PHILLIPS (1962) found a "sodium pump inhibitor" in cholera stools during the Bangkok epidemic of 1960. A capillary permeability factor has been detected in cholera stool by BASU MALLICK and GANGULI (1964) and CRAIG (1965 a). Positive ileal loop response to cholera stool filtrate was noted by DUTT (1965) while BASU MALLICK et al. (1969) have demonstrated that filtrates of some cholera stools possessed a thermolabile cytotoxic factor when tested on primary monkey cell culture, organ culture of mouse intestine and ten day old chick embryos. SCHAFER et al. (1970a) have demonstrated that administration of sterilized filtrates of fluid, obtained from rabbit intestinal loops previously inoculated with *V. cholerae*, to intestinal loops of other rabbits produced a response virtually identical to that produced with crude enterotoxin produced *in vitro*. FRETER *et al.* (1961) were unable to establish the presence of vibrio endotoxin in cholera stools. FINKELSTEIN *et al.* (1963), however, did demonstrate such a substance in the feces and showed that it did not cause cholera in the rabbit.

Many terms have been used to describe the diarrheagenic factor produced by the *Vibrio cholerae*. DE (1959) originally ascribed the term enterotoxin to this factor. The thermolabile factor produced by cholera vibrios, as noted by DUTTA *et al.* (1959), was called "Pro-choleragen A" by FINKELSTEIN *et al.* (1964). It produced fluid enterosorption in experimental animals only in the presence of a thermostable factor also present in *V. cholerae* and called "Pro-choleragen B". Later these workers used the term choleragen (FINKELSTEIN *et al.*, 1966a) to describe the combined active moiety. (CRAIG, 1965a) and RICHARDSON (1969) employed the term skin permeability factor because it appeared that the same active component which caused diarrhea also increased capillary permeability. FEELEY and ROBERTS (1969) called it an exotoxin because it had many of the characteristics of an exotoxin. BURROWS and colleagues (1968) used the term type-2 cholera toxin differentiating it from type-1 endotoxin and type-3 sodium transport inhibitor. In this discussion the general term enterotoxin will be employed for simplicity of presentation and because the diarrheagenic factors of all organisms to be discussed have the single common property of evoking fluid exsorption from the gut.

Development of Animal Models of Cholera

The rabbit ileal loop model is suitable for studies with live organisms (DE and CHATTERJE, 1953), cell free preparations of ultrasonic lysates of liquid culture supernatants of vibrios (DE, 1959; DE *et al.*, 1960). They demonstrated that filtrates of cultures grown in 5% peptone/0.5% saline consistently showed the presence of mucinase and enterotoxic activity. The enterotoxic moiety was precipitable with ammonium sulfate, dialyzable, preserved at 2–4° C for 1 week or by freezing and thawing, but destroyed by heat (56° C for 30 min). DUTTA and colleagues (1959) reintroduced and standardized the infant rabbit model and subsequently showed that intragastric inoculation of 9 to 10 day old rabbits with cell-free materials, prepared by dilute acid extraction of vibrios, produced an acute diarrhea indistinguishable from that due to the vibrio infection. OZA and DUTTA (1963) showed that the disease could also be produced with a cell-free ultrasonic lysate of vibrios given intragastrically to the infant rabbit. These observations were confirmed by FINKELSTEIN *et al.* (1964). Enterotoxin containing culture filtrates were reported to produce choleraic manifestations in human subjects (BENYAJATI, 1966) thus making the laboratory animal models more applicable to study of the human disease.

Although the starved and opiated guinea pig proved to be an effective
model (Formal *et al.*, 1961), it has given way to the more suitable and consistently reproducible systems such as the suckling rabbit and the ligated ileal
loop in the adult rabbit. The most recent model to be widely utilized is the
Thiry-Vella loop in the dog (Sack and Carpenter, 1969).

Production of Enterotoxin

Source

The majority of the so-called classical and El Tor strains of *Vibrio cholerae*
exhibit low toxigenicity. The Inaba 569 B strain was brought to high virulence by
serial animal passage with high toxigenicity for the infant rabbit by Dutta
and Habbu (1955), and has been most widely used in studies of choleragenic
toxins. Other strains used include *Vibrio cholerae 12* (Ogawa) (Evans and
Richardson, 1968), *Vibrio Cholerae B-1307* (Richardson and Noftle, 1970;
Heckly and Wolochow, 1970) and *V. cholerae 3083-13* (Finkelstein *et al.*,
1966 b).

Methods

The first demonstration of a diarrheagenic moiety as an extracellular product of *V. cholerae* was by De (1959) and De *et al.* (1960). However, not all
strains of *V. cholerae* produced enterotoxin under the growth conditions employed by these authors (Richardson, 1969; Finkelstein *et al.*, 1966 b). The
classic strain, *V. cholerae* Inaba 569 B, is the most widely used because it
produces large amounts of enterotoxin under simpler and more varied growth
conditions than do other strains. Irrespective of the strain of origin the enterotoxin appears to be similar. Those produced by Inaba and Ogawa serotypes and
by classical and El Tor biotypes are identical on agar gel double diffusion
precipitin testing (Finkelstein *et al.*, 1966 b). Growth of Inaba 569 B occurs
on Syncase media (contains casamino acids, sucrose and various salts) (Finkelstein and Lo Spalluto, 1969; Evans and Richardson, 1968). Altering
the salt composition of the medium permitted enterotoxin production by
many other strains of *V. cholerae* (Richardson, 1969). A simple medium containing as few as four amino acids, yeast extract and salts will support enterotoxin production by Inaba 569 B (Richardson and Noftle, 1970).

Vigorous aeration of the medium appears to enhance enterotoxin production
(Coleman *et al.*, 1968; Evans and Richardson, 1968) though it is also produced
by stationary cultures (Craig, 1966). Enterotoxin production is also influenced
by temperature and pH. It is greater at lower (25–30 °C) than at higher
temperatures and at pH 7.0 to 7.8 than at more alkaline pH (Kasuma and
Craig, 1970; Richardson, 1969). Enterotoxin produced by strains of *V.
cholerae* other than by Inaba 569 B in agitated cultures is unstable in the
growth medium, the quantity declining rapidly after peak production is
achieved (Kasuma and Craig, 1970; Richardson, 1969).

The enterotoxin is an extracellular product and is demonstrable early in the log phase of growth, reaching a peak between the end of log and the commencement of stationary phase growth (RICHARDSON, 1969). Similar observations have been made concerning staphylococcal enterotoxin production (FRIEDMAN and WHITE, 1965). RICHARDSON (1969) has shown that cells lysed before entry into the exponential growth phase possessed no detectable enterotoxin and that its production appeared to be a function of conditions which prevailed during the log phase of growth.

Purification of Cholera Enterotoxin

The past decade saw continuous attempts at purification of cholera enterotoxin by several groups of investigators (FINKELSTEIN et al., 1964; FINKELSTEIN et al., 1966a, b; COLEMAN et al., 1968). Modifications by FINKELSTEIN and LoSPALLUTO (1969) included the use of ammonium sulfate precipitation of the centrifuged supernatant followed by DEAE ion exchange chromatography, gel filtration, Sephadex G-75 column chromatography and ultrafiltration. RICHARDSON and NOFTLE (1970) and RICHARDSON and EVANS (1968) precipitated the toxin from the millipore filtrate using dextran sulfate and ammonium sulfate followed by gel filtration and ion exchange chromatography on DEAE Sephadex A25. Both of these preparations appeared pure by immunological, ultracentrifugal, immunoelectrophoretic and disc electrophoretic techniques. FINKELSTEIN and LoSPALLUTO (1969) have also described the concurrent purification of an antigenically identical but smaller molecule without the biological activities of the cholera enterotoxin and considered it to be a naturally occurring toxoid which they called "choleragenoid".

DUHAMEL et al. (1970) submitted the millipore filtered supernatant to pressure dialysis through polymeric membranes (Amicon UM-10 and XM-50) followed by gel filtration (Sephadex G-150) and ion-exchange chromatography. These author's observations on the resultant enterotoxin were in close agreement with those of FINKELSTEIN and LoSPALLUTO (1969) but it had a higher molecular weight than that obtained by COLEMAN et al. (1968).

LEWIS and FREEMAN (1969) using crude toxin from *V. cholerae* strain Inaba 569B reported that Sephadex QAE ion-exchange chromatography could produce enterotoxin free of permeability factor. This observation has been confirmed by GRADY and CHANG (1970). However, KAUR and BURROWS (1969) provided data suggesting that the fractions said to be toxic by LEWIS and FREEMAN were, in fact, non-enterotoxic.

Because of the inherent difficultues in large scale application of sequential exclusion chromatographic and membrane concentration procedures (FINKELSTEIN and LoSPALLUTO, 1969), and of dialysis of large columns of crude toxin prior to the dextran sulfate precipitation methods used by others (RICHARDSON, 1969), the application of aluminum compound gels was used by SPYRIDES and

Feeley (1970). Though absolute purification apparently was not obtained, the absorption onto and elution from these gels was simple and showed good concentration together with immunological and chemical purification of the toxin.

Properties of Purified Cholera Enterotoxin

Cholera enterotoxin is heat labile (56° C), non-dialyzable and acidlabile, destroyed by pronase, but trypsin resistant (Dutta and Oza, 1963). It is antigenic, and produces neutralizing antibodies in response to parenteral inoculation. It causes fluid loss from the gut in man (Benyajati, 1966), infant rabbit (Dutta and Habbu, 1955), ligated rabbit intestinal loop (De and Chatterje, 1953) and canine small bowel (Sack and Carpenter, 1969). It also causes increased vascular permeability and skin induration following intracutaneous inoculation in rabbit and guinea pig (Craig, 1965a, b), an effect which can be neutralized by convalescent sera from cholera patients. Recent reports by Lewis and Freeman (1969) and Grady and Chang (1970) claim that the skin permeability factor may be separable from the diarrheagenic moiety. If these claims prove to be true, there would be an added significance since some investigators currently utilize the skin permeability factor in assays for both cholera enterotoxin and antitoxin activity because the skin permeability factor and enterotoxin are presumed to be identical.

The purified enterotoxin contains no carbohydrate, less than 1 % lipid and up to 92 % protein; its molecular weight as estimated by comparison of elution volumes on Sephadex G-75 to those of proteins of known molecular weight indicate a value of 61,000 (Finkelstein and LoSpalluto, 1969, 1970). More recent estimations based on the use of equilibrium centrifugation suggest that the molecular weight of the enterotoxin is 90,000 and that of its naturally occurring toxoid (choleragenoid) is 60,000 (LoSpalluto and Finkelstein, 1971). These investigators found the sedimentation coefficient values of these two proteins to be 5.54 S and 4.25 S and their diffusion constants to be 4.9×10^{-7} cm²/sec and 7.0×10^{-7} cm²/sec respectively. Calculations based on these values indicated that the molecular weights of the two proteins were 100,000 and 56,000. Partial specific volume values estimated by amino acid analysis were 0.722 ml/g and 0.731 ml/g and molecular weights calculated by the Yphantis meniscus depletion method were 84,000 and 56,000 respectively. Treatment with glycine buffer, pH 3.6, reduced both proteins to subunits of approximately 1.5 S and molecular weights of 13,000 to 15,000 indicating that enterotoxin may be a hexamer and "choleragenoid" a tetramer of one or more types of subunit.

Pierce et al. (1970a) have shown that the purified enterotoxin is antigenic when given parenterally to animals. The antitoxic antibody protects against the biological, including diarrheagenic, properties of the enterotoxin (Finkelstein et al.,1966b; Finkelstein, 1970). Parenteral immunization of dogs with enterotoxin produces significant protection against subsequent intestinal challenge with viable *V. cholerae* and the degree of protection parallels the serum antitoxin titer (CURLIN *et al.*, 1970) and lasts at least 9 months (PIERCE *et al.*, 1971a). FEELEY and ROBERTS (1969) observed that purified cholera enterotoxin could be converted into toxoid without loss of antigenic potency. It appears that at last a vaccine specifically stimulating antitoxic immunity may become generally available.

Convalescent sera can neutralize the diarrheagenic effect of cholera enterotoxin when administered with the enterotoxin into rabbit ileal loops (PIERCE *et al.*, 1970b; MOSLEY *et al.*, 1970a; KASAI and BURROWS, 1966). They are also capable of neutralizing some non-intestinal effects of the enterotoxin such as the production of increased vascular permeability (CRAIG, 1965a; MOSLEY *et al.*, 1970a) and lipolysis of rat epididymal fat cells (GREENOUGH *et al.*, 1970a).

Site of Action of Cholera Enterotoxin

Local

The current belief is that the effect of cholera enterotoxin is mediated by its immediate action on the epithelial cell of the small intestinal mucosa with resultant fluid and electrolyte loss. Though there is a delay (2–3 hours) between administration of enterotoxin and observed biological effect, the pathogenetic mechanism appears to start almost immediately since attempts to flush out enterotoxin or to neutralize it with antitoxic antiserum within 1 min of its administration into a canine jejunal loop fail to alter the enterotoxin effect (CARPENTER, 1971).

Some recent observations from this department provide evidence that the luminal aspect of the intestinal epithelium is the site of action of cholera enterotoxin. KAO *et al.* (1970) using immunofluorescent techniques have shown that various preparations of cholera enterotoxin are detectable in the apical portions of both villous and crypt epithelium of washed rabbit ligated loops. The specific fluorescence was seen as early as 5 minutes after instillation, reached a maximum at 2 hours, and disappeared from the epithelial cytoplasm by 4 hours after administration (KAO, personal communication). It was also seen in mucosal macrophages wherein it persisted from 2 to at least 18 hours. SHEAHAN and SPRINZ (1971) found that injection of enterotoxin into the wall of the intestine, provoked an intense inflammatory reaction without significant evidence of luminal fluid accumulation indicating that direct toxin-epithelial cell interaction is required to cause diarrhea. Supporting these findings are studies showing that enterotoxin has no effect when applied to the serosal aspect of stripped viable rabbit ileal mucosa in a dose which induces characteristic changes in ion transport and short circuit current when applied to the mucosal surface (FIELD *et al.*, 1969). BAYLESS *et al.* (1971) observed that exposure of the jejunum of 5 day old rats to cholera toxin failed to produce net secretion whereas it did occur in the adult rat. These authors speculated that the failure to respond in the young rat was caused by the absence or poor developmental state of the intestinal crypts and suggested that the crypt epithelium is associated with fluid secretion in response to cholera toxin.

Systemic

Certain observations have suggested that cholera enterotoxin may be absorbed from the intestine and produce its effect either directly via parenteral routes on distal receptor sites or by inducing the formation of a secondary circulating "messenger" substance which then acts on the receptor sites. Serebro et al. (1968a) using *crude* cholera enterotoxin reported that the usual response was elicited by instillation into one rabbit ileal loop, but was accompanied by a significant reduction in isotonic fluid absorption in a second loop which had not been exposed to enterotoxin. It is of interest that Sussman et al. (1970) showed similar effects in the dog with staphylococcal enterotoxin B. Pierce et al. (1971c) demonstrated that gastric acid production in response to histamine was reduced by 70 % in dogs after jejunal exposure to cholera enterotoxin and suggested that the response was due to a blood-borne jejunal product.

Inoculation of live *V. cholerae* organisms into an isolated segment of jejunum caused a lethal diarrhea in infant rabbits in the absence of any contamination of the patent bowel (Vaughan-Williams et al., 1969). Using cross circulation techniques cholera infection of one infant rabbit was associated with increased exsorption of intestinal fluid by its noninfected partner (Vaughan-Williams and Dohadwalla, 1969). Though these latter studies are interpreted as suggesting that cholera enterotoxin may produce its effects subsequent to absorption it should be remembered that *crude* cholera enterotoxin and live vibrios organisms were used in these experiments. Thus factors other than pure cholera enterotoxin may well play some role in the production of these results. The intense interest in enterotoxin has tended to overshadow the fact that the disease is caused by the interaction of a susceptible host with the vibrio and that the vibrio produces several toxic and antigenic moieties, the interaction of which is still uncertain.

Pathophysiology

Cholera causes a rapid loss from the gastrointestinal tract of an isotonic fluid which is low in protein, with a mean bicarbonate concentration twice that of normal plasma and a mean potassium concentration four times that of plasma (Watten et al., 1959). The amount of fluid lost per day by some cholera patients far exceeds that which is normally secreted and absorbed each day (Carpenter et al., 1966). All the clinical signs and metabolic derangements in cholera result from this fluid loss which rarely exceeds the rate of one liter per hour. The severe acidosis which occurs in cholera is due to bicarbonate loss (Carpenter et al. 1964). The site of fluid loss is the small intestine since no gastric, pancreatic, hepatic or colonic dysfunction has been detected (Sack and Carpenter, 1969; Carpenter et al., 1968). No colonic fluid accumulation was noted by LEITCH and BURROWS (1968). The *Vibrio cholerae* enterotoxin causes net secretion by all segments of the small bowel in the rabbit and dog experimental models (LEITCH *et al.*, 1967; SACK and CARPENTER, 1969).

CARPENTER *et al.* (1968) studied the time course of response in the Thiry-Vella jejunal loop in the dog. Isotonic fluid production begins within two hours after enterotoxin inoculation into the loop, becomes maximal by four hours and is maintained through the tenth hour, thereafter decreasing to cease entirely within twenty-four hours after challenge. Though all segments of the small bowel secreted isotonic fluid, the output per unit length of bowel was greatest in the duodenum and least in the ileum. The electrolyte composition of the secreted intestinal fluid differed from that of plasma and showed a bicarbonate content lower than plasma in the duodenum and a three-fold higher content in the ileum (CARPENTER *et al.*, 1968). Similar observation has been made in human cholera (BANWELL *et al.*, 1970).

These fluid and electrolyte alterations are not accompanied by significant histological changes in either man or the experimental animal (GANGAROSA *et al.*, 1960; NORRIS and MAJNO, 1968; ELLIOTT *et al.*, 1970). Current observations suggest that increased movement of water and electrolyte from plasma to gut lumen is largely responsible for the fluid loss in clinical (BANWELL *et al.*, 1970) and experimental cholera (IBER *et al.*, 1969; HENDRIX and BAYLESS, 1970). Neither glucose absorption nor glucose enhancement of sodium absorption is impaired in either clinical (HIRSCHHORN *et al.*, 1968) or experimental cholera (SEREBRO *et al.*, 1968b). These observations have permitted a direct practical clinical application enabling better fluid and electrolyte control in the therapy of the disease (PIERCE *et al.*, 1969).

In clinical cholera purging continues despite the patient's hypovolemia and hypotension and because there is no significant osmotic gradient between plasma and luminal fluid the filtration pressure which is equivalent to the hydrostatic pressure (CARPENTER *et al.*, 1968) appears unrelated to the fluid production. SEREBRO *et al.*, (1968b) noted that the absorption of glucose was unrelated to the net fluid movement changes during transition from absorption to secretion. Filtration through enlarged pores cannot explain the differing anion concentrations found in jejunal and ileal fluids in cholera both of which differ considerably from those present in the plasma. GORDON (1969) found that mannitol and sodium were not cleared from the blood by the small intestine at the same rates in cholera, whereas (HAKIM and LIFSON (1969) found that with increased serosal pressure *in vitro* the clearance of glucose and sodium were almost identical indicating that the pathways of fluid loss in cholera and in states of increased hydrostatic pressure were not identical.

Pathogenesis of Fluid Exsorption

In the absence of an observable anatomic defect in the epithelial integrity of the small intestine, three major hypotheses were formulated in recent years to explain the loss of fluid into the intestinal lumen (HENDRIX and BANWELL,

1969). These were: 1) Failure of absorption from the intestine due to "poisoning" of the sodium pump. 2) Increased filtration due to hydrostatic pressure or vascular permeability changes and 3) increased intestinal secretion implying an active energy dependent step.

1. Failure of Absorption

This concept appeared very attractive until was shown that several absorptive functions of the small intestine appear to be unimpaired in cholera (GREENOUGH et al., 1970b). Glucose absorption is not changed in either clinical or experimental cholera (PIERCE et al., 1968; SEREBRO et al., 1968). Unidirectional flux studies have shown that the influx of sodium from lumen to plasma both in the presence and absence of added glucose is unaltered by cholera toxin-induced fluid production (IBER et al., 1969; LOVE, 1969; LOVE et al., 1970).

A theory invoking the inhibition of intestinal sodium transport as the causitive mechanism of cholera was originally suggested by various workers (FUHRMAN and FUHRMAN, 1960; HUBER and PHILLIPS, 1962; FUHRMAN et al., 1962; WATTEN et al., 1959). BURROWS and his colleagues (1944) demonstrated the increased permeability of frog skin and increased exsorption of small intestinal fluid of the guinea pig and rabbit in the presence of cholera vibrio cell substances. Later investigations indicated that the cholera enterotoxin and the sodium pump inhibitor were separable on the basis of heat lability, and non-dialyzability (BURROWS, 1968). LEITCH et al. (1967) showed that a dialysate of ultrasonic lysate toxin did not cause fluid accumulation in ileal loops though it reduced transmural potentials in such loops *in vivo* and reduced short circuit current in bowel tissue exposed to toxin both *in vivo* and *in vitro*. This indicated that the fluid exsorptive effect was not mediated by factors which altered the sodium pump.

In 1966 RICHARDSON showed that a heat labile factor from peptone culture filtrates of *V. cholerae* strain VC-12 (Ogawa) inhibited an ion translocase complex isolated from the rabbit intestinal mucosa. The specific inhibition of the ion translocase enzymes *in vitro* was consistent with the sodium transport inhibition theory. However, this inhibitor was shown to be a vibrio mucinase and failed to elicit choleraic diarrhea when injected directly into the small intestines of infant rabbits although viable cells of the VC-12 strain were lethal for these animals (EVANS and RICHARDSON, 1967). Other workers have also provided evidence indicating that the inhibition of sodium transport is not a causitive factor of fluid production in experimental cholera (LING, 1965; FINKELSTEIN et al., 1966a).

The mucinase component has been separated from the choleragenic and vascular permability factors by modifying conditions of growth of *V. cholerae* strain VC-12 (Ogawa) (EVANS and RICHARDSON, 1968). The former was isolated from alkaline peptone cultures at 37° C whereas the latter two were detected in peptone cultures grown at pH 6.5 at 29° C. FINKELSTEIN et al. (1966a) obtained a similar separation of permeability and mucinase factors of choleragen from *V. cholerae* strain 569 B using physical means.

2. Increased Filtration

The second hypothesis to account for increased fluid exsorption in cholera in the face of a physiologically and anatomically intact intestinal epithelial lining assumed a direct effect on the vasculature of the mucosa. It postulated that diarrheal fluid resulted from increased filtration due to hydrostatic pressure or vascular permeability changes. The presumed hydrostatic pressure difference between the plasma and the gut lumen in cholera has not been measured but cannot be higher than the pressure in the intestinal capillaries or lymphatics. In fact, the intracapillary pressure is so low that it alone cannot account for the increased exsorption (FORDTRAN, 1967). Experimental studies using *in vitro* preparations of canine intestinal mucosa have demonstrated that luminal pressures, in excess of those which occur in cholera or diarrhea of other etiology, did not increase mucosal absorption. However, when similar pressures were applied to the serosal aspect, there was an increase in volume flow from serosal to luminal aspect (HAKIM and LIFSON, 1969). These serosal pressures were lower than those previously calculated (FORDTRAN, 1967) to lead to secretory filtration by the intestinal mucosa. The contribution of increased serosal pressures to the pathogenesis of clinical infectious diarrheal diseases, however, appears of limited significance.

Circumstantial evidence has indicated that the capillary permeability factor may be implicated in the genesis of fluid exsorption by altering the permeability of intestinal capillaries and thereby conceivably increasing the interstitial pressure with resultant intestinal secretion. While there is some anatomic evidence of altered capillary permeability (MERRILL and SPRINZ, 1966; DALL-DORF *et al.*, 1969), this has not been confirmed by ELLIOTT *et al.* (1970) nor by NORRIS and MAJNO (1968), nor do the physiologists believe this to be the case.

a) Permeability Factor

Associated with the choleragenic moiety is a vascular permeability factor (CRAIG, 1965 a, b; CRAIG, 1966). This factor like the choleragenic component is heat labile, non-dialyzable and can be neutralized by specific antisera. BASU MALLICK and GANGULI (1964) first showed that cholera stool filtrates produced an immediate increase in skin vascular permeability but also found reactivity of a lesser degree in non-cholera stool filtrates. No specific neutralization of the effect was reported. CRAIG (1965 a) injected millipore (450 mμ) filtrates of cholera stool supernatants into the skin of albino guinea pigs and rabbits and showed marked induration and erythema beginning at 6–8 hours, peaking at 18–24 hours and persisting for 4–5 days. No such reaction was obtained from similar preparations of non-cholera acute diarrheal stools. Stools from convalescent cholera patients did not contain a permeability factor.

Filtrates of vibrio cultures grown in 5 % Difco "Bacto-Peptone", pH 7.3, used by DE *et al.* (1962), evoked identical responses in the skin of both rabbits and guinea pigs (CRAIG, 1965 a). However, living vibrios did not produce a response. Permeability factors were not isolated from similar cultures of

Shigella B, enteropathogenic *E. Coli*, non-typable *E. Coli* and non-cholera vibrio, Heiberg Group II.

Convalescent sera from confirmed cholera cases were capable of neutralizing the permeability factor effects from both cholera cultures and stool filtrates (CRAIG, 1965a). A skin antitoxin titration test has been developed in rabbit and guinea pig skin (CRAIG, 1965a) and has been used by BENENSON *et al.* (1968a) to assay neutralizing antibodies to permeability factor in cases of cholera.

Many observations have suggested that the permeability and choleragenic factors are identical. Like the diarrheagenic factor, the permeability factor was absent from 2 hour shallow cultures at 37° C, was detectable at 4 hours, reached a maximum at 24–48 hours and began to wane after 72 hours incubation (CRAIG, 1965a). These two moieties of cholera enterotoxin are simultaneously detectable in culture filtrates and in cholera stools (CRAIG, 1965a; FINKELSTEIN *et al.*, 1966b). They considered the increased permeability of intestinal capillaries to be related to the factor causing production of the cholera stool. Using several strains of *V. cholerae*, EVANS and RICHARDSON (1968) found that both factors were consistently produced under a wide variety of growth conditions. Recently MOSLEY *et al.* (1970a) have demonstrated, using toxin-antitoxin titration procedures in both the rabbit skin and ileal loop assay systems, that there is a striking similarity between titers of antibodies against permeability factor in the skin system and of those against choleragenic factor in the ileal loop system. PIERCE *et al.* (1970b) found that the titers of antitoxin and anti-permeability factor antibodies were similar in convalescent cholera patients. Factors which influenced one titer caused similar alterations in the other titer but affected vibriocidal antibody titers in different fashion, if at all. While this finding suggested that a single antigen-antibody reaction was being studied and that the ileal loop toxin and permeability factor were identical, this interpretation is not accepted by all (BURROWS, 1968; BURROWS *et al.*, 1965; KAUR *et al.*, 1969).

b) Mechanism of Action of Permeability Factor

The time response of delayed onset and prolonged duration common to many effects of cholera enterotoxin resembles that due to thermal injury (COTRAN and MAJNO, 1964) or that due to other bacterial permeability factors (ELDER and MILES, 1957). Substances such as bradykinin, serum kallikrein and histamine have been shown to cause increased capillary permeability in guinea pig and rabbit skin (BHOOLA *et al.*, 1960). Though these compounds cause an immediate effect, it is not yet clear whether cholera enterotoxin mediates its delayed effect on capillary permeability by direct specific action, or indirectly through activation of endogenous mediators such as kallikrein, bradykinin, or histamine. The involvement of adenyl cyclase may be considered a likely but not yet proven mediator in the genesis of increased vascular permeability.

There is good anatomic evidence that increased vascular permeability occurs in the skin after cholera enterotoxin inoculation (FINKELSTEIN *et al.*,

1966c). However, no incontrovertible evidence exists which demonstrates an anatomic defect in intestinal capillaries after intraluminal instillation of enterotoxin (DALLDORF *et al.*, 1969; ELLIOTT *et al.*, 1970; NORRIS and MAJNO, 1968).

There are additional aspects of cholera which make it unlikely that its pathogenesis is related to the effect of increased vascular permeability. The isotonicity and low protein concentrations of choleraic fluid (WEAVER *et al.*, 1948) coupled with the established morphological integrity of the noninflamed mucosa do not incriminate an exudative process in the pathogenesis of cholera. The absence or low concentrations of protein and polymorphonuclear neutrophils in the cholera stool or loop effluent and lack of mucosal inflammation is characteristic, whereas increased permeability and induration in the skin is associated with both protein and polymorphonuclear exudative response (FINKELSTEIN *et al.*, 1966c; SHEAHAN and SPRINZ, 1971). The suggestion of KEUSCH *et al.* (1967) that cholera toxin provokes the leakage of a protein rich fluid from the villous capillary into the lamina propria from which only the crystalloids and fluid escape into the intestinal lumen appears untenable and has been challenged by BASU MALLICK *et al.* (1969). If this hypothesis were valid, it would have to explain how the protein poor fluid reaches the intestinal lumen against the colloid osmotic pressure of the presumed protein rich fluid in the extracapillary tissues of the lamina propria.

There is no disputing the fact that the fluid exsorbed from the intestine in cholera originates from plasma Though the effect of permeability factor on skin capillaries is dramatic, it is equivocal, at best, on the intestinal vasculature after intraluminal inoculation. The reasons for this difference are unknown but may include possible differences in the capillary beds of the two sites or possible modification of the permeability factor by the intestinal epithelial lining which prevents the enterotoxin reaching the capillary or alternatively permitting it to reach the capillary in a relatively ineffective form. It must be recognized that the amount of enterotoxin absorbed and transported to the intestinal capillary per unit time is infinitesimally smaller than that which is directly applied to the capillary bed of the skin after a single inoculum. There remains the possibility that a non-specific acute inflammatory reaction with its attendant increase in vascular permeability may be evoked by the single bulk inoculum of foreign protein into tissues, a situation unlikely to occur after intestinal absorption of enterotoxin with its resultant diffuse distribution in diluted concentrations throughout the mucosal tissues.

c) The Role of Mesenteric Blood Flow

CARPENTER *et al.* (1969a) studied the relationship between the rate of fluid loss into the intestinal lumen and the blood flow rate and pressure in the mesenteric circulation. They found that dogs maintained in a normal state of hydration after intralumenal challenge with cholera enterotoxin showed no change in superior mesenteric artery flow rates. In dehydrated animals the superior mesenteric artery blood flow generally fell to less than 30% of control levels after orogastric enterotoxin challenge and that, though an increase in thoracic duct lymph flow occurred after challenge with enterotoxin, the total concentration of protein in thoracic duct lymph was not altered to any significant degree (Carpenter *et al.*, 1968). They also demonstrated that reduction of the mean superior mesenteric artery blood pressure to less than 30% of control values did not affect the cholera enterotoxin-induced fluid exsorption into canine jejunal loops.

Though morphological examination has demonstrated dilatation of villous tip capillaries in contrast to the reduced size of those in the crypt region (Elliott *et al.*, 1970), such observations cannot be interpreted as reflecting enterotoxin induced hemodynamic changes in mucosal blood flow. Indeed it is doubtful that such vascular changes alone would be sufficient to account for the enormous loss of fluid seen in clinical cholera. Further, it is also questionable whether the interpretation of flow rates and pressure in the superior mesenteric artery truly reflects the hemodynamics of the intramucosal capillary vasculature.

Indeed, evidence that changes in mucosal blood flow rates may not be required has been provided by Norris and Sumner (1971). They found no significant differences in initial clearance rates of Xenon-133 between choleraic and control loops over a seven hour period following intraluminal instillation of choleragen. In addition, measurements of the total small bowel blood flow rates in control and choleraic loops indicated that an increase in total mucosal blood flow was not required for the choleraic loop to produce its usual effluent volume.

Sheahan and Sprinz (1971) have provided preliminary evidence that the site of introduction of cholera enterotoxin may play just as important a role in the histogenesis of reaction as do the biological properties of the toxin itself. They showed that inoculation of cholera toxin into the wall but not into the lumen of ligated rabbit ileal loops, produced an intense acute inflammatory reaction and apparent edema in the wall similar to that produced in the rabbit skin. There was, however, no significant fluid exsorption into the lumen in contrast to that seen with intraluminal instillation of similar amounts of toxin. Assuming the fluid exsorption to be related to the increased permeability of the vascular beds in both skin and intestinal wall, it appears significant that fluid exsorption did not occur into ligated ileal loops. Sheahan and Sprinz (1971) have interpreted these observations as reflecting the necessity for toxin-epithelial cell interaction before fluid exsorption into the lumen can occur and that the site of inoculation plays a significant role in the tissue response to cholera enterotoxin. The validity of the attempt to explain cholera diarrhea on the basis of increased vascular permeability remains open to question.

3. Increased Secretion

Recent research has focused on fundamental alterations of the mucosal epithelial cell at the molecular level as the pathogenetic mechanism of intestinal fluid exsorption in cholera.

There is increasing evidence that the absorptive and secretory functions of the small intestine may reside in different anatomic areas of the mucosal epithelium. Absorption is well known to occur across the villous columnar epithelium. Secretion has been demonstrated as a function of the crypt epithelium (TRIER, 1964; SHEAHAN *et al.*, 1970). Evidence exists that this epithelium is implicated in the fluid loss induced by cholera enterotoxin. BAYLESS *et al.* (1971) have demonstrated in the rat that there is no secretory response to cholera enterotoxin in the absence of well-developed intestinal crypts. Cycloheximide which damages crypt cells by inhibiting protein synthesis and causing mitotic arrest (VERBIN and FARBER, 1967) also inhibits cholera enterotoxin induced fluid exsorption without depressing glucose absorption (HARPER *et al.*, 1970; SEREBRO *et al.*, 1969; GRAYER *et al.*, 1970).

Recent data obtained during *in vitro* studies suggest that cholera toxin may increase intestinal secretion by elevating levels of cyclic adenosine $3',5'$ monophosphate (cAMP). The addition of cAMP or theophylline to the serosal side of normal gut segments leads to increased intestinal secretion (FIELD *et al.*, 1968). Theophylline has been shown to inhibit the enzymatic breakdown of cyclic AMP to $5'$-AMP by cyclic nucleotide phosphodiesterase (BUTCHER and SUTHERLAND, 1962). The theophylline effect on short circuit current was significantly reduced in tissue pretreated with cholera enterotoxin indicating that both agents were acting on the same secretory mechanism (FIELD *et al.*, 1969). Studies of isolated stripped segments of rabbit and human ileal mucosa suspended in modified Ussing chambers and bathed by isotonic fluid have shown that the normal electrogenic active absorption of sodium and of chloride is changed by the addition of cholera enterotoxin to the mucosal side of the tissue and results in active electrogenic secretion of chloride and decreased active absorption of sodium (FIELD *et al.*, 1969; AL-AWQATI *et al.*, 1970a).

Evidence also exists that cholera enterotoxin may directly stimulate mucosal cell adenyl cyclase, the enzyme which catalyses the synthesis of cyclic $3',5'$ AMP from ATP. SHARP and HYNIE (1971) showed that a homogenate of gut mucosal tissue exposed to cholera enterotoxin had a highly significant increase in adenyl cyclase activity as compared to controls within three hours after exposure to the enterotoxin without change in phosphodiesterase activity. CHEN *et al.* (1971) have further demonstrated that homogenates of jejunal mucosa fron cholera patients showed significantly increased levels of adenyl cyclase activity as compared to that seen in convalescence. The authors maintained that no new synthesis of mucosal adenyl cyclase occurs during cholera. The mechanism for the gradual increase in adenyl cyclase activity is unknown. The incubation of viable rabbit intestinal epithelial scrapings with cholera enterotoxin demonstrated significantly increased levels of cyclic AMP in small intestinal epithelial cells several hours after exposure to cholera enterotoxin (KIMBERG *et al.*, 1971; SCHAFER *et al.*, 1970b).

Prostaglandins also stimulate mucosal cell adenyl cyclase activity (KIMBERG *et al.*, 1971; SHARP and HYNIE, 1971). It is possible that the diarrhea associated with prostaglandin secreting tumors such as medullary carcinoma of the thyroid gland (Williams, 1966; Williams *et al.*, 1968) and some non-beta cell tumors of the islets of Langerhans (Kraft *et al.*, 1970) may be mediated through intestinal mucosal adenyl cyclase stimulation.

Prostaglandin E_1 produced the same changes in sodium and chloride movement as observed with cyclic AMP, theophylline and cholera enterotoxin (Al Awqati *et al.*, 1970b). Similar observations have been made by Kimberg *et al.* (1971). Butcher and Baird (1968) have shown that prostaglandins raised cyclic AMP levels in tissues by direct stimulation of adenyl cyclase activity. Using the canine Thiry-Vella small bowel loop model, superior mesenteric artery perfusion of prostaglandin F2 α at a rate of 2 μg per minute and of theophylline at the rate of 22 mg/minute produced fluid and electrolyte movement similar to that produced by cholera enterotoxin (Greenough *et al.*, 1969). Pierce *et al.* (1971 b) extended these data and showed that theophylline and many prostaglandins (PGE, PGA, and $PGF_2α$) caused loss of water and electrolytes into canine small bowel lumen following their infusion into the superior mesenteric artery. They also noted that theophylline and $PGF_2α$ acted synergystically to induce intestinal fluid loss indicating that their actions may have been on different components of the secretory mechanism.

These observations are consistent with the concept that increased levels of cyclic AMP in gut epithelium may be directly involved in the mediation of the gut fluid secretion caused by cholera enterotoxin. The toxin may either stimulate adenyl cyclase activity or alternatively may mimic the actions of cyclic AMP. Further supportive evidence of this concept stems from the observation that a highly significant reduction in the volume of fluid produced by the small bowel in response to enterotoxin challenge can be caused by ethacrynic acid, a known adenyl cyclase inhibitor (Carpenter *et al.*, 1969b).

It is of interest that enterotoxin applied to the intestinal lumen fails to show stimulate adenyl cyclase activity in tissues other than the small intestine. This is presumably due to the fact that the enterotoxin itself does not penetrate beyond the gut mucosa or if it does that it is absorbed systemically in a state which does not evoke adenyl cyclase stimulation.

Despite the similarity of effect, there are some differences: 1) cyclic AMP, prostaglandins, and theophylline exert immediate effects in contrast to the delayed onset of cholera enterotoxin effect and 2) the effects of cyclic AMP, theophylline and prostaglandins exert their effect when applied to the serosal aspect of the mucosa or via mesenteric artery perfusion while cholera enterotoxin mediates its effect only through the luminal aspect of the mucosa. The time lag between mucosal contact with toxin and fluid exsorption suggests that direct enterotoxin interaction with a specific receptor on the luminal aspect of the mucosa is a prerequisite to fluid secretion since large amounts of toxin added to the serosal side of the intestine or inoculation directly into the intestinal wall are without effect (Field, 1971; Sheahan and Sprinz, 1971). The nature of this receptor is not unique to the intestinal epithelial cell because cholera enterotoxin also causes cyclic AMP-like effects on other tissues (Vaughan *et al.*, 1970; Zieve *et al.*, 1970).

Effects on other Tissues

The study of the effects of cholera enterotoxin on tissues other than the intestine has broadened the concept of its action at the cellular level. Most, if not all of these effects to be described, are also associated with increased levels of cyclic AMP.

Isolated Fat Cells

Crude or purified enterotoxin incubated with isolated rat epididymal fat cells caused, after 2 hours, increased lipolysis by these cells as measured by the increase in the rate of release of glycerol into the incubation medium (VAUGHAN et al., 1970). This effect can be inhibited by boiling the enterotoxin or by ethacrynic acid. It can also be neutralized with cholera antitoxin (GREENOUGH et al., 1970a). CURLIN and CHEN (1971) have indicated that this effect of increased lipolysis by enterotoxin is mediated through an increase in adenyl cyclase activity. HEWLETT and GREENOUGH (1971) have indicated that cholera enterotoxin increases both adenyl cyclase activity and cyclic AMP in fat cells.

Skin Capillaries

An established effect of purified cholera enterotoxin is a marked and sustained increase in skin capillary permeability which can be inhibited by antitoxic antibodies (FINKELSTEIN and LoSPALLUTO, 1970; CRAIG 1965a; CRAIG, 1970). Because the effects of other biologically active amines, such as histamine, serotonin, and prostaglandins which cause increased capillary permeability, are known to be mediated by cyclic AMP, it is reasonable to postulate that the capillary permeability effect of the cholera enterotoxin will also prove to be mediated by this cyclic nucleotide.

An allied response has been demonstrated following injection of cholera enterotoxin into the rat food pad. After a 2–4 hour delay, a reversible prolonged local edema is manifest which is dose dependent and lasts for 5 or more days (FINKELSTEIN et al., 1969). This effect is also inhibited by antitoxic antibodies (FINKELSTEIN and HOLLINGSWORTH, 1970).

Hepatic Cells

Intravenous injection of purified enterotoxin causes increased serum levels of alkaline phosphatase of hepatic origin in dogs (GRAYBILL et al., 1970). There was little evidence of hepatic cell damage and BAKER et al. (1971) have shown in the rat that the raised phosphatase values are due to increased synthesis of the enzyme by hepatic cells. Adenyl cyclase activity was also noted to be raised in this experimental model. No effect on bile flow or electrolyte concentration in the bile of the rat was noted (BAKER et al., 1971).

Hepatic and Platelet Glycogenolysis

Purified enterotoxin caused hyperglycemia in dogs after intravenous injection (GRAYBILL et al., 1970). In mice intravenous injection of purified enterotoxin markedly increased hepatic glycogenolysis. Similar increases in the rate of glycogenolysis occur in human platelet sonicates and rat liver homogenates after *in vitro* incubation with enterotoxin, suggesting that enterotoxin enhances glycogenolysis by stimulating phosphorylase *a* activity in these cells (ZIEVE *et al.*, 1970). In these cells cyclic AMP accelerates the activation of phosphorylase kinases, which enables phosphorylase *b* to be converted to phosphorylase *a*, which in turn accelerates glycogen metabolism to produce glucose. Because cholera enterotoxin has no direct effect on free glycogen but does increase glycogenolysis in disrupted cells in association with elevated levels of phosphorylase *a*, it may mediate its effect in this system by increasing cyclic AMP due to increased adenyl cyclase activity.

The earlier onset of enterotoxin effect on cell fragments noted in some of these *in vitro* studies suggests that the usual delay in onset noted in intact cellular models of experimental cholera may be related to an enterotoxin—cell membrane interaction. Theoretically, the delay in the effect of cholera enterotoxin on intact cells in contrast to its more immediate effect on disrupted cells indicates that the cell membrane receptor-enterotoxin interaction is an important step in the pathogenetic mechanism of fluid production as well as the other enterotoxin effects. The immediate effects of agents such as cyclic AMP, theophylline, and prostaglandins which act through the serosal aspect of the intestinal wall or by the intravascular route in contrast to the ineffectivity of cholera enterotoxin by such routes suggest that cholera enterotoxin must initiate a series of epithelial membrane bound metabolic interactions before it can mediate its effect on the intestinal cellular mechanism which triggers fluid secretion.

Pharmacological Modification
of Experimentally Induced Cholera

The experimental animal intestinal loop response to cholera enterotoxin has been modified in many ways. The effects of ethacrynic acid and cycloheximide have already been briefly mentioned. Ethacrynic acid, a known adenyl cyclase inhibitor, reduces the cholera enterotoxin induced intestinal secretion of fluid and electrolytes (CARPENTER *et al.*, 1969 b), inhibits the increase in short circuit current across isolated, stripped, viable rabbit ileal mucosa (AL AWQATI *et al.*, 1969) and the release of glycerol by rat epididymal fat cells (VAUGHAN *et al.*, 1970).

A similar prevention of fluid exsorption results from prior treatment of rabbits with intravenous cycloheximide, a potent protein synthesis inhibitor (SEREBRO *et al.*, 1969; MORITZ *et al.*, 1971). It causes mitotic arrest in the crypt epithelium because the protein deficient cells cannot proceed from prophase to metaphase stages of the cycle (VERBIN and FARBER, 1967). At a dose causing such effects cycloheximide inhibits the intestinal fluid production normally induced by cholera enterotoxin without depressing glucose absorption

(HARPER *et al.*, 1970; SEREBRO *et al.*, 1969). Calculated bidirectional fluxes of sodium indicate that the cycloheximide effect is attributable to inhibition of the enterotoxin induced increase in blood to lumen sodium flux (GRAYER *et al.*, 1970; HARPER *et al.*, 1970). When administered after enterotoxin challenge, it reduced the fluid production rate during subsequent hours. With both pre- and post-challenge treatments, there was a decrease of the sodium flux from plasma to gut lumen with unaltered lumen to plasma sodium flux without any effect on active glucose absorption. Though MORITZ *et al.* (1971) observed that pretreatment with cycloheximide abolished the cholera enterotoxin effect, they found that administration of cycloheximide $4^1/_2$ hours after cholera entero-toxin challenge evoked little effect on intestinal water or ion fluxes in the sub-sequent 2 hours. The increased net absorptive rate together with the normal villous function and degenerative changes in crypt cells with arrested mitosis indicated that cycloheximide interfered with a protein synthetic dependent step responsible for establishing and maintaining cholera enterotoxin induced fluid exsorption. This would also correlate with the usual time lapse between exposure to toxin and observed fluid accumulation. Using the rat intestinal everted sac model, STROMBECK (1971) found that neither acetazolamide nor cycloheximide produced an inhibitory effect on cholera toxin induced fluid production but that cycloheximide inhibited normal intestinal sodium transport both *in vivo* and *in vitro*. The apparently contradictory results in the rat may represent species differences in the effect of cycloheximide on intestinal crypt epithelium. However, no histological evidence of crypt epithelial damage was provided in these latter studies. FINKELSTEIN *et al.* (1969) have shown preven-tion and reversal by cycloheximide of the local edema of the rat food pad after injection of cholera enterotoxin.

The quantity and type of ligated ileal loop fluid effluent was noted by NORRIS *et al.* (1969) to be altered by the intraluminal addition of various compounds. Sodium acetazolamide (Diamox) reduced fluid output and in addition caused a decrease of sodium and bicarbonate secretion and an increase in chloride absorption. Glucose increased sodium chloride absorption and decreased fluid output without observable effect on bicarbonate secretion. The combination of these two compounds caused cessation of net secretion with return to normal ileal net absorption in the experimental animals. However, though the therapeutic efficacy of glucose in cholera has been established; the role of Diamox in the prevention of fluid exsorption in this disease remains to be demonstrated.

Following the observation of CHOWDHURY and DATTA (1965) that erythrose inhibited the *in vitro* growth of *Vibrio cholerae* this sugar was also shown to prevent dilatation of intestinal loops of adult rabbits as well as diarrhea and death in infant rabbits given prior infections of viable *Vibrio cholerae* (BHATTA-CHARYA *et al.*, 1965). Viable vibrios could still be isolated from the intestines of both experimental animals despite the absence of gross intestinal hyperemic reaction. It is not yet established that erythrose has a specific inhibitory effect on enterotoxin activity.

Pathology of Cholera

A lack of significant mucosal epithelial alteration in the intestine coincident with massive out-pouring of fluid into the intestinal lumen is a characteristic phenomenon of clinical cholera in man and of cholera-like states in experimental animals. Remarkably, this was not widely appreciated until about 10 years ago when Gangarosa *et al.* (1960), Sprinz (1962) and Sprinz *et al.* (1962) demonstrated conclusively in biopsy studies that the small bowel epithelium remained intact during this disease. They showed by light microscopy engorgement of the mucosal capillaries and dilatation of the central lacteal without evidence of an acute inflammatory response. The epithelial lining of the small intestine remained intact but some degenerative changes were seen in the basement membrane with formation of microscopic vacuoles and spaces. These changes were suggested to be the precursors of the non-specific subepithelial edema noted by Goodpasture (1923) and the detachment of the epithelium from the basement membrane (Stoerk, 1916) and possibly of the denudation of epithelium as originally noted by Virchow (1879), Koch (1893), Fraenkel (1893), and Deycke (1892) in autopsy examinations of patients with cholera. It is indeed likely that the intestinal contents, despite the early introduction of fixative material into the intestinal lumen, can have serious deleterious effects on the intestinal epithelial lining after death. Dutt *et al.* (1964) observed extensive epithelial denudation in the intestinal lumen in such circumstances. Dutt (1966) in a subsequent study showed that inoculation of the rabbit gut loop with live *V. cholerae* or its culture filtrate did not produce epithelial alterations in the early hours but was demonstrable at later times. This was presumably due to the anoxic changes due to loop distention.

Confirmation of the observations of Gangarosa *et al.* (1960) were obtained in human cholera (Fresh *et al.* ,1964) and also in experimental animal models. Formal *et al* (1961) using the ligated rabbit loop exposed to *V. cholerae* and Norris *et al.* (1965) using the infant rabbit exposed to live vibrios and their cell-free products observed an intact epithelial lining with vascular congestion, mild transient polymorphonuclear infiltrate and accumulation of proteinaceous edema fluid in the lamina propria and a decrease in the height of the crypt epithelial cells.

These observations had a two-fold effect. They set to rest the time honored "denudation theory" originally championed by Virchow (1879). Secondly, they were the corner stones on which was built the dramatic increase in knowledge concerning cholera and like diseases during the last decade. As a result of this and the knowledge that the cholera vibrio produced an extracellular moiety capable of producing the disease, research activities were directed towards study of the physiological alterations caused by the organism and its products.

These studies left open the question whether the effect of the observed toxic moiety is restricted to the intestinal mucosa or not. It is not possible to differentiate on histologic appearance the effects of acidosis and oligemia from possible direct effects of cholera toxins on tissues such as heart, liver, and pancreas.

The acute (hypokalemia) and late (ischemic nephrosis) effects on the kidney were well known (STOERK, 1916) at the turn of the century and have been re-evaluated by GOLDSTEIN *et al.* (1966).

Ultrastructural Studies

In the elegantly controlled studies of ELLIOTT *et al.* (1970), serial jejunal and ileal biopsies were obtained for up to 20 hours after cholera infection in dogs which were maintained in normal hydration. Arterial pressure, PO_2 and PCO_2 were also maintained within physiological ranges to eliminate possible secondary artifacts due to shock and/or poor tissue oxygenation.

No significant differences were noted by light microscopy between control tissues and those from jejunum or ileum of dogs at any stage of the diarrheal state studied. The epithelium remained intact. The mesenchymal elements of the lamina propria appeared more edematous but did not appear to change in number other than a slight increase of pericryptal polymorphonuclear leucocytes. Slight dilatation of the capillaries was seen in villous tips. The crypts appeared dilated, presumably due to flattening of the epithelium and loss of goblet cell mucus as confirmed by Alcian Blue stains.

Ultrastructurally, cholera vibrios were seen in close proximity to the fuzzy coat of the epithelial brush border but never within the mucosal tissue or crypt lumina. No alterations of the microvilli or their fuzzy coat were seen. Villous and crypt epithelial columnar cells of infected animals were comparable to those of control animals in terms of the number and appearance of mitochondria, lysosomes, ribosomes, endoplasmic reticula and Golgi systems. The intercellular junctions were also similar in both groups of animals. Changes resembling those described by FREEMAN (1962) as typical during active synthesis and release of mucus by goblet cells were seen in cholera infected animals. The capillary endothelial cells were thinned due to distension of mucosal vessels but otherwise no changes were noted from control material in endothelial junction sites, membrane covered fenestrae, the underlying basement membrane or adjacent pericytes. The presence of interstitial edema was indicated by separation of collagen bundles. Neither the epithelial basement membrane not the collagen fibers were affected by cholera infection. These observations thus confirm the earlier light microscopic ones and are in close agreement with those of NORRIS and MAJNO (1968).

Other electron microscopic studies of the intestinal mucosa in choleraic states have shown similar integrity of the epithelium (PATNAIK and GHOSH, 1966; NORRIS and MAJNO, 1968). The studies of GOLDSTEIN *et al.* (1966) on opiated starved guinea pigs, however, indicated a toxic degenerative effect on the mitochondria and Golgi system of endothelial cells and to a lesser extent on the endoplasmic reticulum and Golgi apparatus of epithelial cells. Associated with these intestinal changes, focal degenerative and necrotic changes were seen in heart, liver and pancreas with minimal changes in the kidney. The possible role that starvation and/or opiation may have played in the production of these changes is not known. The fact that live vibrios and not enterotoxin were used in this study and that the response of the guinea pig to cholera may differ from strain to strain of guinea pigs and from other animals are further factors for consideration in the explanation of these results.

PATNAIK and GHOSH (1966) described a widening of the spaces between endothelial cells; only the basement membrane lay between the vascular lumen and perivascular space. MERRILL and SPRINZ (1966) reported focal endothelial damage in one strain of guinea pigs and in two human subjects. These observations have not been confirmed by other investigators.

Vascular Labelling Studies

The introduction of permeability markers permitted study of the possible role which alterations of the endothelial lining may play in the production of choleraic fluid. FINKELSTEIN *et al.* (1966c) with the use of carbon black first demonstrated increased permeability in the capillaries of rabbit and guinea pig skin following intradermal inoculation of cholera enterotoxin. It should be noted that there was a severe acute inflammatory reaction associated with the skin lesion in contrast to the noninflamed appearances of the intestine after intraluminal administration. This may, at least in part, account for the failure of KEUSCH *et al.* (1967) to reproduce the pattern of carbon black permeability in the intestinal mucosal of rabbits exposed to cholera toxin. However, these authors using light microscopy claimed that ferritin, a molecule of 150000 Mol. Wt., did in fact permeate intestinal capillaries of such animals. This observation was confirmed by DALLDORF *et al.* (1969) who studied electron microscopically the passage of intravascularly administered cadmium free ferritin across the endothelial lining of intestinal capillaries of rabbits following exposure to purified cholera enterotoxin. There was, however, no morphological alteration of the endothelial cells other than the presence of ferritin granules within the cytoplasm or their intercellular spaces and these authors concluded that the ferritin molecule passed directly through the endothelial cell to the perivascular spaces. At no stage within the 24 hour study period were the ferritin molecules observed to penetrate the tight junctions between epithelial cells or seen within the lumen of the intestine. NORRIS and MAJNO (1968) failed to demonstrate ultrastructural evidence of passage of saccharated iron oxide particules into the extravascular spaces of rabbit ileal mucosa. Again, the endothelial cells appeared unchanged. There is no ready explanation for these apparent discrepant results. Species differences in animals, differences in the potency of enterotoxin lots or differences in the manner by which endothelial cells transport different marker molecules may be contributory.

Radioactively labelled macromolecules (^{131}I-labelled polyvinyl pyrrolidone and ^{51}Cr-labelled albumin) do not appear in greater concentration in the stools of actively purging cholera patients than in normal stools (GORDON, 1962).

Histochemistry

Low or absent alkaline phosphatase and low leucine aminopeptidase activities were demonstrated in the villous epithelium of the small bowel of autopsied cases of human cholera in Asia (FRESH *et al.*, 1963). However, over 50% of non-diarrheal patients showed absence of alkaline phosphatase activity in intestinal biopsy specimens indicating the importance of knowledge of the natural state of the mucosa prior to cholera infection. Nevertheless, these authors did demonstrate that these enzyme activities were lowered or disappeared completely in epithelial tissues from ligated loops of experimental adult animals exposed to cholera organisms in contrast to normal activities in loops inoculated with isotonic saline or heat-killed cultures (FRESH *et al.*, 1963).

In a subsequent study of intestinal biopsy material from cholera patients, a significant number demonstrated a reduced or absent enzyme activity in the brush border zone (FRESH *et al.*, 1964). The most severe alterations were found in biopsies taken within 14 hours of the onset of diarrhea.

Mucin histochemistry has been employed in the study of cholera mainly to confirm mucin loss from the intestinal crypt epithelium both in the canine model (ELLIOTT *et al.*, 1970) and in rabbit ligated intestinal loop (PATNAIK and GHOSH, 1966). Preliminary observations by SHEAHAN (unpublished data) have indicated subtle changes in the mucin histochemical reactivity of the brush border of the small bowel epithelium suggesting some loss of acidic mucosubstances.

Immunology

Exposure to *V. cholerae* organisms evokes vibriocidal, agglutinating and antitoxin antibodies. The somatic antigens specific to cholera vibrios are heat stable and are designated by letter. The group specific 0 antigen is designated A, and the type specific antigens of Ogawa and Inaba serotypes are designated B and C respectively. The Hikojima serotype contains both type specific antigens as well as the group specific antigen. Because of cross reactivity, the type specific antigens can only be distinguished by cross-absorption studies. GANGAROSA *et al.* (1967) have noted that changes in serotype from Ogawa to Inaba do occur both *in vivo* and *in vitro*.

Most field trial vaccines used since 1963 in East Pakistan have been bivalent. MOSLEY *et al.* (1970b) tested monovalent whole cell Inaba and Ogawa vaccines as well as a purified Inaba antigen during a cholera (Inaba serotype) outbreak in East Pakistan in 1968. Their observations indicated that vaccine induced protection depends on type specific immunity. Because the currently used vaccines, which contain no detectable enterotoxin and provoke vibriocidal and agglutinin antibodies with little antitoxic effect, have been shown to be protective in field trials (OSEASOHN *et al.*, 1965) the true protective value of the antienterotoxic antibodies produced in the above studies cannot be truly evaluated even though protection correlated with antitoxic titers.

Investigations in Dacca, East Pakistan showed a relationship between the rise in vibriocidal titer and the decrease in attack rate with age suggesting that a rising vibriocidal titer reflected increasing immunity (Mosley *et al.*, 1968a and b). Non-vaccinated Pakistanis who showed the presence of vibriocidal antibodies in direct proportion to age and to the degree of exposure to *V. cholerae*, demonstrated a four fold rise in titer of such antibodies after cholera infection (Benenson *et al.*, 1968b). However, Gangarosa *et al.* (1970) cautioned that the vibriocidal antibody levels alone may not serve as indication of exposure to the antigens of *V. cholerae* because high titers and four fold rises in titer were noted in humans and in rabbits never exposed to such antigens. This was explained by the demonstrated marked cross reactivity between antigen of *V. cholerae* and those of the Brucella species and to a lesser extent the Citrobacter species.

Antibacterial Immunity

This form of immunity can be induced in man by natural infection and by parenteral vaccines containing killed whole cells or lipopolysaccharide. Its level has been defined in several field trials and has been correlated with the serum vibriocidal antibody titer. It can be mediated by three different antigens, the lipopolysaccharide preparation of Watanabe and Verwey (1965), the K-S lipopolysaccharide (Kaur and Shrivastava, 1965) and the V-antigen of Kaur and Burrows (1969). The V-antigen, a protein antigen, present in the supernatant of young liquid cultures of vibrios and separable by column chromatography, gives an *in vitro* identity reaction with K-S lipopolysaccharide on immunodiffusion and is highly immunogenic in forming vibriocidal antibody in the rabbit. It is non-toxic to the mouse. This antigen is three times more immunogenic than the reference lipopolysaccharide preparation (Burrows, 1970).

Freter (1956, 1964) has demonstrated the protective effect of antibacterial antibody in the intestinal lumen against live vibrio organisms. Though resistance to intraluminal challenge has been associated with circulating antitoxin, there is no evidence that the neutralization of the enterotoxin actually occurs in the vascular compartment. The site of antitoxin production is not known but presumably resides to some extent at least in the immunocompetent cells of the lamina propria of intestinal mucosa. In some preliminary evidence from this department, Kao and Sprinz (1971) indicate that local antitoxic immunity plays some role in the defense against cholera diarrhea. These investigators have shown that cholera enterotoxin evokes an IgG anti-enterotoxin antibody response which is demonstrable in the crypt but not villous epithelium. However, the protective effect induced in these animals seemed to be rate-limited and was easily overwhelmed by the intestinal administration of large doses of enterotoxin.

Antitoxic Immunity

Separation of enterotoxin from peptone supernatants gives an elution pattern in deionized water from DEAE A 24 Sephadex showing three incompletely separated peaks (BURROWS, 1970). The first, subfraction 1, contains almost all the toxic activity; subfraction 2 contains almost all the immunogenicity and the last peak is inactive. Thus, the toxic moiety could be separated into a non-immunogenic component and an immunogenic protein, designated T antigen. The latter is non-choleragenic as assessed by the ileal loop response and is nonreactive in mouse tests in doses of 10 mg. A dose of only 10 μg of subfraction 1 elicits a positive loop response. T antigen is formed by vibrios in the absence of toxic activity when the peptone concentration of the culture medium is reduced or when its pH is reduced to 6.5. The efficaciousness of this nontoxic immunogen as a vaccination agent must await evaluation.

A rising titer of circulating antitoxin directed against cholera enterotoxin occurs in convalescent cholera patients (CRAIG, 1965a; KASAI and BURROWS, 1966; DUTT, 1967; BENENSON et al., 1968a; PIERCE et al., 1970b). The magnitude of the antitoxic antibody response in convalescence is directly related to the duration of exposure to the enterotoxin. Prompt tetracycline therapy in cholera patients is associated with significantly lower antitoxic responses and may be related to reduced enterotoxin production subsequent to cessation of vibrio growth. Such treatment has no effect on vibriocidal antibody response (PIERCE et al., 1970b).

Many species of experimental animal have been studied in efforts to elucidate the immunological aspects of cholera enterotoxin with a view to developing an effective vaccine. These studies have indicated the importance of using antigenically pure enterotoxin preparations, the route of antigen administration employed, and the recognition that antibody activity may not correlate with protection against subsequent challenge.

FINKELSTEIN and ATTHASAMPUNNA (1967) showed that their preparation of cholera enterotoxin produced antitoxic antibodies in rabbits which increased resistance to the fluid producing effects of enterotoxin and live vibrio organisms and to the increased skin permeability effect of enterotoxin. Because this preparation was apparently contaminated with somatic antigen as indicated by a rise in agglutenin titers the protective role of antitoxic antibody against vibrio challenge remained in dispute. The sera from these immunized animals also neutralized enterotoxin *in vitro* but had little effect when given intraperitoneally to suckling rabbits 18 hours prior to challenge. Because the toxin-antitoxin ratios were different in these two situations the true role of passively transferred immunity was not elucidated. FEELEY and ROBERTS (1969) showed that commercially prepared vaccines did not evoke antitoxic antibody response in rabbits and guinea pigs. On the other hand culture filtrates experimentally prepared as crude vaccines produced antitoxic as well as agglutenin and vibriocidal antibodies. Formalinized toxoids prepared from these filtrates were noted to be 3–5 times more antigenic than untreated toxin when tested in guinea pigs and rabbits. Again the contamination with somatic antigen in these preparations does not permit an understanding of the specific role which antitoxic antibody may play in immunity against cholera.

Studies with the canine model have shown that repeated intraluminal challenge with cholera enterotoxin in doses sufficient to caused marked fluid loss did not produce either detectable circulating antitoxin or increased resistance to subsequent challenge (CARPENTER et al., 1968, 1969 b; CARPENTER and GREENOUGH, 1968; CURLIN and CARPENTER, 1970). These observations differed from those noted in man (KASAI and BURROWS, 1966). Though it is not yet known why such differences exist between man and dog, they may be related to the larger antigenic doses in clinical than in experimental cholera or to possible species differences in the capability to absorb antigenically intact enterotoxin. CURLIN et al. (1970) showed that parenteral immunization of dogs with crude culture filtrates of cholera organisms produced increased resistance to intraluminal challenge with enterotoxin as well as with living vibrios. However, the crude filtrate evoked circulating vibriocidal and agglutinating antibodies in addition to antitoxic antibodies.

FELSENFELD et al. (1968) showed that parenteral or oral immunization of chimpanzees or patas monkeys with the dialysand of a crude filtrate of an early liquid peptone culture of Inaba 569 B strain produced serum antitoxic activity. In the recently developed chinchilla experimental model for cholera (BASU and PICKETT, 1969) the animals were protected with live but not with killed vaccine against challenge with 1×10^{10} live vibrios (BASU et al., 1970). Both groups of treated animals, however, showed similar agglutinin and vibriocidal antibody titers.

The explanation for the required prolonged antigenic exposure to promote antitoxic response may lie in the poor accessibility of the enterotoxin to sites that form circulating antibody either because it is poorly absorbed (Mol. Wt. 90,000) (LoSPALLUTO and FINKELSTEIN, 1971) or because the toxin is avidly bound to the intestinal mucosal epithelial cells (CURLIN et al., 1968) or is rapidly metabolized. The finding that titers of circulating antitoxin may be sustained for longer periods of time (6–18 months) than vibriocidal antibody titers suggests that protection associated with circulating antitoxin may be greater than that currently mediated by whole cell cholera vaccines, which do not stimulate significant production of antitoxin (BENENSON et al., 1968 c). Very high antitoxin titers have been produced in repeatedly immunized rabbits (PIERCE et al., 1970 a) suggesting that parenteral enterotoxin immunization may more efficiently produce systemic antitoxin production and hopefully confer longer lasting protection as suggested by the recent demonstration by (CURLIN et al., 1970) that high circulating levels of antitoxin conferred protection against challenge with live V. cholerae in dogs.

The permeability factor produced by the cholera organism is also antigenic. Patients with cholera developed antibodies capable of neutralizing permeability factor in vitro (CRAIG, 1965 a, b; BENENSON et al., 1968 a). VERNON and CRAIG (1967) showed that cholera patients became resistant to the effects of intracutaneous injection of permeability factor during the first week after the onset of diarrhea. This factor when administered as toxoid increased immunogenicity (FEELEY and ROBERTS, 1969). Toxoid immunization was found to be more effective than that with commercially prepared vaccines in the prevention of increased skin permeability in both guinea pigs and rabbits after intracutaneous injection of permeability factor (CRAIG, 1971) and was associated with raised antitoxin titers as compared to the absence of such antitoxin in vaccine recipients. CRAIG (1970) showed that the administration of anti-permeability factor antibodies into the circulation of guinea pigs had a limited effect on the response to an intracutaneous injection of permeability factor. However, the antigen concentration at inoculation sites was probably more than sufficient to overcome the neutralization effect of circulating antibodies at the local level.

Current commercially prepared vaccines do not contain enterotoxin or permeability factor. The inclusion of enterotoxin in parenteral vaccines may enhance their effectivity of causing protection. Parenteral routes of vaccination appear superior for evoking both antitoxic and antibacterial immunity. Current parenteral vaccines give better and more sustained vibriocidal antibody response than that following clinical cholera indicating that antibacterial immunity is poorly produced by the oral route (CURLIN and CARPENTER, 1970). Recent epidemiological studies reveal that in an endemic area, children may be infected year after year indicating that one oral immunization does not provide sufficient protection against subsequent challenge. The results of current investigations to determine the efficaciousness of a toxoid vaccine will be awaited with interest.

Immunochemistry — Cholera Bacterial Antigens

The antigenic specificity of the serotype antigens is apparently determined by lipopolysaccharide moieties of high molecular weight and considered to be endotoxin. They occur in supernates of liquid cultures of cholera vibrio only when autolysis has taken place and they evoke mouse protective and vibriocidal antibody. FINKELSTEIN (1970) has indicated that only a single antigenic type of enterotoxin is produced by pathogenic strains of *V. cholerae*. However, BURROWS (1970) has claimed that the antigens of the choleragenic toxin and the associated nontoxin protein which occur in the intracellular substance and not in the cell wall of the vibrio can be separated by ion exchange chromatography. The toxic moiety (subfraction 1) was eluted first and was not immunogenic. Subfraction 2 eluted from DEAE Sephadex in 0.5 M sodium chloride sodium was immunogenic but was non-toxic. Both fractions were lipoproteins, subfraction 1 containing 25–30% of lipid as glycerides and subfraction II 6–8% as serine based lipid. Each subfraction contained 3% carbohydrate and the remainder was protein of conventional amino acid composition. Further purification of the toxic subfraction by cold alcohol-ether precipitation indicated a molecular weight of approximately 10,000.

Relationship of Antibodies to Immunity

The role of the respective antigenic moieties in the pathogenesis of cholera must be first discerned before reliable conclusions can be drawn concerning the significance of serum or intestinal lumen antibody levels. The vibrio-vibriocidal antibody interaction must take place within the gut lumen and the relationship of serum antibody levels to those in intestinal fluids in the vibriocidal system is not yet clear. Vibriocidal antibodies as currently measured include IgA, IgG and IgM and are from serum which contains all the components of complement up to C'9, lysozyme and other factors. Intestinal IgG has been demonstrated in the crypt epithelium of rabbits immunized against cholera toxin and found to have limited protective effect (Kao *et al.*, 1970). Recent interest has focused on the non-complement dependent component IgA as playing a possible role in local immunity. It is not yet established that it does play a significant role at this level. However, the results of studies exploring whether this immunoglobulin may exhibit local vibriocidal and/or antitoxin effect will be awaited with interest as their significance will obviously extend to other diarrheic states of bacterial origin.

The significance attached to the neutralization of cholera enterotoxin by serum antitoxin in the isolated rabbit intestinal loop or in the skin remains questionable because the antigens used have not been sufficiently pure and serum levels of antitoxin may not reflect those in local secretions. Further, high levels of serum antitoxin may reflect an immune response to clinically manifest cholera but not necessarily bear any direct relationship to the degree of colonization of the gut by virulent vibrios. On the other hand, high levels of vibriocidal antibody even with low levels of antitoxin could exist assuming that the level of vibriocidal immunity prevented significant multiplication of vibrios thereby reducing the amount of antigenic toxin formed. In addition, serum vibriocidal antibody levels may not necessarily reflect the levels of vibriocidal antibody in the intestinal secretions wherein vibrio multiplication occurs.

Anti-vibrio antibody was detected, though inconstantly, in all three IgA, IgG and IgM immunoglobulins in jejunal aspirates of cholera patients. In the serum of these patients IgG and IgM antibody rose early in the disease while IgA rose only when *V. cholerae* had disappeared from the intestine (Northrup and Hossain, 1970). The irregular detection of antibody activity in intestinal immunoglobulins may be related to their degradation by intestinal enzymes (Northrup *et al.*, 1970). It was suggested that the relationship between the appearance of serum IgA antibody and the disappearance of *V. cholerae* from the intestine may reflect an absorption of all the available IgA antibody by the *V. cholerae* antigen thereby preventing its early detection in the serum. Assuming that the serum IgA antibodies are produced by intestinal lymphoid cells, their delayed appearance may thus be explained. In support of this Crabbé *et al.* (1969) showed that after oral immunization of germfree mice with ferritin, the mucosal cells produced IgA antiferritin antibody followed by serum IgA antibodies.

Many aspects of cholera immunity are not yet understood. Some people develop cholera despite the presence of serum antibody levels generally associated with resistance to cholera. On the other hand, the diarrheal syndrome in cholera appears attributable to enterotoxin yet protection can be conferred by vaccines devoid of toxin antigen. Factors predisposing to enhanced or reduced resistance to cholera infection are similarly poorly understood. The possible effects of chronic malnutrition, pregnancy, passive immunization and role of maternal antibody require further study.

Staphylococcal Enterotoxin

Introduction

Staphylococcal food poisoning is the classical example of diarrhea mediated by a bacterial enterotoxin and has been well documented (DACK, 1956). The symptoms of staphylococcal food poisoning in humans may result from proliferation of the organism in the intestinal tract, but are much more commonly due to the ingestion of preformed enterotoxin contaminating foodstuffs. The disease is characterized by vomiting and diarrhea within 2–6 hour of ingestion and is rarely fatal in man. Most laboratory animals are much less susceptible than man to peroral challenge with staphylococcal enterotoxin (DACK, 1956). Though oral and intravenous administration of staphylococcal enterotoxin may produce many similar symptoms including both vomiting and diarrhea, the relationship of the effects produced by parenteral administration to those associated with food poisoning is not known.

Staphylococci cause both superficial and deep wound infection and are commonly isolated from patients with septicema, pulmonary, cardiac and urinary tract infections. No specific role has been attributed to enterotoxin in the pathogenesis of these diseases. Staphylococcal pseudomembranous enterocolitis, which is seen in patients after antibiotic therapy, is similar in several respects to staphylococcal food poisoning. Because of these similarities the enterotoxin was suggested as the causitive agent in both diseases (DACK, 1956; PROHASKA et al., 1956). Despite the isolation of potent enterotoxin producing strains from patients suffering from enteritis after antibiotic therapy (SURGALLA and DACK, 1955; HALLANDER and KÖRLOF, 1967) and the fact that enteritis was produced in chinchillas given antibiotics for several days followed by a pure culture of enterotoxigenic strain of staphylococcus (TAN et al., 1959) there is to date no specific evidence which has identified staphylococcal enterotoxin as the causitive agent of pseudomembranous enterocolitis.

Identification, Purification, and Properties of the Enterotoxins

Staphylococcus aureus produces numerous toxic components. Though not all strains of staphylococci are enterotoxigenic, current estimates, based on the use of presently available sensitive means of detection, indicate that more

Table 1. *Staphylococcal strains associated with the production of various enterotoxins*

Strain	Enterotoxin
100	A
196E	A
S6	B
C-243	B
137	C
361	C
483	C
494	D
293	C and D
315	D
L16	D
224	E

than 50% of strains tested produce enterotoxins. Some strains may produce more than one detectable form of enterotoxin (Table 1). The difficult and insufficiently reliable animal tests used in earlier studies to assess the incidence of enterotoxigenicity among coagulase positive staphylococci proved inconclusive (Dolman, 1934; Evans *et al.*, 1950). The introduction of serological methods permitted the more rapid and specific identification of various enterotoxins designated A, B, C, etc., from specific strains of *staphylococcus aureus* (Casman *et al.*, 1963) (Table 1). To date enterotoxins A (Casman, 1960), B (Bergdoll *et al.*, 1959), C (Bergdoll *et al.*, 1965) and D (Casman *et al.*, 1967) have been identified and enterotoxin E has been tentatively identified (Bergdoll, 1970).

The various enterotoxins produced by the organism are apparently metabolic products formed at the cell surface and released into the surrounding medium (Friedman and White, 1965). They are chemically, physically, and biologicaly distinct from endotoxin (Martin and Marcus, 1964). Close similarity exists between the physical and biological properties of the various purified enterotoxins (Table 2). They occur as white fluffy powders in the lyophilized state and are readily soluble in aqueous solution. They are resistant to proteolytic enzymes and are capable of producing emesis in young rhesus monkeys in doses as low as 5 µg. Their molecular weights are in the range of 34 000 to 35 300. During recent years successful attempts have been made to purify some of these enterotoxic substances. Because enterotoxin B has been most extensively studied, it will be discussed first.

Enterotoxin B

The early attempts to purify enterotoxin B (Bergdoll *et al.*, 1959; Frea *et al.*, 1963) produced only milligram amounts of toxin. Schantz *et al.*, (1965) using column chromatography employing carbocyclic acid resins isolated a highly purified preparation in high yield. This substance appeared homo-

Table 2. *Properties of staphylococcal enterotoxins*

Property	Strain S100 Entero-toxin A (Chu et al., 1966)	Strain S6 Entero-toxin B (Schantz et al., 1965)	Strain 137 Entero-toxin C_1 (Borja and Bergdoll, 1967)	Strain 361 Entero-toxin C_2 (Avena and Bergdoll, 1967)
Nitrogen content %	16.5	16.1	16.2	16.0
Sedimentation coefficient ($S^o_{20,w}$), S	3.04	2.89	3.00	2.90
Diffusion coefficient ($D^o_{20,w}$), $\times 10^{-7}$ cm^2 sec^{-1}	7.94	7.72	8.10	8.10
Reduced viscosity (ml/g)	4.07	3.92	3.4	3.7
Isoelectric point	6.8	8.6	8.6	7.0
Partial specific volume ml/g	0.726	0.743	0.732	0.742
Maximum absorption (mμ)	277	277	277	277
Extinction ($E^{1\%}_{1\,cm}$)	14.3	14.0	12.1	12.1
Molecular weight	34,700	35,300	34,100	34,000
Toxicity (MED), μg	5	5	5	5–10
Effect of heat 60° 30 min	labile	stable	stable	moderately stable
Appearance (lyophilized powder)	white fluffy	white fluffy	white fluffy	white fluffy
Resistant to proteolytic enzymes	yes	yes	yes	yes
Solubility in water and salt solutions	yes	yes	yes	yes

geneous when subjected to several kinds of ultracentrifugal analysis, to be stable over a wide pH range (5–10 at least) and in physical solution for long periods of time at room temperature (Wagman *et al.*, 1965). It was separated into two main protein fractions by starchgel electrophoresis (Baird-Parker and Joseph, 1964). These two fractions were shown to differ only in charge and toxicity, but not in size or serological specificity. Such differences were attributed to variations in the secondary or tertiary molecular configuration of the two fractions and not to the effects of purification methods employed.

Amino acid analysis (Spero *et al.*, 1965) showed the toxin to consist solely of amino acid arranged as a single polypeptide chain, rich in aspartic acid and lysine, with glutamic acid as the N-terminal residue and lysine as the C-terminal residue with no free sulfhydryl groups and only one disulfide bridge. Reduction cleavage of the disulfide bridge and alkylation of the resulting SH groups with both iodacetamide and iodacetate produced derivatives which had the same emetic activity and immunological properties as the native enterotoxin (Dalidowicz et al., 1966). Chemical modification of amino groups of enterotoxin B by nitration (Chu, 1968) or by guanidation of as many as 90 % of the lysine residues had no effect on its toxic or serological properties in contrast to reduction of both activities seen with acetylation and succinylation of these groups (Chu et al., 1969). The toxin lost some of its ability to precipitate antibody within 8 hours of being toxoided with formalin (Silverman et al., 1966). By 48 hours the toxoid gave a reaction of partial identity when compared to toxin in the Ouchterlony double gel diffusion test but still retained its emetic activity in monkeys after intravenous administration. It thereafter decreased and after 9 days of formalin treatment was devoid of emetic activity. Bergdoll (1966) considered this action to be non-specific and unrelated to specific modification of amino groups.

Enterotoxin A

Staphylococcal enterotoxin A was highly purified using chromatography on carboxymethyl cellulose and gel filtration with Sephadex G-100 and G-75 (Chu et al., 1966). It is a simple protein and essentially homogeneous as determined by ultracentrifugal analysis. In contrast to enterotoxin B which is heat stable (Schantz et al., 1965), enterotoxin A is heat labile showing a 50 % decrease in immunological reactivity after heating at 60° C for 20 minutes, and complete loss of reactivity after heating at 80° C and 100° C for 3 and 1 minutes respectively (Chu et al., 1966).

Enterotoxin C

Two strains (137 and 361) of *staphylococcus aureus* have now been shown to produce enterotoxin C and have been called enterotoxins C_1 and C_2 respectively (Bergdoll et al., 1965). Both have been purified by ion exchange chromatography on carboxymethyl-cellulose and molecular sieving through Sephadex G-75 and G-50 gels (Borja and Bergdoll, 1967; Avena and Bergdoll, 1967). There are slight differences in their electrophoretic mobilities and in their elution patterns from carboxymethyl cellulose columns but they are immunologically similar. Both enterotoxins are simple proteins, antigenic, consist of single polypeptide chains cross linked by single disulphide bridges; and are capable of producing significant emesis (Borja and Bergdoll, 1969). The amino acid analysis of both enterotoxins has been elucidated (Huang et al., 1967); each has glutamic acid as the N-terminal amino acid and glycine as the C-terminal amino acid.

Denaturing agents such as guanidine hydrochloride and urea produced a reversible change in the intrinsic viscosity of the enterotoxin C molecule without observable effect on its serological or emetic properties (Chu et al.,

1969). The serological and toxic properties of enterotoxin C were abolished in alkaline solutions (pH 12–13), were unaffected by acetylation of five tyrosyl groups but were abolished by acetylation, following prior exposure to guanidine hydrochloride, of 21 tyrosyl residues.

Enterotoxin D

CASMAN *et al.* (1967) demonstrated the occurrence of a fourth enterotoxin, enterotoxin D. This enterotoxin was produced by strains which did not produce A, B, or C enterotoxins, was absent from the growth products of non-enterotoxigenic strains and produced emesis in the cat. Its biological activity was neutralized only by a specific antibody and not by those to enterotoxins A, B, and C. Attempts to purify enterotoxin D have provided a low yield of the toxic product and insufficiently reliable tests to establish its purity have been used (CASMAN *et al.*, 1967).

Enterotoxin E

This enterotoxin has only been tentatively identified (BERGDOLL, 1970) and work is currently in progress on its purification.

Incidence of Enterotoxins

In humans, enterotoxin A is more frequently associated with clinical staphylococcal food poisoning than is enterotoxin B. Occasionally, strains producing both enterotoxins A and B have been isolated from the same patient. On the other hand, laboratory animals are more susceptible to enterotoxin B and the disease spectrum can be reproduced by oral administration to monkey, cat, dog and chinchilla (WARREN *et al.*, 1963; WARREN *et al.*, 1964; PROHASKA, 1966; KENT, 1966).

A recent survey of the incidence of the different types of enterotoxins produced by coagulase positive staphylococci isolated from varying sources was determined by use of the slide gel diffusion test (CASMAN *et al.*, 1967). The sources included clinical specimens, apparently healthy individuals, raw milk, mastitic cows, frozen foods and foods incriminated in food poisoning. Entero-toxins A or D occurred most commonly in all categories. Enterotoxin A was produced by almost 50% of "food poisoning" strains, enterotoxin D by approximately 8%, and enterotoxins A and D together by another 25% of these strains. Enterotoxin D appeared to be most commonly produced by strains isolated from milk and frozen foods. Enterotoxins B and C were of much less frequent occurrence from all sources. In addition, as many as 30% of the remaining strains which did not produce enterotoxins A, B, C, or D were found to be positive for enterotoxigenicity in the cat test.

Associations of Enterotoxigenicity

The contamination by staphylococci of cooked rather than raw meat is associated with staphylococcal food poisoning. CASMAN (1965) has shown that staphylococci will grow and produce enterotoxin on the surface of raw and cooked meat relatively free from contamination by other microorganisms but not in ground raw beef so contaminated. He suggested that the non-involvement of raw meat in food poisoning was due to the inability of the staphylococcus to compete with other organisms present in the meat.

Coagulase

It has been generally agreed that coagulase positive staphylococci are the predominant enterotoxigenic strains (EVANS *et al.*, 1950). ZAKARIAN (1967) studied a total of 170 strains of coagulase positive staphylococci. Of this number 106 strains were isolated from children with enterocolitis, 36 from washings, vomitus and food products associated with food poisoning and 28 from feces of normal healthy children. Only 12 of the strains isolated from children with staphylococcal enterocolitis produced an enterotoxin whereas all the strains associated with food poisoning were enterotoxigenic. Coagulase negative, enterotoxin producing strains have also been described (THATCHER and SIMON, 1956; OMORI and KATO, 1959; BERGDOLL *et al.*, 1967). A recent outbreak of staphylococcal food poisoning due to coagulase negative *staphylococcus epidermidis* was described by BRECKENRIDGE and BERGDOLL (1971) and enterotoxin A, which produced emesis in monkeys, was identified in cultures of the isolant.

Bacteriophage

No phage pattern could be associated with enterotoxins A or B (CASMAN, 1965). Lysogeny with temperate phages from strain PS42D which produces enterotoxin A (CASMAN, 1965) conferred enterotoxicity A to some 31 non-toxigenic strains.

Methicillin Sensitivity

DORNBUSCH *et al.* (1969) reported that 37 of 41 methicillin resistant strains were enterotoxin B producers. Because both these factors were cotransducible and were lost after acriflavine treatment, these authors suggested that both these characters may be extrachromosomally determined. This was not confirmed by workers from New Zealand (JARVIS and LAWRENCE, 1970) who did, however, point out that methicillin was not extensively used in that country.

Other Staphylococcal Factors

No correlation has been noted between enterotoxin production and other products of the staphylococcus organism such as hemolysins, penicillinase, nuclease or phosphatase (BERGDOLL, 1970). However, the prolonged lag phase and the decreased production of coagulase, nuclease, and phosphatase have been noted in association with the almost 20-fold increase in enterotoxin A production by the last mutant strain following serial exposure of the parent enterotoxigenic A strain 100 of *staphylococcus aureus* to the mutagenic agent N-methyl, N[1]-nitro-N-nitrosoguanidine (FRIEDMAN and HOWARD, 1971).

Enterotoxin Production

Media

The most commonly used media for enterotoxin production are meat infusion broths (CASMAN and BENNETT, 1963; McLEAN *et al.*, 1968) and simpler media such as proteose peptone, casein hydrolysate (DOLMAN and WILSON, 1938; FAVORITE and HAMMON, 1941) or pancreatic digests of casein (SEGALOVE, 1947; SURGALLA *et al.*, 1951; KATO *et al.*, 1966). Supplements were found necessary for optimal growth of staphylococci especially on the simpler media and included peptone, glucose, thiamine and niacin (BERGDOLL, 1970; REISER and WEISS, 1969; MARKUS, 1969). Small volumes of staphylococcal enterotoxin were obtained with growth on semi-solid agar (CASMAN and BENNETT, 1965) and with aerated growth (SURGALLA *et al.*, 1951) in brain heart infusion and casein hydrolysate media. However, earlier and increased production of staphylococcal enterotoxin with the use of aerated cultures was noted by others (STARK and MIDDAUGH, 1969; McLEAN *et al.*, 1968). Four to eight times higher titers of enterotoxins A, B and C were obtained by growth of strains 100, S-6, and 361 respectively in "cellophane over agar" cultures (HALLANDER, 1965; JARVIS and LAWRENCE, 1970). Growth appears best with incubation at 37° C. The pH of the medium influences both the cell growth rate of *staphylococcus aureus* and the toxin synthesis and release (MARKUS and SILVERMAN, 1969). Increasing concentrations of sodium chloride and lowered incubation temperatures decreased enterotoxin production (STARK and MIDDAUGH, 1969).

Cellular Source of Enterotoxin

FRIEDMAN and WHITE (1965) using immunofluorescent techniques demonstrated the presence of enterotoxin B in the cell surface of unwashed cells cultured for 8 hours but not in those in the early log phase (3 hours). The immunofluorescent pattern was easily removed by washing with water, which indicated a loose binding of the water soluble enterotoxin to the bacterial cell wall. These observations support those of HARTMAN and GOODGAL (1959) who suggested that the enterotoxin had the characteristics of a bacterial cell surface constituent.

Relationship to Cell Growth

There is evidence that the functions of cell growth and toxin production are not directly related to one another. McLEAN *et al.* (1968) using *staphylococcus aureus* strain ATCC 14458 showed that enterotoxin B production was independent of cell growth and that low concentrations of curing salts as well as decreased temperatures lowered enterotoxin production to a greater degree than cell growth.

In the standard casein hydrolysate medium the formation of enterotoxin B by *staphylococcus aureus* strain S-6 occurred only during the postexponential phase when total protein synthesis was arithmetic (Morse *et al.*, 1969). The rate of toxin synthesis was greater than the rate of total protein synthesis. Cellular growth per se is not necessary for toxin production since 95 % of the enterotoxin B produced by the S6 strain of *staphylococcus aureus* occurs during the latter part of exponential phase of growth (Markus and Silverman, 1969). Under their experimental conditions, toxin production proceeded without increase of DNA, RNA or cell protein (Markus and Silverman, 1968). Toxin was also produced into a nitrogen-free medium indicating the presence of endogenous toxin precursors. Toxin production occurred only when the washed stationary phase cultures are shaken to establish aerobic conditions.

Cell respiration poisons such as 2,4-dinitrophenol or sodium azide caused 90 % to 100 % inhibition of toxin excretion which suggests that toxin excretion is an energy dependent process (Markus and Silverman, 1968). Metabolic inhibitors, including those with action on the cell wall, prevent toxin formation in growing cells (Friedman, 1966, 1968; Morse *et al.*, 1969) but not in non-replicating cells (Markus and Silverman, 1968). Staphylococcal enterotoxin production from strains ATCC 13565, ATCC 14458, S6, and S100 was inhibited by streptomycin but not by penicillin (Cotillo, 1967). Similar observations were made by Rosenwald and Lincoln (1966). The addition of glucose to the medium represses the oxidative abilities of *staphylococcus aureus* (Strasters and Winkler, 1963) and has been found to repress the rate of toxin synthesis independently of pH changes (Morse *et al.*, 1969). These observations were interpreted as suggesting that toxin synthesis was regulated by catabolite repression.

Methods of Assay of Staphylococcal Enterotoxins

Biological

The most common biological assay procedures are the intraperitoneal or intravenous injections of cats and kittens (Dolman and Wilson, 1940) and the feeding of young rhesus monkeys (Surgalla *et al.*, 1953). The latter is the most reliable since only the enterotoxins produce predictable and reproducible emesis in these animals. Vomiting within 5 hours of feeding in at least 2 of 6 animals constitutes a positive result. Other assay methods including the effect of enterotoxins on tissue cultures have not proven generally satisfactory (Bergdoll, 1970) though Schaeffer *et al.* (1966) did report positive results with human embryonic intestinal cells using large amounts of enterotoxin.

Immunological

Many different methods have been used. Precipitation and gel diffusion techniques have become well established for the quantitative assay of staphylococcal enterotoxins but are limited in terms of their sensitivity and speed (HALL *et al.*, 1965). Qualitative detection is also possible by these methods and is considered superior to that obtained by biological assay methods. The recent introduction of the use of erythrocytes sensitized with staphylococcal enterotoxin antitoxin was found to be of advantage (SILVERMAN *et al.*, 1968). SALOMON and TEW (1968) also showed that the use of latex particles coated with specific antitoxin provided a method which was simple, rapid, with an increased sensitivity. The test was capable of detecting 2×10^{-4} µg of staphylococcal enterotoxin B per ml of sample. Immunofluorescent methods have also been used but are not as sensitive as the hemagglutination procedures (FRIEDMAN and WHITE, 1965; GENIGEORGIS and SADLER, 1966a, 1966b).

Immunology

The purification of the various staphylococcal enterotoxins enabled the production of specific precipitating antibodies and the specific immunization of experimental animals which in turn indicated that the enterotoxins were antigenically distinct from one another. Staphylococcal enterotoxin B and its toxoid are immunogenic, the former being the more effective antigen, by either the intracutaneous or the oral route (SILVERMAN *et al.*, 1969a). Such immunizations provided relatively high levels of antibody titer and protection for period of at least one year in monkeys. Complete protection against emesis and death was only provided by intracutaneous inoculation with enterotoxin at low dosage levels. Parenteral immunizations of rabbits with either toxin or toxoids showed no differences in their protective effects (SILVERMAN *et al.*, 1969b).

The only reported attempts at oral immunization using crude enterotoxin against staphylococcal food poisoning were unsuccessful (DACK *et al.*, 1931; DOLMAN, 1943). The presence of antibodies to enterotoxin in the serum of humans resistant to enterotoxin was claimed by FELSENFELD and NASUNIYA (1964) but because of the use of impure preparations as reference material there was no definite proof that the precipitation lines obtained were specifically due to enterotoxin-antienterotoxin reactions.

The detection of an anamnestic reaction in monkeys with specific antitoxin antibodies in their serum illustrates the necessity of testing animals prior to experimental usage. Up to 50% of monkeys tested showed the presence of antibodies ranging in titer from the usual of below 1:80 to 1:2500 in some animals. The immunogenicity of the toxin by the oral route and their continued exposure to toxin contaminated food in their native habitat may explain why such animals may become immune. Minor infection is, of course, another. It may be interesting to study the role which nasal carriers contribute to antitoxin titers or if there exists a relationship between the carrier state and the host immune response.

Specific antibodies have not been demonstrated in serum of humans resistant to staphylococcal food poisoning (Bergdoll, 1970). However, Dolman (1944) showed that volunteers given several subcutaneous injections of crude enterotoxoid became resistant to toxin thereby indicating some possible protective antibody formation. Similarly, monkeys fed enterotoxin B repeatedly became resistant to 200 minimum emetic doses of toxin but serum precipitating antibodies were not demonstrable (Bergdoll, 1966). Nevertheless, the serum did provide some degree of passive immunity when administered to other monkeys given 10 MED of enterotoxin *per os* indicating the presence of serum antitoxin in resistant monkeys. Monkeys could be actively immunized against very high doses of enterotoxin by intramuscular enterotoxoid immunization. The presence of serum antibodies in immunized animals was demonstrated by the failure of monkeys to react to oral partially purified enterotoxin treated with antisera from rabbits (Surgalla *et al.*, 1954).

Pathogenesis

Diarrhea

Attempts at understanding the diarrheagenic mechanisms of these enterotoxins have been concentrated on the study of intestinal morphology and motility induced by the enterotoxin in experimental animals. The pathogenesis of fluid exsorption in staphylococcal food poisoning as in most other instances of diarrhea remains unknown. Hayama and Sugiyama (1964) observed that removal of the cecum facilitated the production of diarrhea in rabbits given enterotoxin intravenously but not *per os*. Though this effect is not understood, it suggested that the portions of the gastrointestinal tract proximal to the cecum may be a site of action of intravenously given enterotoxin. Shemano *et al.* (1967) have provided evidence in the dog that the intravenous injection (100 µg/kg) of purified staphylococcal enterotoxin causes emesis, diarrhea, and a decrease of small intestinal tone and contractility. Intestinal bolus transport was inhibited and gastric emptying time was delayed as observed in X-ray studies. Neither bilateral vagectomy nor chemical sympathectomy influenced these effects of enterotoxin. In similar fashion the spontaneous contractility and tone of the isolated rabbit ileum was unaffected in a concentration of up to 10 µg/ml of staphylococcal enterotoxin. These effects suggest indirectly that diarrheagenic mechanisms may be associated with alterations of fluid fluxes in the bowel, perhaps aided by the delayed transit time allowing better toxin-epithelial surface interaction.

Some evidence exists that such mechanisms may be contributory. Sullivan (1969) has shown *in vitro* that enterotoxin inhibits the net absorption of water and solutes in the everted sac of rat small intestine. Transport processes rather than metabolic disturbances are suggested as more likely since oxygen uptake and lactic acid production were unchanged. The net water transport from mucosal to serosal surface was two thirds reduced with similar inhibitions of transport of sodium, potassium, and glucose. Chloride transport appeared most severely affected and lactic acid transport to the least extent.

Similar to the situation which exists in cholera, SUSSMAN *et al.* (1970) found impaired net absorption of sodium and water in Thiry-Vella fistulae of jejunum or ileum in dogs following administration of up to 1 mg of highly purified enterotoxin B into such loops. There was no effect on potassium handling and no histological change was seen. The mean change was a net secretion of water and sodium. In some tests with dosages exceeding 0.25 mg of toxin the absorption of sodium and water in the control fistula was also reduced suggesting that enterotoxin was absorbed from one fistula and acted on the other. It is of interest that similar observations have been made in the infant rabbit with crude cholera toxin (SEREBRO *et al.*, 1968) and with live vibrio organisms (VAUGHAN-WILLIAMS *et al.*, 1969).

SHEAHAN *et al.* (1970) noted a decrease in the sulfated mucosubstances of the apical granules of the crypt epithelium of the monkey intestine associated with crypt hyperplasia within 4–8 hours after oral ingestion of staphylococcal enterotoxin B. Though evidence for increased secretion of these granules was seen, it is not yet established that the crypt epithelium is the only area of the small bowel which is specifically concerned with fluid and electrolyte exsorption in this animal model. Nevertheless, it is significant that the crypt epithelium also appears to be implicated in cholera fluid exsorption (KAO *et al.*, 1971; SEREBRO *et al.*, 1969).

Current work in this laboratory has demonstrated that the intraluminal instillation of staphylococcal enterotoxin B causes fluid accumulation in the ligated jejunal loop in the monkey (SHEAHAN unpublished observations). The ileum and colon were refractory within the limits of dosage and experimental incubation periods (1 mg/ml and from 2–18 hours respectively). Both ileal and jejunal loops were unreactive in the rabbit. Thus, it appears that staphylococcal enterotoxins may possess some capability to evoke intestinal fluid exsorption but differ from other enterotoxins in that much greater doses are required to produce comparable effects. In addition, preliminary observations have shown evidence for a skin permeability factor in enterotoxin B as assessed in the rabbit dermis (SHEAHAN unpublished observations).

SUGIYAMA (1966) has suggested that the pathogenetic mechanisms of staphylococcal food poisoning are due to the primary effect on the gastrointestinal tract. Because many endotoxin-like actions have been demonstrated following administration of enterotoxin (SUGIYAMA, 1966; SUGIYAMA and McKISSIC, 1966) it was proposed that the illness was due either to the direct endotoxin-like properties of the enterotoxin itself or to an alteration of the gut permitting the endotoxin of the indigenous flora of the gastrointestinal tract to mediate its effect. A further possibility was a tissue enterotoxin interaction producing products capable of evoking endotoxin-like response. Nevertheless, since the enterotoxins used were described as being only 95 % pure, the possibility of contamination with endotoxin has not been excluded in these studies.

^{14}C radioisotopic staphylococcal enterotoxin B has been prepared (BOWDEN, 1968). This substance was found to be similar to the unlabelled compound in terms of assay of serological specificity, ultracentrifugal analysis, and emetic responsiveness in monkeys. The application of radiolabelled enterotoxin B may permit more specific approaches to the study of the pathogenetic mechanisms by which it produces diarrhea and possibly some of its other effects.

Emesis

The monkey is less susceptible to the emetic action of enterotoxin than is man (DACK, 1956). This may be due to the lesser tendency of monkeys to vomit rather than to a decreased sensitivity of monkey tissues to enterotoxin.

The site of emetic action of staphylococcal enterotoxin has been studied in the cat and monkey (SUGIYAMA *et al.*, 1961; CLARKE *et al.*, 1962). Vagotomized monkeys developed a low refractoriness to the vomiting stimulus of intravenous administration of enterotoxin (SUGIYAMA and HAYAMA, 1964), but were highly resistant to intragastric emetic challenges (SUGIYAMA and HAYAMA, 1965). Similar observations were made in the cat (CLARKE *et al.*, 1962). Surgical ablation of the chemoreceptor trigger zone (area postrema in the floor of the fourth ventricle) in the monkey resulted in abolition of emetic response to intragastric or intravenous administration of enterotoxin but not of oral copper sulfate, an agent which acts through gastrointestinal receptors (SUGIYAMA *et al.*, 1961). The reason is because the sacro-lumbo-thoraco-bulbar tracts which innervate the abdominal viscera have terminations near the area postrema (KURU and SUGIHARA, 1955) and that ablation of this area interrupts the impulse pathways from the abdominal viscera to the vomiting center which are required to cause vomiting (SUGIYAMA and HAYAMA, 1965). Lateral cerebroventricular injection of enterotoxin failed to elicit vomiting indicating that it is not elicited by direct action of enterotoxin on the vomiting center (SUGIYAMA and HAYAMA, 1965).

Abdominal sympathectomy alone had no effect on the emetic response in monkeys but when coupled with a low intrathoracic vagotomy, producing complete deafferentiation of the abdominal viscera, the monkey was rendered completely refractory to the emetic stimulus of enterotoxin given by either route as well as to intragastric copper sulfate (SUGIYAMA and HAYAMA, 1965). However, such animals retained the capability of vomiting after Veriloid suggesting an intact vomiting center. These observations have been interpreted as evidence that the site of emetic action in the Rhesus monkey is in the abdominal viscera, that the sensory emetic stimulus reaches the vomiting center via the vagus and sympathetic nerves and that staphylococcal enterotoxin has no apparent direct action on the central nervous system.

Pathology

Enterotoxin B administered orally to three human volunteers (RAJ and BERGDOLL, 1969) produced typical symptoms of staphylococcal food poisoning. The effective dose utilized was equivalent to 20–25 µg of purified toxin thereby establishing that the human is more sensitive to the effect of this enterotoxin than the monkey. The clinical disease was characterized by normal temperature and blood pressure, vomitus and stools free of blood and mucus, and reversal to normal health in a short period of time.

The studies of PALMER (1951) which described the lesion in peroral biopsies of the gastric mucosa in patients with staphylococcal food poisoning, appear to be the only contribution to the knowledge of the morphological response in the human. Studies in laboratory animals have been more extensive. Next to man and chimpanzee the monkey has been found to be the most susceptible laboratory animal (WILSON, 1959; DACK, 1956). WARREN et al. (1964) and PROHASKA (1963) produced a severe enteritis in dogs and PROHASKA et al. (1959) in cats and chinchillas by the intrajejunal instillation of crude staphylococcal extract. Repeated oral doses of enterotoxin B produced enterocolitis in monkeys (KENT, 1966) and in chinchillas (WARREN et al., 1963).

The pathological appearances of the sequential changes occurring in the gastrointestinal tract of the Rhesus monkey following a single oral dose of 150 µg of enterotoxin B have been described by KENT (1966). Emesis and/or diarrhea was produced in almost all animals, usually occurring within 3–4 hours of challenge. The diarrhea was accompanied by the passage of mucus in many instances. No gross lesions were detectable other than congestion and edema throughout the gastrointestinal tract. Microscopically the gastric lesions consisted of an acute inflammatory response chiefly in the cardiac (periesophageal) and pyloric areas of the mucosa and was most prominent between 4 and 8 hours after challenge. There appeared to be some associated loss of mucus from the epithelial cells.

In the small intestine the mucosal response was characterized by an intense acute inflammation, villous blunting and crypt elongation, which was maximal between 4 and 8 hours after challenge. The reaction was more severe in the duodenum and jejunum than in the ileum. Slight elongation of crypts appeared to be the sole residuum of effect 72 hours after challenge. A slight leucocytic exudate with loss or mucus from surface cells at six and eight hours after challenge were the only changes seen in colonic mucosa. The emetic and diarrheal effects of repeated daily doses of staphylococcal enterotoxin appear to be related to gastric mucosal emptying time because, with high diluent volumes, four of six animals had diarrhea after the first dose in contrast to the 10 animals given small volumes who had no diarrhea or emesis after the second or subsequent daily doses.

Enzyme Histochemistry

Studies of oxidative, hexokinase and phosphatase enzyme changes in the experimental model have been studied (KENT et al., 1966). At the height of the lesion there was a slight reduction of enzyme activity in surface mucous epithelium of the stomach and a slight increase in acid phosphatase activity in chief cells. In the jejunum a rapid decrease and recovery of enzyme activity occurred which correlated well with structural alterations already noted. Similar but less conspicuous changes were seen in the ileum. An interesting observation was the altered pattern of lipid (presumed absorbed) distribution from normal. The loss of lipid from villous jejunal epithelial cells occurred between 2–8 hours with recovery by 12 hours. The later disappearance of these lipid droplets—after 24 hours—in the ileum was interpreted by these investigators as failure of the jejunal mucosa to absorb lipid at the height of the lesion. The delayed disappearance of lipid from the ileal mucosa may be related to a delayed transit time and/or dilution effect.

Mucin Histochemistry

The epithelial mucosubstances of the small intestinal epithelium and most specifically of the jejunum were shown to be markedly altered at the same time as the structural morphological and histoenzymatic changes were most evident, namely between 4 and 8 hours post-challenge (Sheahan *et al.*, 1970). These changes were also reversible and had returned to near normal within 48 to 72 hours of initial insult. In addition to goblet cell mucin discharge there was a marked depletion of acid mucosubstances, in particular of sulfomucins, from the apical granules of the crypt epithelium. These authors suggested a relationship between the depletion of sulfated mucosubstances from the crypt epithelium and the crypt cell proliferation indicating that sulfated mucosubstances may exert a controlling influence on cell regeneration and that their absence may permit increased cell proliferation in the intestinal crypt epithelium.

Electron Microscopy

Ultrastructural evidence of the small intestinal epithelial cellular damage due to staphylococcal enterotoxin ingestion appeared confined to the mitochondrial components which became swollen and showed dislocated cristae (Merrill and Sprinz, 1968). These changes were associated with cytoplasmic vacuolations of villous and crypt epithelial cells with lesser involvement of the intestinal microvilli. Both merocrine and apocrine secretion of the apical granules of small bowel crypt epithelium was stimulated by the influence of staphylococcal enterotoxin B (Sheahan *et al.*, 1970). However, this evidence of secretory capacity by crypt cells cannot as yet be interpreted as evidence for fluid secretion by these cells.

Cytopathogenicity

Hallander and Bengtsson (1967) showed that staphylococcal delta-lysin and to a lesser extent alpha-lysin exerted strong toxic actions on human erythrocytes, granulocytes, and kidney cells in tissue culture. Other toxins and enzymes including enterotoxin B failed to show any cytopathogenic effects.

However, SCHAEFFER *et al.* (1966) did report that enterotoxin B was cytopathic *in vitro* to human embryonic intestinal cells and that the effect could be neutralized with specific antisera or by prior trypsin treatment of the cell culture (SCHAEFFER *et al.*, 1967). The latter observation may indicate the presence of a trypsin sensitive component on the embryonic cell surface which is required for enterotoxin interaction with the cell.

Thus staphylococcal enterotoxin appears to have the capability of altering some of the metabolic functions of both the villous absorptive and the crypt secretory epithelium particularly in the upper small bowel. This is also the site of fluid exsorption in ligated intestinal loop of the monkey in response to toxin exposure (SHEAHAN unpublished observations). TRIER (1964) has provided evidence in the human that secretion occurs in the crypt epithelium. The mucin histochemical and ultrastructural evidence of apical granule secretion in the monkey indicate that staphylococcal enterotoxin does stimulate secretion and suggests that the crypt epithelium of this animal species also possesses a secretory capacity. However, the mechanism by which such secretion is stimulated remains to be ascertained. The possibility that staphylococcal enterotoxin may mediate its cellular action by stimulating adenyl cyclase as cholera enterotoxin does is being currently investigated.

Systemic Effects of Staphylococcal Enterotoxin

Despite the advances in purification of these substances, the effects of their administration by other than the oral route requires careful interpretation because products of the staphylococcus other than enterotoxin may cause symptoms similar to those caused by enterotoxin.

Oral administration of staphylococcal enterotoxin produced leucocytosis within thirty minutes, peaked at three hours and returned to normal by 28 hours (SUGIYAMA and McKISSIC, 1966). When given intravenously (SUGIYAMA and McKISSIC, 1966; CRAWLEY *et al.*, 1966a, 1966b), an initial leucopenia preceded the neutrophilic leucocytosis. Serum glutamicoxaloacetic acid transaminase is raised following intravenous injection of 25 µg/kg of enterotoxin B to Rhesus monkeys (CRAWLEY *et al.*, 1966a). SUGIYAMA *et al.* (1958) noted similar changes following oral administration of crude enterotoxin to monkeys.

Highly purified staphylococcal enterotoxin B produces shock and death in monkeys after intravenous administration (CRAWLEY *et al.*, 1966b). RHODA *et al.* (1970) demonstrated that the shock associated with staphylococcal enterotoxemia is accompanied by pooling of blood in peripheral vessels without major shifts of volume between different fluid compartments of the body. Studies of the fate of intravenously administered staphylococcal enterotoxin labelled with radioiodine have indicated that it is rapidly removed from the

circulation by the kidney (Crawley *et al.*, 1966b; Morris *et al.*, 1967). Normann *et al.* (1969) showed by immunofluorescent means that 75 % of the injected dose rapidly localized in the proximal renal tubules, probably by glom-
erular filtration and tubular reabsorption, in both the monkey and the rat.
Within 15 seconds the label was demonstrable in the region of the brush
border of the tubular epithelium, and at 30 minutes the whole cell had become
fluorescent with subsequent total disappearance at 8 hours The only other site
in which the enterotoxin was detectable by immunofluorescent means was the
Kuppfer cell of the liver in the rat. These authors also employed radioiodinated
enterotoxin in tracer studies of bilaterally nephretomized rats and showed
that, in addition to the major localization in the liver, significant amounts
of radioactivity occurred in the gastrointestinal tract, lung and skin. Though
localization of toxin occurs in the kidney, no evidence as yet exists which im-
plicates the kidney as playing a role in mediating its toxicity (Staab *et al.*,
1969). The failure to demonstrate toxin localization in the brain was evidence
that at least its emetic effect is not mediated directly on the vomiting center.

These observations were not in agreement with those of Crawley *et al.*
(1966b) who noted that the lung was a major site of toxin localization. Finegold (1967) observed that the morphological alterations which occurred within
45—55 hours after intravenous enterotoxin administration to monkeys were
limited to the capillary and venous endothelium and interstitial tissues of the
lung and that no morphological changes were seen in other tissues. However,
these latter observations alone do not specifically indicate the quantitative
localization of toxin in any particular organ.

Escherichia Coli Enterotoxin

Introduction

Bacteriological study of the gastrointestinal content has established the
existence of a normal microbial flora and recently has been reviewed by Gorbach (1971). *Escherichia Coli* organisms have long been considered to be a
constituent of the normal bowel flora and nonpathogenic while resident in the
bowel. Past failure to associate these organisms with enteric disease reflects
the original preoccupation with causation of bacterial disease and the relative
neglect of the role played by the host response.

Certain strains of *Escherichia Coli* designated enteropathogenic (EEC) are
associated with infantile gastroenteritis (Neter, 1959; Taylor, 1966). The most
common EEC serotypes which have been associated with epidemic diarrhea
in infants include 026:B6, 055:B5, 086:B7, 0111:B4, 0119:B14, 0124:B17,
0125:B15, 0126:B16, 0127:B8 and 0128:B12 (Ewing *et al.*, 1963). Striking
quantitative differences were noted between the bowel flora of the infant with
E. Coli gastroenteritis and the healthy carrier. In addition to the often pure
fecal culture, the small bowel including the duodenum of the infant was heavily

populated with the offending organism (THOMSON, 1955a, 1955b). This was confirmed by KOYA *et al.* (1954) in adult volunteers given these organisms by mouth. However, despite the continued diligent search for both viral and bacterial pathogens the majority of cases of gastroenteritis in infants less than two years of age remains unexplained (CRAMBLETT *et al.*, 1971).

Acute inflammatory changes occurred in the mucosa of rabbit intestinal loops exposed to some strains of EEC (TAYLOR *et al.*, 1958; McNAUGHT and ROBERTS, 1958; YAHAGI *et al.*, 1967) whereas other strains dilated intestinal loops without mucosal inflammatory reaction (DE *et al.*, 1956; TAYLOR *et al.*, 1961). Both living and chloroform killed cultures of EEC strains isolated from babies with infantile diarrhea dilated rabbit intestinal loops, but not those of the same 0 serogroups isolated from other sources (TAYLOR and BETTELHEIM, 1966). These authors concluded that the gut dilatatory effects were due to an active labile substance produced by the organism. The value of this observation was obviated by the finding that injection of chloroform containing preparations into porcine intestinal ligated loops caused fluid accumulation and dilatation even in the absence of bacteria or their products from the inoculum (SMITH and HALLS, 1967b; GYLES and BARNUM, 1969).

Sporadic outbreaks of gastroenteritis in adults have also been associated with some serotypes of enteropathogenic *E. Coli*. The isolants from adult patients were reported as *E. Coli* 0124:B72 (LANYI *et al.*, 1959), 086:B7 (COSTIN *et al.*, 1964), 0111:B4, 026:B6 and 0128:B12 (BENGTSSON *et al.*, 1966) and 0111:B4 (SCHROEDER *et al.*, 1968). There was no conclusive serological response to infection in these outbreaks which may be attributable, amongst other factors, to the fact that some individuals were symptom-free carriers of some of these organisms as was observed in the study of rectal cultures from presumed healthy adults (DANIELSSON *et al.*, 1965; ROSNER, 1966). Experimental production of diarrheal disease by some of these organisms in children and adults was occasionally associated with a rise in serum agglutinins for the specific organism (KIRBY *et al.*, 1950; BRAUN and HENCKEL, 1952; FERGUSON and JUNE, 1952; JUNE and FERGUSON, 1953; FUKUMI and KOSAKAI, 1954; KOYA *et al.*, 1954; NAKANISHI *et al.*, 1956; SAKAZAKI and NAMIOKA, 1957).

Acute diarrhea in adults has been recently associated with strains of *E. Coli* not previously recognized as being enteropathogenic. Certain strains of *E. Coli* have been isolated from children and adults with a shigella-like diarrheal disease whereas others were isolated from patients with a salmonella-like illness (SAKAZAKI *et al.*, 1967). Most strains of the former group (028, 0112, 0124, 0136, 0143, 0144) were non-motile, had biochemical properties resembling shigella organisms, produced keratoconjunctivitis in guinea pigs (SERENEY, 1955), dilated rabbit intestinal segments causing acute inflammation of the mucosa, and multiplied within Hela cells (OGAWA *et al.*, 1968). The remaining strains of the group studied (026, 044, 055, 086, 0111, 0119, 0125, 0126, 0127, 0128, 0146) failed to produce any of these latter three effects. Invasive properties were also associated with *Escherichia Coli* strains of serotypes 0115 (TRABULSI and DE TOLEDO, 1969) and 0136:K78 (B22) (DE TOLEDO and

Table 3. *Serotypes of E. Coli organisms, strains of which are associated with enterotoxin mediated diarrhea in humans*

| E. Coli | Serotype | | Source | Rabbit gut loop reaction | | Author |
O	K	H		filtrate or lysate	live organism	
148	?	28	human	+	+	Dupont *et al.* (1971)
6	?	16	human	+	+	Dupont *et al.* (1971)
15		11	human	+		Gorbach *et al.* (1971)
78		12	human	+		Gorbach *et al.* (1971)
126	?	12	human	+		Gorbach *et al.* (1971)
6		16	human	+		Gorbach *et al.* (1971)
Untypable		27	human	+		Gorbach *et al.* (1971)
25		42	human	+		Gorbach *et al.* (1971)
126	B16	12	human	+		Gorbach *et al.* (1971)
148	?	28	human	NT		Rowe *et al.* (1970)
8[a]	87, 88ab	19	pig (Moon, H.)			Dupont *et al.* (1971)

[a] Mild diarrhea with oral feeding of 10^{10} live organisms to volunteers.

Trabulsi, 1969) isolated from patients with acute febrile diarrhea in South America.

Recent investigations have demonstrated that certain strains of *E. Coli*, also previously unrecognized as enteropathogenic, which were isolated from adult patients with acute diarrhea, possessed the capability to produce an enterotoxin (Table 3). Glew *et al.* (1969) observed that culture filtrates of *E. Coli* strains isolated from the small bowel of patients with acute diarrhea were capable of evoking fluid exsorption into and dilatation of rabbit intestinal loops. Rowe *et al.* (1970) isolated an untypable strain of *E. Coli*, since designated 0148:K?28, from the stool of 54% of British troops with "traveller's diarrhea" in Aden but not from those of healthy soldiers. Studies in Calcutta, India have shown that 50% of adult patients with undiagnosed diarrheal disease harbored large numbers of *E. Coli* in the small bowel and fecal effluent which often consisted of a single serotype (Gorbach, 1970; Gorbach *et al.*, 1971). Some strains elaborated an enterotoxin which dilated rabbit intestinal loops. This enterotoxin (Sack *et al.*, 1967) appears to be similar to that associated with *E. Coli* diarrhea in calves and swine (Smith and Halls, 1967b; Smith and Gyles, 1969; Kohler, 1968; Gyles and Barnum, 1968; Moon *et al.*, 1970).

Diarrheal diseases mediated by strains of *E. Coli* which differ serologically from those isolated from humans occur in neonatal domestic animals (Smith, 1962; Smith and Jones, 1963; Smith and Halls, 1967a, b; Nielsen and Sautter, 1968). As in the human, *E. Coli* organisms capable of invading intestinal tissues (Table 4) or of producing an enterotoxin (Table 5) have been

Table 4. *E. Coli strains with evidence of invasive qualities*

Strain	Authors	Criteria of invasion			
		sereney test	hela cell	rabbit gut loop	infection in man
0115	TRABULSI and DE TOLEDO (1969)	+ 8/8	NT	NT	+ 1/1
0144:K ? (B)	OGAWA *et al.* (1968)	+ 7/7	+ 5/5	+ 5/5	NT
0143:K ? (B)	OGAWA *et al.* (1968)	+ 1/1	+ 1/1	+ 1/1	NT
0136:K78	OGAWA *et al.* (1968)	+ 3/3	+ 3/3	+ 1/1	NT
0124:K72	OGAWA *et al.* (1968)	+ 3/4	+ 2/4	+ 1/1	NT
028ac:K73	OGAWA *et al.* (1968)	+ 1/1	+ 1/1	NT	NT
0124:K72:H	DUPONT *et al.* (1971)	+ 3/4	+ 4/4	+ 4/4	+ 1/5
0143:K ?:H	DUPONT *et al.* (1971)	+ 4/4	+ 4/4	+ 4/4	+ 5/8
0144:K ?:H	DUPONT *et al.* (1971)	+ 4/4	+ 4/4	+ 4/4	+ 3/5
0136:K78(B22)	DE TOLEDO *et al.* (1969)	+ 13/13	NT	NT	NT

associated with acute diarrhea. Intestinal epithelial penetration by certain strains of *E. Coli* has been demonstrated in the germfree and gnotobiotic neonatal pig (KENWORTHY, 1970; DREES and WAXLER, 1970; STALEY *et al.*, 1969b), in the neonatal conventional pig (STALEY *et al.*, 1969a), in the neonatal foal (STALEY *et al.*, 1970), and in the ligated rabbit intestine (DRUCKER *et al.*, 1967). In most instances there was an attendant mucosal acute inflammatory response.

Certain other strains of *E. Coli* are associated with enteric colibacillosis, an acute diarrheal disease of swine which resembles human cholera in many respects (NIELSEN and SAUTTER, 1968). To establish their pathogenicity, as in the human, the organisms proliferated in the anterior (upper) small bowel and produced an enterotoxin with resultant fluid and electrolyte movements into the lumen (SMITH and HALLS, 1967a, 1967b; GYLES and BARNUM, 1969; MOON *et al.*, 1970; KOHLER and CROSS, 1969). The absence of tissue invasion and acute inflammation in the natural (SMITH and JONES, 1963) or in experimentally induced disease (SMITH and HALLS, 1967b) attested to its enterotoxic pathogenesis.

The observations on humans and on experimental animals indicated that the heretofore considered "normal flora" may indeed harbor diarrheagenic organisms and that some of many strains of *E. Coli* which were capable of causing diarrhea may, by currently used diagnostic procedures, be untypable or may be serotypes not previously considered to be enteropathogenic. In addition, there are apparently at least two mechanisms by which these organisms produce diarrhea. This is of particular significance in cholera endemic areas and represents a factor to be considered in epidemiological studies of diarrhea. The possibility that such organisms may cause disease in temperate climates also warrants close scrutiny. GOLDSTEIN *et al.* (1971) have preliminary evidence

Table 5. *Serotypes of E. Coli organisms, strains of which are associated with enterotoxin mediated diarrhea in domestic animals*

E. Coli Serotype			Animal source	Gut loop reaction								Author
O	K	H		filtrate or lysate				live organism				
				pig	calf	lamb	rabbit	pig	calf	lamb	rabbit	
8	87; 88ab	19	pig	33/40	—	—	—	+	—	—	—	Gyles and Barnum (1969)
8	87; 88ab		pig	—	—	—	—	8/8	1/1	1/1	1/1	Smith and Halls (1967a)
8	87; 88ab	19	pig	+	—	—	+	—	—	—	3/15	Moon *et al.* (1970)
8	87; 88ac	19	pig	10/13	—	—	—	+	—	—	—	Gyles and Barnum (1969)
8	87; 88ac	?	pig	3/5	—	—	—	+	—	—	—	Gyles and Barnum (1969)
8	87; 88ac	?	pig	4/7	—	—	—	+	—	—	—	Gyles and Barnum (1969)
8	87; 88ac		pig	—	—	—	—	9/9	1/1	1/1	0	Smith and Halls (1967a)
8	87; (B)		pig	+	—	—	—	+	—	—	—	Truszezynski and Pilaszek (1969)
8	?;		calf	—	—	—	—	0	+	—	—	Smith and Halls (1967b)
138	81;	?	pig	0/10	—	—	—	+	—	—	—	Gyles and Barnum (1969)
138	81; 88ac	19	pig	7/8	—	—	—	+	—	—	—	Gyles and Barnum (1969)
138	81;		pig	+	+	—	—	36/37	13/14	1/1	0	Smith and Halls (1967a)
138	81; 88ac		pig	—	—	—	—	4/4	—	—	—	Smith and Halls (1967a)
138	81; (B)		pig	+	—	—	—	+	—	—	—	Truszezynski and Pilaszek (1969)
141	85ab, ac	4	pig	7/7	—	—	—	+	—	—	—	Gyles and Barnum (1969)
141[a]	85ab, ac		pig	—	—	—	—	17/18	4/5	2/2	0	Smith and Halls (1967a)

141	85 ab; 88 ac	4	pig	3/5	—	—	—	+	—	—	—	GYLES and BARNUM (1969)
141	85 ab; 88 ab		pig	+	+	—	—	13/13	4/4	3/3	4/4	SMITH and HALLS (1967a)
141	85 ac; 88 ab	4	pig	5/5	—	—	—	+	—	—	—	GYLES and BARNUM (1969)
141	85 ac;		pig	—	—	—	—	13/13	2/2	1/1	0	SMITH and HALLS (1967a)
141	85 ab (B)		pig	+	—	—	—	+	—	—	—	TRUSZEZYNSKI and PILASZEK (1969)
147	89; 88 ac	19	pig	4/5	—	—	—	+	—	—	—	GYLES and BARNUM (1969)
147	89; 88 ac		pig	—	—	—	—	9/9	1/1	2/2	2/2	SMITH and HALLS (1967a)
147	?; 88 ac	19	pig	6/6	—	—	—	+	—	—	—	GYLES and BARNUM (1969)
147	?; 88 ac	19	pig	6/6	—	—	—	+	—	—	—	GYLES and BARNUM (1969)
149	91; 88 ac	10	pig	8/10	—	—	—	+	—	—	—	GYLES and BARNUM (1969)
115[b]	?; 88 ac	10	pig	4/5	—	—	—	+	—	—	—	GYLES and BARNUM (1969)
139[c]	82; (B)		pig	+	—	—	—	+	—	—	—	TRUSZEZYNSKI and PILASZEK (1969)
101	u460 A	NM	pig	—	—	—	+	—	—	—	5/15	MOON et al. (1970)
101	?		calf	—	—	—	—	3/3	1/1	0	0	SMITH and HALLS (1967b)
9	9		calf	0	+	—	—	2/2	2/2	0	0	SMITH and HALLS (1967b)
9	?		pig	—	—	—	—	2/2	2/2	2/2	0	SMITH and HALLS (1967a)
A1	Al; 88 ac		pig	—	—	—	—	28/28	1/1	2/2	—	SMITH and HALLS (1967a)
45	?; 88 ac		pig	—	—	—	—	8/8	4/4	—	—	SMITH and HALLS (1967a)

[a] SMITH and HALLS found only 1/23 positive responses with strains of this serotype (filtrate).
[b] Related to this strain.
[c] ?Plasmid transmitted.

that chronic diarrhea can be associated with over-population of the upper small bowel by *E. Coli* organisms. Some of these patients had clinical, roentgenographic, and morphological changes consistent with tropical sprue.

Production of E. Coli Enterotoxin

SMITH and HALLS (1967b) cultured enterotoxigenic *E. Coli* strains on soft agar, with glucose added, for 24 hours at 37° C with straining of fluid through muslin followed by centrifugation and acetone precipitation of the supernatant. The deposit when dissolved in water represented the enterotoxin. KOHLER (1968) cultured strains in Syncase broth for 18 hours; the filtered broth supernatant represented the heat stable enterotoxin and the filtered supernatant of the sonic lysate of centrifuged cells represented the heat labile enterotoxin. GYLES and BARNUM (1969) used agitated 3 % peptone water, with glucose and buffer (pH 7.8) salts added, and incubated growth for 7 hours at 37° C followed by centrifugation and filtration through 0.45-μ membrane filters. MOON *et al.* (1970) used both agitated and stationary trypticase soy broth and media with incubation for 20 hours at 37° C followed by centrifugation and filtration through 0.45 μ millipore membrane filters. Enterotoxin production varied with the incubation time, the greatest extracellular amount being present after $1/_2$–3 days incubation and then decreasing until there was little present after 8 days incubation (SMITH and HALLS, 1967b).

Properties of E. Coli Enterotoxin

Two forms of enterotoxin, one heat stable and the other heat labile, have been described (GYLES and BARNUM, 1969; SMITH and GYLES, 1970a). The heat stable enterotoxin was mainly an extracellular product and its pig intestinal loop dilatation properties were not neutralized by specific antisera; the heat labile enterotoxin was more consistently associated with bacterial cell lysates than with culture supernatants and was neutralized by specific antisera (SMITH and HALLS, 1967b).

All strains of *E. Coli* enteropathogenic for pigs produced heat stable toxin but only those naturally possessing the K88 antigen produced heat labile enterotoxin (SMITH and GYLES, 1970a). Because production of both of these enterotoxins was controlled by a transmissable plasmid (Ent) which always transmitted both enterotoxins together to recipient strains and because there was no essential difference in the pig intestinal loop responses or in the diarrheal syndrome with oral feeding to piglets following the administration of either type of enterotoxin, these authors concluded that the heat stable and the heat labile enterotoxins were essentially two different forms of the same enterotoxin. Contrary to these findings are the observations that a greater proportion of enteropathogenic strains of *E. Coli* produced heat labile rather than heat stable enterotoxins (GYLES and BARNUM, 1969). Similarly, not all entero-pathogenic strains studied by TRUSZEZYNSKI and PILASZEK (1969) were observed to produce heat stable enterotoxin. It is conceivable that strain variations or the different enterotoxin production methods employed by the various investigators may have contributed to these discrepant results.

Differences have been noted between heat stable and heat labile enterotoxins (SMITH and GYLES, 1970b; KOHLER, 1971). The heat labile enterotoxins prepared from *E. Coli* strains which were enteropathogenic for pigs, produced a stronger rabbit gut dilatatory effect than that with the heat stable forms (SMITH and GYLES, 1970b). The heat labile enterotoxin appears to be a larger molecule and to cause death by endotoxic shock in contrast to the inability of the small molecular sized heat stable enterotoxin to produce endotoxin poisoning (KOHLER, 1971). Neither of the two forms of enterotoxin were observed to cause significant morphological changes following intragastric administration to gnotobiotic pigs (KOHLER and CROSS, 1969).

Both enterotoxins are resistant to trypsin and to absorption by Kaolin and aluminium oxide. The heat stable enterotoxin is resistant to methanol treatment but is susceptible to ethanol, acetone, chloroform and butanol treatment (KOHLER, 1971). The heat-labile enterotoxin is non-dialyzable and precipitable with ammonium sulfate (GYLES and BARNUM, 1969). Properties ascribed to different enterotoxin preparations are shown in Table 6. No enterotoxin effects were attributable to endotoxic extracts, the polysaccharide K antigen or to the K88 antigen (GYLES and BARNUM, 1969).

Skin permeability factors have not been detected in the heat labile enterotoxins of *E. Coli* strains isolated from humans with severe acute diarrheal disease (GLEW *et al.*, 1969; SACK *et al.*, 1971) nor in the heat stable enterotoxins enteropathogenic for pigs (SMITH and HALLS, 1968; MOON and WHIPP, 1971). However, a crude, heat-labile enterotoxin preparation of strain *E. Coli* 263-BA serotype 08:K87, K88a, b:H19, in addition to causing enterosorption of fluid in pigs, rabbits and dogs, also caused both increased vascular permeability in rabbit dermis with an associated acute inflammatory response and rat foot edema (MOON and WHIPP, 1971). This crude preparation may have contained some endotoxin which is known to have some skin toxicity under certain conditions (LARSON *et al.*, 1960). However, in contrast to endotoxin which is heat stable, the dermal toxicity of the enterotoxin preparation from *E. Coli* strain 263-BA was heat labile presumably indicating the activity is not due to endotoxin.

Transmissability of Ent Factor

A transmissable genetic factor (ENT), responsible for enterotoxin production, occurs in some strains of *E. Coli* of porcine origin (SMITH and HALLS, 1968). This factor could be transmitted independently of other transmissable factors such as drug resistance (SMITH, 1966; SMITH and ARMOUR, 1966) and hemolysin (SMITH and HALLS, 1967a). It is capable of being transmitted from

Table 6. *Properties of E. Coli enterotoxin*

	Sack et al. (1971)	Smith and Halls (1967b)	Gyles and Barnum (1969)	Moon et al. (1970)	Kohler (1971)
Enteric activity	yes	yes	yes	yes	yes
Skin activity	none	NT	NT	yes[c]	
Dialyzability	none	none	none	none	
Heat susceptibility	labile	stable: 100° 30° labile: 121° 2 hr.	labile[b]	labile	stable and labile
Ammonium sulfate precipitation	yes		yes	NT	
Immunogenic	yes		yes[a]	NT	
Lethal effect (mice)		none			
Trypsin sensitivity			None		
Effect of lyophilization				none	

NT = Not tested.

[a] Cross reacts with V. cholerae enterotoxin.

[b] One strain gave heat labile and heat stable enterotoxins.

[c] Moon and Whipp 1971 (1 strain only).

enterotoxigenic *E. Coli* strains to other strains of the same species as well as to *Salmonella typhimurium* and *S. cholerasuis* by conjugation in mixed culture (Smith and Halls, 1968).

(Ent) is probably another example of a plasmid. Possession of it by an organism is a stable characteristic; it is not lost during laboratory cultivation, acriflavine treatment or residence in the alimentary tract of pigs or mice (Smith and Halls, 1968). Ent⁺ organisms could not be differentiated from Ent⁻ ones, morphologically, culturally or antigenically. However, Ent⁺ *E. Coli* organisms produced diarrhea in piglets but Ent⁻ organisms of the same strain did not. Non-enterotoxigenic strains of *E. Coli, S. typhimurium* and *S. Cholerasuis* given Ent⁺, as well as the individual donor strains, provoked a positive loop response in pig and calf intestine but not in those of rabbit or mouse (Smith and Halls, 1968).

Pathogenesis

Since recognition of the role of enterotoxin in the pathogenesis of cholera (Dutta *et al.*, 1959), similar interest has developed in *E. Coli* mediated diarrhea (Taylor *et al.*, 1958; Taylor *et al.*, 1961) and many investigators have provided laboratory evidence that some enteropathogenic strains produce enterotoxins whereas non-enteropathogenic strains do not (SMITH and HALLS, 1967; KOHLER, 1968; GYLES, 1968; GYLES and BARNUM, 1968, 1969; KOHLER and CROSS, 1969; TRUSZEZYNSKI and PILASZEK, 1969; MOON *et al.*, 1970). However, not all enteropathogenic strains of *E. Coli* produce their enteropathogenicity by the formation of enterotoxins. Some *E. Coli* organisms produce their effects as a result of their invasive capabilities (SAKAZAKI *et al.*, 1967; OGAWA *et al.*, 1968; FORMAL *et al.*, 1971; DUPONT *et al.*, 1971). The latter organisms produce a shigella-like disease, cross react with shigellae (EDWARDS and EWING, 1962) and have biochemical properties similar to shigellae (DUPONT *et al.*, 1971; OGAWA *et al.*, 1968; SAKAZAKI *et al.*, 1967).

The very recent studies of DUPONT *et al.* (1971) and FORMAL *et al.* (1971) in experimental animals and in volunteers attempt to clarify some concepts of the pathogenesis of *E. Coli* mediated diarrhea. These authors have provided evidence both *in vitro* and *in vivo* that some strains of *E. Coli* have the capability to invade the intestinal mucosa and produce diarrhea associated with a febrile enteritis similar to that seen in dysentery but without apparent proliferation of the organism in the upper small bowel. Other strains produce a diarrhea which is not associated with fever or enteritis, is associated with the organisms capability to proliferate in the upper small bowel and to produce an enterotoxin. The latter resembles that situation which obtains in cholera enterotoxin mediated diarrhea in that it is a non-febrile disease without observable changes in the intestinal mucosa associated with over-population of the upper small bowel by the organism.

Similarly, there are insufficient pathological changes to explain the mechanism of fluid loss in enteric infection due to certain strains of *E. Coli* which are enteropathogenic for young pigs and serologically different from strains pathogenic for humans (SMITH and JONES, 1963; KOHLER and BOHL, 1966a; KOHLER, 1967; KOHLER and CROSS, 1969; MOON *et al.*, 1966; MOON *et al.*, unpublished data). The pathogenetic mechanism involved was originally suggested to be anaphylactic (THOMLINSON, 1963) but STEVENS (1963) considered that the diarrhea was related to toxic products of the organism which GYLES (1966) indicated were not likely to be endotoxin. Endotoxic extracts (GYLES and BARNUM, 1969; SMITH and HALLS, 1967b; TRUSZEZYNSKI and PILASZEK, 1969) and intact K88 antigen (GYLES and BARNUM, 1969) failed to produce a positive rabbit loop response. SMITH and HALLS (1967a) and MOON *et al.* (1966) demonstrated the enteropathogenicity of the live organisms in the ligated anterior but not posterior intestinal loops of pigs, calves and lambs but only occasionally in the rabbit. The enteropathogenicity of the organisms was subsequently shown by many investigators to be associated with their capability to produce an enterotoxin (SMITH and HALLS, 1967b; GYLES and BARNUM, 1969; MOON *et al.*, 1970; KOHLER and CROSS, 1969) without attendant morphological changes in the intestinal mucosa. This is in contrast to the acute inflammatory changes noted in the intestinal mucosa of domestic animals after exposure to invasive strains of *E. Coli* (STALEY *et al.*, 1969a, b, 1970; KENWORTHY 1970); DRUCKER *et al.*, 1967).

Thus, it is apparent that *E. Coli* mediated acute diarrheal disease in both the domestic and experimental animal may be caused by two distinct mechanisms with distinctly differing effects on the intestinal mucosa; one due to the invasive properties of the organism and the other due to its capability to over-populate the upper small bowel and to produce an enterotoxin.

Pathology

The effects of the *E. Coli* enterotoxigenic strains on human intestinal function are self-limited and are as follows: 1) extensive replacement of the normal bowel flora and population of the upper small bowel by the offending organism, 2) patients with toxigenic strains in their small bowel have net secretion and fluid accumulation into the small intestinal lumen, and 3) the toxigenic strains disappear from the bowel, sometimes within 24–36 hours after the onset of diarrhea; the bowel flora returns to normal composition and distribution and the mucosa regains its normal absorptive function by 6–8 days after onset of the disease (Gorbach *et al.*, 1971; Banwell *et al.*, 1971; Dupont *et al.*, 1971). Net intestinal secretion of isotonic fluid occurred in approximately 50% of patients with acute "undifferentiated" diarrhea studied by Banwell *et al.* (1971) and was seen to be greater in the jejunum than in the ileum and also greater in those patients with specific enterotoxigenic strains of *E. Coli* than in those with mixed *E. Coli* organisms as their predominant intestinal flora. In both groups of patients there was upper jejunal overgrowth by the respective groups of *E. Coli* organisms and no morphological changes were seen in mucosal biopsies of jejunum, ileum, or rectum.

Little pathological change has been described in the intestinal mucosa as a result of exposure to *E. Coli* enterotoxins. Dupont *et al.* (1971) failed to observe any significant histopathological change in the guinea pig ileum or conjunctiva, rabbit intestinal loop, monkey intestine or human rectal biopsy following administration of enterotoxigenic strains or of their enterotoxins. This was in sharp contrast to the effects seen with those *E. Coli* strains which mediated their pathogenicity through their invasive qualities in which the mucosa was severely damaged in all experimental models. An intense acute inflammatory reaction occurred within 7 hours, confirming the earlier observations of Ogawa *et al.* (1968).

Moon *et al.* (unpublished data) found no significant light or electron-microscopic evidence of change in either the pig jejunum or rabbit ileum following exposure to the enterotoxin prepared from the strain *E. Coli* 08:K87, K88a, b:H19 or to *Vibrio cholerae* enterotoxin other than goblet cell discharge. No evidence of epithelial or endothelial cell damage was seen. Kohler and Cross (1969) also observed the absence of histopathological change in gnotobiotic pigs which developed diarrhea after being fed bacterial free broth filtrates of *E. Coli* strain 09:K?:NM. These morphological responses resemble those seen in experimental animals following intestinal exposure to *V. cholerae* enterotoxin (DALLDORF *et al.*, 1969; ELLIOTT *et al.*, 1970; NORRIS and MAJNO, 1968).

Broth culture supernatants of *E. Coli* isolated from patients with acute diarrhea caused net fluid production in rabbit jejunal loops (GLEW *et al.*, 1969; SHERR *et al.*, 1971). Unidirectional flux measurements showed that the enterotoxin containing supernatant caused an increase of mucosal to lumen flux of both sodium and water but had no effect on lumen to mucosal flux (SHERR *et al.*, 1971). The effluents of both rabbit and pig intestinal loops in response to *E. Coli* enterotoxin were similar in composition (MOON *et al.*, 1970). They were not ultrafiltrates of plasma, having a higher pH and higher sodium, potassium, and bicarbonate concentrations than those of plasma. These observations resemble those concerning the characteristics of the fluid secreted by the rabbit intestinal loops in response to cholera enterotoxin (LEITCH and BURROWS, 1968; NORRIS and MAJNO, 1968).

Thus the similar lack of morphological response and the similar electrolyte concentrations of the secreted fluid in response to both *E. Coli* and *V. cholerae* types of enterotoxin suggests that the pathogenetic mechanisms accounting for fluid exsorption in response to both of these enterotoxins may be similar. The observation of SHERR *et al.* (1971) that the fluid response to both of these enterotoxins may be inhibited by cycloheximide further indicates that the site of fluid loss in *E. Coli* mediated acute diarrhea may also involve the crypt epithelium of the small bowel.

Immunology

Relatively little is yet known concerning the antigenic characteristics of *E. Coli* enterotoxins. This must await their chemical purification and characterization. Current crude preparations appear to be weaker antigenically than *V. cholerae* enterotoxin and show little immunological cross reactivity (SACK *et al.*, 1971). GYLES and BARNUM (1969), however, indicated some immunological cross reactivity between *V. cholerae* and *E. Coli* enterotoxins; the enterotoxicity of *V. cholerae* lysate being neutralized by an antiserum prepared against living organisms of strain *E. Coli* 08:K87, 88a, b:H19.

Strains of *E. Coli* enteropathogenic for pigs produced an antigenic heat labile enterotoxin and a non-antigenic heat stable enterotoxin (GYLES and BARNUM, 1969; SMITH and GYLES, 1970a). Antisera prepared against these strains neutralized the gut dilatatory effects of these organisms and appeared to be bactericidal rather than antitoxic in character. These antisera also neutralized the effects of the heat labile but not heat stable enterotoxins of these organisms (SMITH and GYLES, 1970a). Human enteropathogenic strains of *E. Coli* appear to produce immunologically distinct enterotoxins in contrast to the apparently identical serological nature of enterotoxins produced by pig enteropathogenic strains (SMITH and GYLES, 1970b). GYLES and BARNUM (1969) found no such immunological differences in specificity between the

homologous and heterologous antisera prepared against the enterotoxins produced by various strains of *E. Coli* but did observe that antisera prepared
against nonenteropathogenic strains, endotoxin, capsular polysaccharide
and K88 antigen did not neutralize the enterotoxic effects of these strains.

Attempts to vaccinate sows with whole cell lysates from enteropathogenic
strains of *E. Coli* have been largely unsuccessful (KOHLER, 1971). Vaccination
of sows with heat stable enterotoxins did not cause passive transfer of protective
antibodies to piglets nursing such sows when the piglets were challenged with
heat stable enterotoxin from the same strain (KOHLER and BOHL, 1966b).
Epidemiological studies currently in progress which are designed to estimate
the prevalence of both invasive and enterotoxigenic strains of *E. Coli* may
determine whether attempts to establish a vaccine for humans will be feasible
as well as practical.

Comparison of E. Coli and V. Cholerae Enterotoxins

In addition to the similarities which exist between the enterotoxins of
E. Coli and *V. cholerae* organisms, there are similarities between the enterotoxigenic diarrheal states mediated by strains of both organisms (Table 7).
The most important of these are the colonization of the upper small intestinal
tract by the organism and the production by the organism of a filterable
toxic moiety which causes a non-febrile, non-inflammatory diarrheal disease
in man, a natural host, and reproduces the pathophysiological fluid exsorption
when instilled into the intestinal lumen of the appropriate experimental animal
without observable changes in the intestinal mucosal architecture. Such
similarities indicate that there may be a common mechanism by which the
small bowel secretes isotonic fluid in response to bacterial enterotoxin stimulation. This is in concert with the apparent limited capacity of the intestine to
respond to injury (SPRINZ, 1969, 1971).

There are also significant differences between acute *E. Coli* diarrhea and
acute cholera. The small volume of diarrheal fluid lost, the lesser severity and
the shorter duration of symptoms establish the former as being a much milder
disease. This may be related to a more rapid clearance of enterotoxigenic
E. Coli organisms from the bowel—sometimes within 24–36 hours as against
4–8 days in cholera (GORBACH *et al.*, 1970). Enterotoxins prepared from
E. Coli organisms appear to be antigenically weaker than those obtained from
various strains of *V. cholerae*. The ileum is considerably less sensitive to *E. Coli*
enterotoxin than is the jejunum in contrast to the effectivity of *V. cholerae*
enterotoxin throughout the small bowel. The genetic factor controlling *E. Coli*
enterotoxicity is transmissable to other species of organism but to date no
such phenomenon has been demonstrated with the *V. cholerae* organism.
However, it remains a distinct possibility that transmissability of the diarrheagenic factor between *V. cholerae*, *E. Coli* and indeed other bacterial species
may occur.

Table 7. Comparison of Clinical Effects and properties of Enterotoxins of *V. Cholerae* and *E. Coli*

	V. Cholerae enterotoxin	*E. Coli* enterotoxin
A. Clinical effects		
Duration of disease	$++++$[a]	$++$[a]
Severity of disease	$++++$	$++$
Diarrhea	$++++$	$++$
Fever	none	none
Dehydration (severe)	common	rare
Shock and death	occasional	no
Upper small bowel colonization	yes	yes
Time of clearance of organism from bowel	4–8 days	24–36 hr.
Intestinal mucosal inflammation	none	none
B. Biological effects		
Fluid production in experimental models	yes	yes
Fluid production inhibited by cycloheximide	yes	yes
Increased skin permeability	yes	no[b]
Effect on other tissues	yes	not tested
Transmissability under genetic control	not tested	yes
Intestinal mucosal alteration	no	no
Characteristics of secreted fluid	similar	similar
C. Properties		
Protein nature	yes	yes
Effect of heat	labile	labile and stable
Dialyzability	yes	yes
Effect of freezing and thawing	no	no
Effect of proteolytic enzymes	no	no
Immunogenicity	yes	yes
Production in vitro	yes	yes

[a] Arbitrary signs of degree.
[b] One strain has been shown to cause increased skin permeability.

Clostridium Perfringens Enterotoxin

C. perfringens is one of the primary causes of food poisoning abroad (HOBBS *et al.*, 1953). In England and Wales where all types of food poisoning outbreaks are reportable, this organism was incriminated in as many outbreaks as was *staphylococcus aureus* (VERNON, 1965). Though food poisoning is not a reportable disease in the United States recent estimates based on reports received by the Center for Disease Control since 1966 indicate that *C. perfringens* is second only to *staphylococcus aureus* in occurrence as a causitive agent of food borne disease outbreaks of bacterial origin (GANGAROSA and DONADIO, 1970). Food poisoning caused by strains of this organism produces a mild diarrhea usually occurring 6—24 hours after ingestion of food containing large numbers of organisms.

Development of Experimental Knowledge

Many pathogenetic mechanisms have been postulated. A transient mild infection was suggested because cell free culture filtrates and cultures heated at 100° C did not produce food poisoning symptoms when fed to human volunteers whereas live cultures or suspensions of one of three cultures did produce symptoms (Dische and Elek, 1957). Dack *et al.* (1954), however, failed to produce symptoms in human volunteers fed culture filtrates or whole broth cultures. Nygren (1962) suggested that phosphorylcholine, a product resulting from the hydrolysis of lecithin in the presence of alphatoxin (lecithinase C) of *Clostridium perfringens* was the etiological agent. Such contentions were not confirmed in mice or monkeys (Weiss *et al.*, 1966), rabbits (Duncan *et al.*, 1968) or lambs (Hauschild *et al.*, 1968) and a 500 mg oral dose produced no ill effects in a human volunteer (Dack, 1964).

Though enteritis has been experimentally produced in humans with cells of *C. perfringens* (Dische and Elek, 1957; Hauschild and Thatcher, 1968), studies of pathogenesis of clostridial food poisoning have been hampered until recently by the lack of a suitable laboratory animal experimental model. Guinea pigs and frogs were found insensitive to intragastric or intraduodenal challenge and oral administration of cultures to monkeys produced only an occasional loose stool (Hobbs *et al.*, 1953). However, the enteropathogenicity of strains of *C. perfringens* isolated from food poisoning outbreaks has been experimentally demonstrated by the production of diarrhea (Duncan and Strong, 1969a; Hauschild *et al.*, 1967) and dilatation of ligated ileal loops (Duncan *et al.*, 1968; Hauschild *et al.*, 1968, 1970b) in both the rabbit and the lamb and there was good correlation in both species between the occurrence of diarrhea and intestinal loop dilatation.

Duncan and Strong (1969b) observed that cell extracts and concentrated culture filtrates as well as the whole cells from which they were derived caused fluid accumulation in rabbit ileal loops and overt diarrhea when injected into normal rabbit ileum. The toxic factor was present in cell free preparations of cells grown in sporulation media but not from those grown in asporogenic media.

Factors Affecting Diarrheagenesis

The capability to produce diarrhea was shown to depend on the strain utilized, since strains isolated from sources other than those associated with food poisoning were not diarrheagenic. The cultural methods employed were also important for production of diarrheagenic properties contained in the organisms and in their extracts. Skim milk was the culture medium which most commonly provided growth of organisms which caused positive reactions while veal broth, fluid thioglycollate, nutrient broth and 5 % tryptone were far less effective media (Duncan *et al.*, 1968). The organisms proliferated within both challenged and control intestinal loops to an extent far in excess of the numbers inoculated, but the fluid accumulation within the loop was

not related to the degree of organism proliferation and negative loop responses
were not due to the organism's failure to survive or proliferate (DUNCAN *et al.*,
1968).

Vegetative and sporulating cells of *C. perfringens* behave differently both
in ligated intestinal segments and whole intestines (HAUSCHILD *et al.*, 1970b).
In both systems vegetative cells which result from growth on Fluid Thioglycollate medium require the presence of fresh medium for their activity
whereas sporulating cells grown on sporulating media do not. Sporulating cells
cause diarrhea within 2 to 2.5 hours of intraduodenal inoculation whereas
with vegetative cells the onset occurs between 6 and 12 hours. This difference
may be attributed to the fact that vegetative cells do not contain appreciable
amounts of preformed enterotoxin but do produce such a factor *in situ* (HAU-
SCHILD *et al.*, 1970a) which may be related to the capability of such cells to
sporulate *in vivo* (HAUSCHILD *et al.*, 1970b). HAUSCHILD *et al.* (1970b) showed
that concentrated supernatant fluids from vegetative cultures had no effect
on ligated lamb intestinal loops but that cell extracts from sporulating cultures
of *C. perfringens* Type A caused extensive accumulation of fluid which was
completely inhibited by rabbit immune sera against these extracts.

Preparation and Properties of Enterotoxin

According to the methods of DUNCAN and STRONG (1969b) strains of
C. perfringens Type A isolated from feces of food poisoning cases or from
incriminated foods were initially activated by culture on Fluid Thioglycollate
medium and then transferred to DS sporulation medium (DUNCAN and STRONG,
1968) and incubated at 37° C for three hours. The extract was prepared either
by sonification of the harvested cells followed by centrifugation and Seitz
filtration or by Seitz filtration of the concentrated culture supernatants and
dialysis against Carbowax 20,000 (polyethylene glycol) at 4° C. Similar methods
were employed by HAUSCHILD *et al.* (1970a). Diarrheagenic factors for rabbits
were contained in sonicated extracts of cells cultured for 3 to 24 hours on
sporogenic media, but only in the supernatants of 24 hour or older cultures
on such media (DUNCAN and STRONG, 1969b). On the other hand, such preparations obtained from cultures grown on Fluid Thioglycollate media were
not enterotoxic.

The enterotoxic activity of organisms grown on sporulation media is non-
dialyzable and heat labile (10 min at 60° C) (DUNCAN and STRONG, 1969b;
HAUSCHILD *et al.*, 1970b). Its protein nature is indicated by the facts that it is
precipitable by ammonium sulfate (HAUSCHILD *et al.*, 1970b) and is destroyed
by pronase (DUNCAN and STRONG, 1969b). It retains its activity when stored
at temperatures between 37° C and −21° C. It has maximal activity between
pH 6.0 and pH 11.0, and is inactive at pH 1.0 and at pH 12.0. It is resistant
to trypsin, lipase and amylase (DUNCAN and STRONG, 1969b). It is of large
molecular weight and is antigenic. Immune sera prepared against the enterotoxic factor from sporulating cells completely inhibit the action of that factor

in ligated intestinal loops but do not inhibit that due to whole cells in the gut lumen (HAUSCHILD *et al.*, 1970b).

Pathology

The histological changes reported by DUNCAN *et al.* (1968) ranged from marked villous destruction to "effacing of villi" in association with inoculation of *C. perfringens* organisms producing fluid accumulation in and dilatation of ligated rabbit ileal loops. These authors did not report on the time sequence relationships of morphological alterations to fluid accumulation and dilatation, thereby obviating the evaluation of possible secondary effects of vascular stasis and pressure necrosis due to long standing dilatation. Such effects have been described in intestinal loops inoculated with *E. Coli* organisms for periods longer than 18 hours (TAYLOR *et al.*, 1958; MOON *et al.*, 1966).

Pathogenesis

The mechanism by which *C. perfringens* enterotoxin causes diarrhea is not known. Strains of *C. perfringens* do produce factors which stimulate adenyl cyclase activity in frog erythrocyte membranes (ROSEN and ROSEN, 1970) and mimic the effects of dibutyryl cyclic 3',5'-AMP, an analogue of cyclic 3',5'-AMP, on the thyroid gland (MACCHIA *et al.*, 1967). There is to date no evidence that the action of *C. perfringens* enterotoxin on the small intestinal mucosa is identical to that of *V. cholerae* enterotoxin. Nevertheless, there is now sufficient indication for further study of cellular mechanisms which incorporate cell bound enzyme pathways potentially involved in intestinal mucosal fluid secretion and which are susceptible to activation by bacterial products of *C. perfringens*.

Shigella Dysenteriae Enterotoxin

Neurotoxicity associated with an infection by *shigella* organisms but independent of their presence in affected tissues was first noted by CONRADI (1903) and confirmed by FLEXNER and SWEET (1906). The neurotoxin was shown to be separate from endotoxin (OLITSKY and KLIGLER, 1920; MCCARTNEY and OLITSKY, 1923) and to be highly potent when purified (VAN HEYNINGEN and GLADSTONE, 1953).

Diarrheal disease associated with *shigella* organisms has generally been considered due to the bacterial invasion of the mucosa (LABREC and FORMAL, 1961; LABREC *et.al.*, 1964; FORMAL *et al.*, 1965, 1966; TAKEUCHI *et al.*, 1965, 1968). Inoculation of ligated rabbit intestinal loops with different serological types of living *Shigella* organisms produced fluid accumulation within 12 hours (ARM *et al.*, 1965). Irrespective of the serological *Shigella* type an acute inflammatory response similar to that in human bacillary dysentery was seen. The tissue response and exudate accumulation preceded demonstrable increase in numbers of *shigella* organisms. The capability of provoking response was noted only with freshly isolated living organisms. The susceptibility was also apparently seasonably variable and positive responses were not elicited during the summer months (ARM *et al.*, 1965). TAYLOR and WILKINS (1961) noted that recently isolated strains of *S. Sonnei* gave a consistent positive intestinal response in contrast to the variable response with *S. flexneri*.

KEUSCH *et al.* (1970) recently observed that at least one strain, designated MK-102, of *Sh. dysenteriae I*, isolated from a patient in Guatemala with severe dysentery, produced an enterotoxin capable of causing fluid exsorption in the rabbit intestinal loop. These authors originally suggested that the mucosal invasion may be required for bacterial growth and consequent enterotoxin production. Since then a partially purified shigella enterotoxin preparation has been isolated.

Production and Purification of Enterotoxin

Enterotoxin production occurred with growth or the strain for 18 hours at 37° C in either aerated Schaedler's broth or a low molecular dialysate of 3 % peptone broth shake culture. It was partially purified by millipore membrane filtration (0.22 µ pore size) of the centrifuged supernatant of broth cultures followed by pressure dialysis through Amicon UM-10 and XM-50 membranes, sephadex G-150 gel filtration and DEAE Sephadex column chromatography (KEUSCH *et al.*, 1970).

Properties

The resultant enterotoxin was heat and acid labile with an indicated molecular size of approximately 50,000. It was an active diarrheagenic agent *in vivo* in submicrogram quantities causing the accumulation of a mucoid fluid in ligated rabbit intestinal loops, the ileum being the most responsive segment of the gut. Concentration of sodium and potassium in secreted fluid did not vary with time, but concentrations of chloride increased and those of bicarbonate and other anions fell. The protein concentration was much higher and volume of fluid response was much lower than that seen with *V. cholerae* enterotoxin under similar circumstances. The enterotoxin possessed heat labile neurotoxicity for mice (lethal dose greater than 50 µg) but did not demonstrate the capability to cause increased skin permeability in rabbit or guinea pig.

The administration of non-invasive enterotoxigenic Shiga vaccine strains was not associated with adverse reaction in volunteers given oral doses of 10^9 to 10^{11} vaccine organisms (LEVINE *et al.*, 1971). These authors concluded that the enterotoxin did not play a major role in the pathogenesis of Shiga dysentery in man and suggested that live attenuated oral vaccines may be more beneficial in the control of dysentery than toxoid vaccines. Nevertheless, too little is known as yet concerning the possible role of *Shigella* enterotoxins to permit sweeping generalized conclusions concerning its role in diarrheagenesis.

When the results of the morphological response of the mucosa following exposure to the toxin are described, investigations concerning the possible relationships between the organism's invasive and enterotoxigenic properties and their dual or sequential effects on the mucosa should be feasible. Clarification of the identity of neurotoxic and enterotoxigenic factors should also be of interest. Neurotoxin had no apparent effect on isolated segments of monkey small or large intestine when 10,000–20,000 monkey intravenous LD_{50} doses were inoculated intraluminally (Branham *et al.*, 1953). Evidence exists that *Shigella Shigae* exotoxin increased the permeability of the blood brain barrier to inorganic phosphate in the mouse, an animal species which is susceptible to the neurotoxic effect, but not in the nonsusceptible rat (Stulc, 1966).

Pseudomonas Aeruginosa Enterotoxin

Pseudomonas aeruginosa has long been implicated in diarrheal disease (Williams and Cameron, 1894). It has been recently suggested that this organism's capacity to cause diarrhea may be related to its capability to produce an enterotoxin. Kubota and Liu (1971) demonstrated that both the 18 hour broth culture of whole organisms and the 10-fold concentrated supernatant of culture fluids of various strains of *Pseudomonas aeruginosa* virulent for mice following intraperitoneal injection, caused dilatation of the rabbit ligated ileal loop. These animals usually died within 24–36 hours. At autopsy there was focal necrosis of the liver, severe pulmonary edema and hemorrhage, and focal hemorrhage in the kidneys. Cardiac blood at death was sterile indicating that tissue damage was caused by extracellular toxins. The morphological response of the intestinal mucosa following exposure to such preparations was not described. Strains which were not virulent for mice and strains which had been heat killed irrespective of the virulence of the live organism gave negative results. The pathological changes in the liver and lungs of rabbits were apparently not due to the enterotoxin alone because they could be produced with purified preparations of the lethal toxin inoculated into the ligated ileal loop without evoking fluid accumulation (Kubota and Liu, 1971).

The crude enterotoxin(s) appeared to be distinct from other toxic moieties of the organism such as hemolysin, protease, lecithinase (phospholipase C) or the lethal toxin, since purified preparations of these materials failed to induce a positive loop response. The enterotoxic activity was precipitable with ammonium sulfate, was abolished by boiling or by treatment with trypsin and the activity was apparently lost during attempts to purify it.

Acknowledgement

The helpful advice, valued criticism and constant support of Helmuth Sprinz, M. D., Director, Division of Experimental Pathology, Walter Reed Army Institute of Research, Washington, D. C., during the preparation of this manuscript is gratefully acknowledged.

References

AL-AWQATI, Q., CAMERON, J. L., FIELD, M., GREENOUGH, W. B. III: Response of human ileal mucosa to choleragen and theophylline. J. clin. Invest. **49**, 2a (1970a).
— FIELD, M., PIERCE, N. F., GREENOUGH, W. B.: Effect of prostaglandin E_1 (PGE$_1$) on electrolyte transport in rabbit ileal mucosa. J. clin. Invest. **49**, 2a (1970b).
— GREENOUGH, W. B., CARPENTER, C. C. J.: Ethacrynic acid inhibits gut fluid loss in cholera. Clin. Res. **17**, 422 (1969).
ARM, H. G., FLOYD, T. M., FABER, J. E., HAYTES, J. R.: Use of ligated segments of rabbit small intestine in experimental shigellosis. J. Bact. **89**, 803–809 (1965).
AVENA, R. M., BERGDOLL, M. S.: Purification and some physicochemical properties of enterotoxin C, *staphylococcus aureus* strain 361. Biochemistry **6**, 1474–1480 (1967).
BAIRD-PARKER, A. C., JOSEPH, R. L.: Fractionation of staphylococcal enterotoxin B. Nature (Lond.) **202**, 570–571 (1964).
BAKER, A. L., KAPLAN, M. M., KIMBERG, D. V., PIERCE, N. F.: Stimulation of rat liver enzyme activity by intravenous cholera toxin. Gastroenterology **60**, 739 (1971).
BANWELL, J. G., GORBACH, S. L., PIERCE, N. F., MITRA, R., MONDAL, A.: Acute undifferentiated human diarrhea in the tropics. II. Alterations in intestinal fluid and electrolyte movements. J. clin. Invest. **50**, 890–900 (1971).
— PIERCE, N. F., MITRA, R. C., BRIGHAM, K. L., CARANASOS, G. J., KEIMOWITZ, R. I., FEDSON, D. S., THOMAS, J., GORBACH, S. L., SACK, R. B., MONDAL, A.: Intestinal fluid and electrolyte transport in human cholera. J. clin. Invest. **49**, 183–195 (1970).
BASU, S., PICKETT, M. J.: Chinchilla: A new host for choleragenic vibrios. Bact. Proc. p. 75 (1969).
— ROBINSON, R. L., PICKETT, M. J.: Preliminary studies on the bioassay of anti-cholera vaccines in chinchillas. J. infect. Dis. **121**, Suppl. S 56–S 57 (1970).
BASU MALLICK, K. C., BANNERJEE, P. L., MALLICK, D. C., GHOSH, E., MONDAL, A.: Active principles in cholera stool. Indian J. med. Res. **57**, 983–987 (1969).
— GANGULI, N. C.: Some observations on the pathogenesis of cholera. Indian J. med. Res. **52**, 894–901 (1964).
BAYLESS, T. M., LUEBBERS, E., ELLIOTT, H. L.: Immature jejunal crypts: Absence of response to stimulus for fluid secretion. Gastroenterology **60**, 762 (1971).
BENENSON, A. S., MOSLEY, W. H., FAHIMUDDIN, M., OSEASOHN, R. O.: Cholera vaccine field trials in East Pakistan. 2. Effectiveness in the field. Bull. Wld Hlth Org. **38**, 359–372 (1968c).
— SAAD, A., MOSLEY, W. H.: Serological studies in cholera. 2. The vibriocidal antibody response of cholera patients determined by a microtechnique. Bull. Wld Hlth Org. **38**, 277–285 (1968b).
— — — AHMED, A.: Serological studies in cholera. 3. Serum toxin neutralization — rise in titre in response to infection with *vibrio cholerae* and the level in the "normal" population of East Pakistan. Bull. Wld Hlth Org. **38**, 287–295 (1968a).
BENGTSSON, S., BERG, R., DANIELSSON, D., LANDMARK, K. M., NORBRING, F., SANDLER, O.: En vattenburen epidemi med enteropatagena *Escherichia* coli. Lakartidningen **63**, 4499–4506, 1966.
BENYAJATI, C.: Experimental cholera in humans. Brit. med. J. **1966 I**, 140–142.
BERGDOLL, M. S.: Immunization of rhesus monkeys with enterotoxoid B. J. infect. Dis. **116**, 191–196 (1966).
— Enterotoxins, In: Microbial toxins: Bacterial protein toxins. Edit. MONTIE, T. C., KADIS, S., and AJL, S. J. Vol. II, p. 265–326. New York: Academic Press 1970.
— BORJA, C. R., AVENA, R. M.: Identification of a new enterotoxin as enterotoxin C. J. Bact. **90**, 1481–1485 (1965).

Bergdoll, M. S., Sugiyama, H., Dack, G. M.: Staphylococcal enterotoxin purification. Arch. Biochem. **85**, 62–69 (1959).
— Weiss, K. F., Muster, M. J.: The production of staphylococcal enterotoxin by a coagulase negative microorganism. Bact. Proc. p. 12 (1967).
Bhattacharya, P. K., Chowdhury, J. R., Datta, A. G.: Studies on the inhibitory effect of erythrose on the development of experimental cholera. Brit. med. J. 2, **1965 II, 1351.**
Bhoola, K. D., Calle, J. D., Schachter, M.: The effect of bradykinin, serum kallikrein and other endogenous substances on capillary permeability in the guinea pig. J. Physiol. (Lond.) **152**, 75–86 (1960).
Borja, C. R., Bergdoll, M. S.: Purification and partial characterization of enterotoxin C produced by *staphylococcus aureus* strain 137. Biochem. (Wash.) **6**, 1467–1473 (1967).
— — Staphylococcal enterotoxin C. II. Some physical, immunological, and toxic properties. Biochemistry **8**, 75–79 (1969).
Bowden, J. P.: A method of preparing small quantities of ^{14}C-labelled staphylococcal enterotoxin B. Biochim. Biophys. Acta (Amst.) **168**, 150–152 (1968).
Branham, S. E., Dack, G. M., Riggs, D. B.: Studies with *shigella dysenteriae* (Shiga). IV. Immunological reactions in monkeys to the toxins in isolated intestinal pouches. J. Immunol. **70**, 103–113 (1953).
Braun, O. H., Henckel, H.: Säuglingsenteritis durch pathogene Colitypen, insbesondere E. Coli 55/B₅. Z. Kinderheilk. **70**, 273–285 (1952).
Breckenridge, J. C., Bergdoll, M. S.: Foodborne gastroenteritis due to coagulase negative staphylococcus. New Engl. J. Med. **284**, 541–543 (1971).
Burrows, W.: Cholera toxins.: Ann. Rev. Microbiol. **22**, 245–268 (1968).
— Toward an effective prophylactic immunity to cholera. J. infect. Dis. **12**, Suppl. S 58–S 61 (1970).
— Musteikis, G. M., Oza, N. B., Dutta, N. K.: Cholera toxins: Quantitation of the frog skin reaction and its relation to experimental enteric toxicity. J. infect. Dis. **115**, 1–8 (1965).
— Wagner, S. M., Mather, A. N.: The endotoxin of the cholera vibrio: Action on living semipermeable membranes. Proc. Soc. exp. Biol. (N.Y.) **57**, 311–314 (1944).
Butcher, R. W., Baird, C. E.: Effects of prostaglandins on adenosine 3'5' monophosphate levels in fat and other tissues. J. biol. Chem. **243**, 1713–1717 (1968).
— Sutherland, E. W.: Adenosine 3'5' phosphate in biological material. I. Purification and properties of cyclic 3'5' nucleotide phosphodiesterase and use of this enzyme to characterize adenosine 3'5' phosphate in human urine. J. biol. Chem. **237**, 1244–1250 (1962).
Carpenter, C. C. J.: Cholera enterotoxin – recent investigations yield insights into transport processes. Amer. J. Med. **50**, 1–7 (1971).
— Barua, D., Sack, R. B., Wallace, C. K., Mitra, P. P., Khanra, S. R., Werner, T. S., Duffy, T. E., Oleinick, A.: Clinical studies in Asiatic cholera. V. Shock producing acute diarrheal disease in Calcutta: A clinical and biochemical comparison of cholera with severe non-cholera diarrhea 1963–1964. Bull. Johns Hopk. Hosp. **118**, 230–242 (1966).
— Chaudhuri, R. N., Mondal, A.: A simple effective therapy of cholera. Indian J. med. Res. **52**, 924–932 (1964).
— Curlin, G. T., Greenough, W. B. III.: Response of canine thiry-vella jejunal loops to cholera exotoxin and its modification by ethacrynic acid. J. infect. Dis. **120**, 332–338 (1969 b).
— Greenough, W. B. III.: Response of the canine duodenum to intraluminal challenge with cholera exotoxin. J. clin. Invest. **47**, 2600–2607 (1968).
— — Sack, R. B.: The relationship of superior mesenteric artery blood flow to gut electrolyte loss in experimental cholera. J. infect. Dis. **119**, 182–193 (1969 a).

CARPENTER, C. C. J., SACK, R. B., FEELEY, J. C., STEENBURG, R. W.: Site and characteristics of electrolyte loss and effect of intraluminal glucose in experimental canine cholera. J. clin. Invest. **47**, 1210–1220 (1968).
CASMAN, E. P.: Further serological studies of staphylococcal enterotoxin. J. Bact. **79**, 849–856 (1960).
— Staphylococcal enterotoxin. Ann. N.Y. Acad. Sci. **128**, 124–131 (1965).
— BENNETT, R. W.: Culture medium for the production of staphylococcal enterotoxin A. J. Bact. **86**, 18–23 (1963).
— — Detection of staphylococcal enterotoxin in food. Appl. Microbiol. **13**, 181–189 (1965).
— — DORSEY, A. E., ISSA, J. A.: Identification of a fourth staphylococcal enterotoxin, enterotoxin D. J. Bact. **94**, 1875–1882 (1967).
— BERGDOLL, M. S., ROBINSON, J.: Designation of staphylococcal enterotoxins. J. Bact. **85**, 715–716 (1963).
CHEN, L. C., ROHDE, J. E., SHARP, G. W. G.: Intestinal adenylcyclase activity in human cholera. Lancet **1971 I**, 939–941.
CHOWDHURY, R. J., DATTA, A. G.: Studies on the growth inhibitory effect of erythrose on *vibrio cholerae*. Biochim. biophys. Acta (Amst.) **104**, 296–298 (1965).
CHU, F. S.: Hydrogen ion equilibria of staphylococcal enterotoxin B. J. biol. Chem. **243**, 4342–4349 (1968).
— CRARY, E., BERGDOLL, M. S.: Chemical modification of amino groups in staphylococcal enterotoxin B. Biochemistry **8**, 2890–2896 (1969).
— THADHANI, K., SCHANTZ, E. J., BERGDOLL, M. S.: Purification and characterization of staphylococcal enterotoxin A. Biochemisty **5**, 3281–3289 (1966).
CLARKE, W. G., VANDERHOOFT, G. F., BORISON, H. L.: Emetic effect of purified staphylococcal enterotoxin in cats. Proc. Soc. exp. Biol. (N.Y.) **111**, 205–207 (1962).
COHNHEIM, J. F.: Lectures on general pathology. A handbook for practitioners and students. Section III. The pathology of digestion (1882) (translated from the second German edition by A. B. MCKEE). New Syndenhan Soc. (Lond.) **133**, 949–960 (1890).
COLEMAN, W. H., KAUR, J., IWERT, M. E., KASAI, G. J., BURROWS, W.: Cholera toxins: Purification and preliminary characterization of ileal loop reactive type 2 toxin. J. Bact. **96**, 1137–1143 (1968).
CONRADI, H.: Über lösliche, durch aseptische Autolyse erhaltene Giftstoffe von Ruhr- und Typhusbazillen. Dtsch. med. Wschr. **29**, 26–28 (1903).
COSTIN, I. D., VOICULESCU, D., GORCEA, V.: An outbreak of food poisoning in adults associated with *E. coli* serotype O 86:B 7:H 34. Path. et Microbiol. (Basel) **27**, 68–78 (1964).
COTILLO, L. G.: Tentativas de inhibicion de la sintesis de enterotoxina estafilococcia por penicilina y estreptomicina. Rev. Saude Publ. S. Paulo **1**, 188–192 (1967).
COTRAN, R. S., MAJNO, G.: The delayed and prolonged vascular leakage in inflammation. I. Topography of the leaking vessels after thermal injury. Amer. J. Path. **45**, 261–181 (1964).
CRABBÉ, P. A., NASH, D. R., BAZIN, H., EYSSEN, H., HEREMANS, J. F.: Antibodies of the IgA type in intestinal plasma cells of germfree mice after oral or parenteral immunization with ferritin. J. exp. Med. **130**, 723–744 (1969).
CRAIG, J. P.: A permeability factor (toxin) found in cholera stools and culture filtrates and its neutralization by convalescent cholera sera. Nature (Lond.) **207**, 614–616 (1965 a).
— The effect of cholera stool and culture filtrates on the skin of guinea pigs and rabbits. In: Proceedings of the Cholera Research Symposium USPHS Publication 1328, p. 153–158. Washington, D. C.: U. S. Government Printing Office 1965 b.
— Preparation of the vascular permeability factor of *vibrio cholerae*. J. Bact. **92**, 793–795 (1966).

CRAIG, J. P.: Some observations on the neutralization of cholera vascular permeability factor *in vivo*. J. infect. Dis. **121**, S100–S110 (1970).
— Cholera toxins. Microbial toxins: Bacterial Protein Toxins, vol. IIA, p. 189–254. New York: Academic Press 1971.
CRAMBLETT, H. G., AZIMI, P., and HAYNES, R. E.: The etiology of infectious disease in infancy with special reference to enteropathogenic *E. coli*. Ann. N.Y. Acad. Sci. **176**, 80–92 (1971).
CRAWLEY, G. J., BLACK, J. N., GRAY, I., BLANCHARD, J. W.: Clinical chemistry of staphylococcal enterotoxin poisoning in monkeys. Appl. Microbiol. **14**, 445–450 (1966a).
— GRAY, I., LE BLANG, W. A., BLANCHARD, J. W.: Bloodbinding, distribution and excretion of staphylococcal enterotoxin in monkeys. J. infect. Dis. **116**, 48–56 (1966b).
CURLIN, G. T., CARPENTER, C. J.: Antitoxic immunity to cholera in isolated perfused canine ileal segmants. J. infect. Dis. **121**, Suppl. S132–S136 (1970).
— CHEN, L. C.: Cholera toxin stimulation of rat lipocyte adenyl cyclase activity. Clin. Res. **19**, 456 (1971).
— CRAIG, J. P., SUBONG, A., CARPENTER, C. C. J.: Antitoxic immunity in experimental canine cholera. J. infect. Dis. **121**, 463–470 (1970).
— SUBONG, A., CRAIG, J. P., CARPENTER, C. C. J.: Antitoxic immunity in experimental canine cholera. Trans. Ass. Amer. Phycns **81**, 314–322 (1968).
DACK, G. M.: Food poisoning. Chicago: Chicago University of Press 1956.
— Microbial Food Poisoning. Food Technol. **18**, 1904–1906 (1964).
— JORDAN, E. O., WOOLPERT, O.: Attempts to immunize human volunteers with staphylococcus filtrates that are toxic to man when swallowed. J. Prevent. Med. (Baltimore) **5**, 151–159 (1931).
— SUGIYAMA, H., OWENS, F. J., KIRSNER, J. B.: Failure to Produce Illness in Human Volunteers Fed *Bacillus Cereus* and *Clostridium Perfringens*. J. infect. Dis. **94**, 34–38 (1954).
DALIDOWICZ, J. E., SILVERMAN, S. J., SCHANTZ, E. J., STEFANYE, D., SPERO, L.: Chemical and biological properties of reduced and alkylated staphylococcal enterotoxin B. Biochemistry **5**, 2375–2381 (1966).
DALLDORF, F. G., KEUSCH, G. T., LIVINGSTON, H. L.: Transcellular permeability of capillaries in experimental cholera. Amer. J. Path. **57**, 153–170 (1969).
DANIELSSON, D., LAURRELL, G., SJOLIN, S.: An outbreak of diarrhea due to enteropathogenic *E. coli* studied by means of fluorescent antibody identification and conventional bacteriological culture. Acta paediat. scand. **54**, 432–438 (1965).
DE, S. N.: Enterotoxicity of bacteria-free culture filtrates of *vibrio cholerae*. Nature (Lond.) **183**, 1533–1534 (1959).
— BHATTACHARYA, K., SARKAR, J. K.: A study of the pathogenicity of strains of *bacterium coli* from acute and chronic enteritis. J. Path. Bact. **71**, 201–209 (1956).
— CHATTERJE, D. N.: An experimental study of the mechanism of action of *vibrio cholerae* on the intestinal mucous membrane. J. Path. Bact. **66**, 559–562 (1953).
— GHOSE, M. L., CHANDRA, J.: Further observations on cholera enterotoxin. Trans. Roy. Soc. Trop. Med. Hyg. **56**, 241–245 (1962).
— — SEN, A.: Activities of bacteria-free preparations from *vibrio cholerae*. J. Path. Bact. **79**, 373–380 (1960).
DEYCKE, G.: Über histologische und bacilläre Verhältnisse im Choleradarm: Dtsch. med. Wschr. **18**, 1048–1049 (1892).
DISCHE, F. E., ELEK, S. D.: Experimental Food Poisoning by *Clostridium Welchii*. Lancet **1957 II**, 71–74.
DOLMAN, C. E.: Ingestion of staphylococcus exotoxin by human volunteers. J. infect. Dis. **55**, 172–183 (1934).
— Bacterial food poisoning. Canad. J. publ. Hlth **34**, 205 (1943).

DOLMAN, C. E.: Antigenic properties of staphylococcus enterotoxin. Canad. J. publ. Hlth 35, 337–351 (1944).
— WILSON, R. J.: Experiments with staphylococcal enterotoxin. J. Immunol. 35, 13–30 (1938).
— — Kitten test for staphylococcus enterotoxin. Canad. pub. Hlth J. 31, 68–71 (1940).
DORNBUSCH, K., HALLANDER, H. O., LOFQUIST, F.: Extrachromosomal control of methicillin resistance and toxin production in *staphylococcus aureus*. J. Bact. 98, 351–358 (1969).
DREES, D. T., WAXLER, G. L.: Enteric *colibacillosis* in gnotobiotic swine: An electron microscopic study. Amer. J. vet. Res. 31, 1160–1171 (1970).
DRUCKER, M. M., YEIVIN, R., SACKS, T. G.: Pathogenesis of *Escherichia coli* enteritis in the ligated rabbit gut. Israel J. med. Sci. 3, 445–452 (1967).
DUHAMEL, R. C., TALBOT, P., GRADY, G. F.: Production, purification and assay of cholera enterotoxin. J. infect. Dis. 121, Suppl. S85–S91 (1970).
DUNCAN, C. L., STRONG, D. H.: Improved Medium for Sporulation of *Clostridium Perfringens*. Appl. Microbiol. 16, 82–89 (1968).
— — Experimental Production of Diarrhea in Rabbits with *Clostridium Perfringens*. Canad. J. Microbiol. 15, 765–770 (1969a).
— — Ileal Loop Fluid Accumulation and Production of Diarrhea in Rabbits by Cell-Free Products of *Clostridium Perfringens*. J. Bact. 100, 86–94 (1969b).
— SUGIYAMA, H., STRONG, D. H.: Rabbit Ileal Loop Response to Strains of *Clostridium Perfringens*. J. Bact. 95, 1560–1566 (1968).
DUPONT, H. L., FORMAL, S. B., HORNICK, R. B., SNYDER, M. J., LIBONATI, J. P., SHEAHAN, D. G., LABREC, E. H., KALAS, J. P.: Pathogenesis of *Escherichia coli* diarrhea. New Engl. J. Med. 285, 1–9 (1971).
DUTT, A. R.: Enterotoxic activity in cholera stool. Indian J. med. Res. 53, 605–609 (1965).
— Study of ligated rabbit-gut segment and its content after introduction of *v. cholerae* and its culture filtrate. Indian J. med. Res. 54, 431–436 (1966).
— Serological studies in cholera. Indian J. med. Res. 55, 299–307 (1967).
— MONDAL, A., DE, S. N.: Some observations on the pathology of cholera intestine. Indian J. med. Res. 52, 902–907 (1964).
DUTTA, N. K., HABBU, M. K.: Experimental cholera in infant rabbits: A method for chemotherapeutic investigation. Brit. J. Pharmacol. 10, 153–159 (1955).
— OZA, N. B.: The effect of gastointestinal enzymes on cholera toxin. Bull. Wld Hlth Org. 28, 307–310 (1963).
— PANSE, M. V., KULKARNI, D. R.: Role of cholera toxin in experimental cholera. J. Bact. 78, 594–595 (1959).
EDWARDS, P. R., EWING, W. H.: Identification of enterobacteriaceae. Second. ed. Minneapolis: Burgess Publishing Co. 1962.
ELDER, J. M., MILES, A. A.: The action of the lethal toxins of gas gangrene clostridia on capillary permeability. J. Path. Bact. 74, 133–145 (1957).
ELLIOTT, H. L., CARPENTER, C. C., SACK, R. B., YARDLEY, J. H.: Small bowel morphology in experimental canine cholera. A light and electron microscopic study. Lab. Invest. 22, 112–120 (1970.)
EVANS, J. B., BEUTTNER, L. G., NIVEN, C. F., JR.: Evaluation of the coagulase test in the study of staphylococci associated with food poisoning. J. Bact. 60, 481–484 (1950).
EVANS, D. J., RICHARDSON, S. H.: Nutritional factors governing the production of an ion translocase inhibitor by *vibrio cholerae*. Bact. Proc. p. 88 (1967).
— — *In vitro* production of choleragen and vascular permeability factory by *vibrio cholerae*. J. Bact. 96, 126–130 (1968).
EWING, W. H., DAVIS, B. R., MONTAGUE, T. J.: Studies on the occurrence of *E. coli* serotypes associated with diarrheal disease. National Communicable Disease Center, Atlanta, Georgia (1963).

Favorite, G. O., Hammon, W. McD.: Production of staphylococcus enterotoxin and alpha hemolysin in simplified medium. J. Bact. **41**, 305–316 (1941).

Feeley, J. C., Roberts, C. O.: Immunological responses of laboratory animals to cholera vaccines, toxin and toxoid. Tex. Rep. Biol. Med. **27**, 213–226 (1969).

Felsenfeld, O., Burrows, W., Kasai, G. J., Greer, W. E., Jiricka, Z.: The cellular immune response of non-human primates to crude type 2 cholera toxin. J. infect. Dis. **118**, 491–499 (1968).

— Nasuniya, N.: Staphylococcal antitoxin values in the sera of permanent residents and visitors in Thailand. J. trop. Med. Hyg. **67**, 300–303 (1964).

Ferguson, W. W., June, R. C.: Experiments on feeding adult volunteers with *Escherichia coli* III, B₄, a coliform organism associated with infant diarrhea. Amer. J. Hyg. **55**, 155–169 (1952).

Field, M.: Intestinal secretion: Effect of cyclic AMP and its role in cholera. New Engl. J. Med. **284**, 1137–1144 (1971).

— Fromm, D., Wallace, C. K., Greenough, W. B. III.: Stimulation of active chloride secretion in small intestine by cholera exotoxin. J. clin. Invest. **48**, 24a (1969).

— Plotkin, G. R., Silen, W.: Effects of vasopressin, theophylline and cyclic adenosine monophosphate on short circuit current across isolated rabbit ileal mucosa. Nature (Lond.) **217**, 469–471 (1968).

Finegold, M. J.: Interstitial pulmonary edema. An electron microscopic study of the pathology of staphylococcal enterotoxemia in Rhesus monkeys. Lab. Invest. **16**, 912–924 (1967).

Finkelstein, R. A.: Antitoxic immunity in experimental cholera: Observations with purified antigens and the ligated ileal loop model. Infect. Immun. **1**, 464–467 (1970).

— Atthasampunna, P.: Immunity against experimental cholera. Proc. Soc. exp. Biol. (N.Y.) **125**, 465–469 (1967).

— — Chulasamaya, M., Charunmethee, P.: Pathogenesis of experimental cholera: Biologic activities of purified procholeragen A. J. Immunol. **96**, 440–449 (1966b).

— Hollingsworth, R. C.: Antitoxic immunity in experimental cholera: Observations with purified antigens and the rat foot edema model. Infec. Immun. **1**, 468–473 (1970).

— Jehl, J. J., Goth, A.: Pathogenesis of experimental cholera: Choleragen induced rat foot edema; a method of screening anticholera drugs. Proc. Soc. exp. Biol. (N.Y.) **132**, 835–840 (1969).

— LoSpalluto, J. J.: Pathogenesis of experimental cholera. Preparation and isolation of choleragen and choleragenoid. J. exp. Med. **130**, 185–202 (1969).

— — Production of highly purified choleragen and choleragenoid. J. infect. Dis. **121**, S64–S72 (1970).

— Mukerjee, S., Rudra, B. C.: Demonstration and quantitation of antigen in cholera stool filtrates. J. infect. Dis. **113**, 99–104 (1963).

— Norris, H. T., Dutta, N. K.: Pathogenesis of experimental cholera in infant rabbits. I. Observations on the intraintestinal infection and experimental cholera produced with cell free products. J. infect. Dis. **114**, 203–216 (1964).

— Nye, S. W., Atthasampunna, P., Charunmethee, P.: Pathogenesis of experimental cholera: Effect of choleragen on vascular permeability. Lab. Invest. **15**, 1601–1609 (1966c).

— Sobocinski, P. Z., Atthasampunna, P., Charunmethee, P.: Pathogenesis of experimental cholera; identification of choleragen (Procholeragen A) by disc immunoelectrophoresis and its differentiation from cholera mucinase. J. Immunol. **96**, 440–449 (1966a).

Flexner, S., Sweet, J. E.: The pathogenesis of experimental colitis and the relation of colitis in animal and man. J. exp. Med. **8**, 514–535 (1906).

Fordtran, J. S.: Speculations on the pathogenesis of diarrhea. Fed. Proc. **26**, 1405–1414 (1967).

Formal, S. B., Dammin, G., Sprinz, H., Kundel, D., Schneider, H., Horowitz, R. E., Forbes, M.: Experimental shigella infections. V. Studies in germ-free guinea pigs. J. Bact. **82**, 284–287 (1961).

— Dupont, H. L., Hornick, R., Snyder, M. J., Libonati, J., Labrec, E. H.: Experimental models in the investigation of the virulence of dysentery bacilli and *Escherichia coli*. Ann. N. Y. Acad. Sci. **176**, 190–196 (1971).

— — Kent, T. H., Austin, S., Labrec, E. H.: Fluorescent—Antibody and histologic study of vaccinated and control monkeys challenged with *shigella flexneri*. J. Bact. **91**, 2368–2376 (1966).

— Kundel, D., Schneider, H., Kunev, N., Sprinz, H.: Studies with *vibrio cholerae* in the ligated loop of the rabbit intestine. Brit. J. exp. Path. **42**, 504–510 (1961).

— Labrec, E. H., Schneider, H.: Pathogenesis of bacillary dysentery in laboratory animals. Fed. Proc. **24**, 29–34 (1965).

Fraenkel, E.: Über Choleraleichenbefunde. Dtsch. med. Wschr. **19**, 157–159 (1893).

Frea, J. I., McCoy, E., Strong, F. M.: Purification of type B staphylococcal enterotoxin. J. Bact. **86**, 1308–1313 (1963).

Freeman, J. A.: Fine structure of the goblet cell mucosus secretory process. Anat. Rec. **144**, 341–345 (1962).

Fresh, J. W., Versage, P. M., Reyes, V.: Intestinal morphology in human and experimental cholera. United States Naval Medical Research Report. MR 005.09 to 1040.1.12, 1–10 (1963).

— — — Intestinal morphology in human and experimental cholera. Arch. Path. **77**, 529–537 (1964).

Freter, R.: Coproantibody and bacterial antagonism as protective factors in experimental enteric cholera. J. exp. Med. **104**, 419–426 (1956).

— Comparison of immune mechanisms in various experimental models of cholera. Bull. Wld Hlth Org. **31**, 825–834 (1964).

— Smith, H. L., Sweeney, F. J.: An evaluation of intestinal fluids in the pathogenesis of cholera. J. infect. Dis. **109**, 35–42 (1961).

Friedman, M. E.: Inhibition of staphylococcal enterotoxin B formation in broth cultures. J. Bact. **92**, 277–278 (1966).

— Inhibition of staphylococcal enterotoxin B formation by cell wall blocking agents and other compounds. J. Bact. **95**, 1051–1055 (1968).

— Howard, M. B.: Induction of mutants of *staphylococcus aureus* 100 with increased ability to produce enterotoxin A. J. Bact. **106**, 289–291 (1971).

— White, J. D.: Immunofluorescent demonstration of cell-associated staphylococcal enterotoxin B. J. Bact. **89**, 1155 (1965).

Fuhrman, F. A., Fuhrman, G. J., Burrows, W.: Action and properties of an inhibitor of active transport of sodium produced by cholera vibrios. J. infect. Dis. **111**, 225–232 (1962).

Fuhrman, G. J., Fuhrman, F. A.: Inhibition of active sodium transport by cholera toxin. Nature (Lond.) **188**, 71–72 (1960).

Fukumi, H., Kosakai, N.: Disease producing effect of coliform organisms. Nikonlji-Shimpo, No 1506, 914 (1954), (cited by Sakazaki et al. 1967).

Gangarosa, E. J., Beisel, W. R., Benyajati, C., Sprinz, H., Piyaratn, P.: The nature of the gastrointestinal lesion in Asiatic cholera and its relation to pathogenesis. A biopsy study. Amer. J. trop. Med. Hyg. **9**, 125–135 (1960).

— Dewitt, W. E., Feeley, J. C., Adams, M. R.: Significance of vibriocidal antibodies with regard to immunity to cholera. J. infect. Dis. **121**, Suppl. S36–S43 (1970).

— Donadio, J. A.: Surveillance of Foodborne Disease in the United States. A Comparison of Data — 1968–1969. J. infect. Dis. **122**, 354–358 (1970).

Gangarosa, E. J., Sanati, A., Saghari, H., Feeley, J. C.: Multiple serotypes of *vibrio cholerae* isolated from a case of cholera. Evidence suggesting *in vivo* mutation. Lancet **1967** I, 646–648.

Genigeorgis, C., Sadler, W. W.: Effect of sodium chloride and pH on enterotoxin B production. J. Bact. **92**, 1383–1387 (1966a).

— — Characterization of strains of *staphylococcus aureus* isolated from livers of commercially slaughtered poultry. Poult. Sci. **45**, 973–980 (1966b).

Glew, R. H., Gorbach, S. L., Sack, R. B., Wallace, C. K.: Gut fluid loss produced by culture filtrates of *E. coli* isolated from the small bowel of patients with acute diarrhea. Clin. Res. **17**, 368–369 (1969).

Goldstein, P., Mandle, R. J., Wirts, C. W., Dammin, G. J.: Chronic "nonspecific" coliform diarrhea in Philadelphia. Gastroenterology **60**, 669 (1971).

— Merril, T. G., Sprinz, H.: Experimental cholera: Morphological evidence of cytotoxicity. Arch. Path. **82**, 54–59 (1966).

Goodpasture, E. W.: Histopathology of intestine in cholera. Philipp. J. Sci. **22**, 413–424 (1923).

Gorbach, S. L.: Acute diarrhea—A "toxin" disease? New Engl. J. Med. **283**, 44–45 (1970).

— Intestinal microflora. Gastroenterology **60**, 1110–1128, 1971.

— Banwell, J. G., Chatterjee, B. D., Jacobs, B., Sack, R. B.: Acute undifferentiated diarrhea in the tropics. I. Alterations in intestinal microflora. J. clin. Invest. **50**, 881–889 (1971).

— Neale, G., Levitan, R., Hepner, G. W.: Alterations in human intestinal microflora during experimental diarrhea. Gut **11**, 1–6 (1970).

Gordon, R. S. Jr.: The failure of Asiatic cholera to give rise to "exudative enteropathy". In: SEATO conference on cholera, Bangkok, p. 54 (1962).

Gordon, R. S.: Intestinal secretory mechanisms in cholera. Symposium on cholera, Unzen, Nagasaki, National Institute of Health, Tokyo, p. 106 (1969).

Grady, G. F., Chang, M. C.: Cholera enterotoxin free from permeability factor? J. infect. Dis. **121**, Suppl. S92–S95 (1970).

Graybill, J. R., Kaplan, M. M., Pierce, N. F.: Hormone-like effects of cholera exotoxin. Clin. Res. **18**, 454 (1970).

Grayer, D. T., Serebro, H. A., Iber, F. L., Hendrix, T. R.: Effect of cycloheximide on unidirectional sodium fluxes in the jejenum after cholera toxin exposure. Gastroenterology **58**, 815–819 (1970).

Greenough, W. B. III, Carpenter, C. C. J., Bayless, T. M., Hendrix, T. R.: The role of cholera exotoxin in the study of intestinal water and electrolyte transport. Progress in gastroenterology, vol. 2 (Jerzy Glass G. B., ed.), p. 236. New York: Grune & Stratton 1970b.

— Pierce, N. F., Al-Awqati, Q., Carpenter, C. C. J.: Stimulation of gut electrolyte secretion by prostaglandins, theophylline and cholera exotoxin. J. clin. Invest. **48**, 32a (1969).

— — Vaughan, M.: Titration of cholera enterotoxin and antitoxin in isolated fat cells. J. infect. Dis. **121**, S111–S113 (1970a).

Gyles, C. L.: The response of ligated loops of pigs intestine to *Escherichia coli*. M. Sc. Thesis, University of Guelph, Canada (1966).

— Enterotoxicity of cell free *Escherichia coli* preparations in ligated segments of pig's intestine. Ph. D. Thesis, University of Guelph, Canada (1968).

— Barnum, D. A.: A heat labile enterotoxin from *Escherichia coli*. Bact. Proc. p. 104 (1968).

— — A heat labile enterotoxin from strains of *Escherichia coli* enteropathogenic for pigs. J. infect. Dis. **120**, 419–426 (1969).

Hakim, A. A., Lifson, N.: Effects of pressure on water and solute transport by dog intestinal mucosa in vitro. Amer. J. Physiol. **216**, 276–284 (1969).

HALL, H. E., ANGELOTTI, R., LEWIS, K. H.: Detection of the staphylococcal enterotoxins in food. Hlth Lab. Sci. 2, 179–191 (1965).
HALLANDER, H. O.: Production of large quantities of enterotoxin B and other staphylococcal toxins on solid media. Acta. path. microbiol. scand. 63, 299–305 (1965).
— BENGTSSON, S.: Studies on the cell toxicity and species specificity of purified staphylococcal toxins. Acta path. microbiol. scand. 70, 107–119 (1967).
— KÖRLOF, B.: Enterotoxin producing staphylococci. Acta path. microbiol. scand. 71, 359–375 (1967).
HARPER, D. T., GRAYER, D. I., YARDLEY, J. H., HENDRIX, T. R.: Reversal of cholera exotoxin-induced jejunal secretion by cycloheximide. Johns Hopk. med. J. 126, 258–266 (1970).
HARTMAN, P. E., GOODGAL, S. H.: Bacterial Genetics (with particular reference to genetic transfer). Ann. Rev. Microbiol. 13, 465–504 (1959).
HAUSCHILD, A. H. W., NIILO, L., DORWARD, W. J.: Experimental enteritis with food poisoning and classical strains of Clostridium Perfringens type A in lambs. J. Inf. Dis. 117, 379–386 (1967).
— — — Clostridium Perfringens type A infection of ligated intestinal loops in lambs. Appl. Microbiol. 16, 1235–1239 (1968).
— — — Enteropathogenic factors of food poisoning Clostridium Perfringens type A. Canad. J. Microbiol. 16, 331–338 (1970a).
— — — Response of ligated intestinal loops in lambs to an enteropathogenic factor of Clostridium Perfringens type A. Canad. J. Microbiol. 16, 339–343 (1970b).
— THATCHER, F. S.: Experimental food poisoning with heat-susceptible Clostridium Perfringens type A. Canad. J. Microbiol. 14, 705–709 (1968).
HAYAMA, T., SUGIYAMA, H.: Comparative resistance of vagotomized monkeys to IV Vs. Intragastric staphylococcal enterotoxin challenges. Proc. Soc. exp. Biol. (N.Y.) 115, 243–246 (1964).
HECKLY, R. J., WOLOCHOW, H.: Characterization and purification of cholera toxin. J. infect. Dis. 121, Suppl. S80–S84 (1970).
HENDRIX, T. R., BANWELL, J. G.: Pathogenesis of cholera. Gastroenterology 57, 751–755 (1969).
— BAYLESS, T. M.: Digestion: Intestinal secretion. Ann. Rev. Physiol. 32, 139–164 (1970).
HEWLETT, E. L., GREENOUGH, W. B. III.: Purified cholera enterotoxin (CT) increases adenyl cyclase (ACY) and adenosine 3'5' cyclic monophosphate (CYAMP) in fat cells. Clin. Res. 19, 459 (1971).
HIRSCHHORN, N., KINNIE, J. L., SACHAR, D. B., NORTHRUP, R. S., TAYLOR, J. O., AHMAD, Z., PHILLIPS, R. A.: Decrease in net stool output in cholera during intestinal perfusion with glucose containing solutions. New Engl. J. Med. 279, 176–181 (1968).
HOBBS, B. C., SMITH, M. E., OAKLEY, C. L., WARRACK, G. H., CRUICKSHANK, J. C.: Clostridium Welchii Food Poisoning. J. Hyg. (Lond.) 51, 75–101 (1953).
HUANG, I. Y., SHIH, T., BORJA, C. R., AVENA, R. M., BERGDOLL, M. S.: Amino acid composition and terminal amino acids of staphylococcal enterotoxin C. Biochemistry (Wash.) 6, 1480–1484 (1967).
HUBER, G. S., PHILLIPS, R. A.: Cholera and the sodium pump. SEATO Conference on Cholera, Dacca. E. Pakistan SEATO, Bangkok, Thailand, p. 37–40 (1962).
IBER, F. L., McGONAGLE, T. J., SEREBRO, H. A., LUEBBERS, E. H., BAYLESS, T. M., HENDRIX, T. R.: Unidirectional sodium flux in small intestine in experimental canine cholera. Amer. J. med. Sci. 258, 340–350 (1969).
JARVIS, A. W., LAWRENCE, R. C.: Production of high titers of enterotoxins for the routine testing of staphylococci. Appl. Microbiol. 19, 698–699 (1970).

June, R. C., Ferguson, W. W., Worfel, M. T.: Experiments in feeding adult volunteers with *Escherichia coli* 55, B$_5$, a coliform organism associated with infant diarrhea. Amer. J. Hyg. **57**, 222–236 (1953).

Kao, V. C. Y., Sprinz, H.: Cholera toxin: Localization of immune response in ligated loops of rabbit ileum. Fed. Proc. **30**, 572 (1971).

— — Burrows, W.: Experimental cholera: Immunohistochemical observations on the localization of toxin in the intestinal mucosa. Gastroenterology **58**, 965 (1970).

Kasai, G. J., Burrows, W.: The titration of cholera toxin and antitoxin in the rabbit ileal loop. J. infect. Dis. **116**, 606–614 (1966).

Kasuma, H., Craig, J. P.: Production of biologically active substances by two strains of *vibrio cholerae*. Infec. Immun. **1**, 80–87 (1970).

Kato, E., Khan, M., Kujovich, L., Bergdoll, M. S.: Production of enterotoxin A. Appl. Microbiol. **14**, 966–972 (1966).

Kaur, J., Burrows, W., Cervavski, L.: Cholera toxins: Immunogenicity of the rabbit ileal loop toxin and related antigens. J. Bact. **100**, 985–993 (1969).

— Shrivastava, J. B.: Further studies on the KS preparation of vibrio polysaccharides. In: Proceedings of the Cholera Research Symposium. PHS Publication 1328, p. 248–253. Washington, D. C.: U.S. Government Printing Office 1965.

Kent, T. H.: Staphylococcal enterotoxin gastroenteritis in rhesus monkeys. Amer. J. Path. **48**, 387–407 (1966).

— Jervis, H. R., Kuhns, J. G.: Enzyme histochemistry of acute staphylococcal enterotoxin gastroenteritis in rhesus monkeys. Amer. J. Path. **48**, 667–681 (1966).

Kenworthy, R.: Effect of *Escherichia coli* on germfree and gnotobiotic pigs. J. comp. Path. **80**, 53–63 (1970).

Keusch, G. T., Atthasampunna, P., Finkelstein, R. M.: A vascular permeability defect in experimental cholera. Proc. Soc. exp. Biol. (N.Y.) **124**, 822–825 (1967).

— Mata, L. J., Grady, G. F.: Shigella enterotoxin: Isolation and Characterizasion. Clin. Res. **18**, 442 (1970).

Kimberg, D. V., Field, M., Johnson, J., Henderson, A., Gershon, E.: Stimulation of intestinal mucosal adenyl cyclase by cholera enterotoxin and prostaglandins. J. clin. Invest. **50**, 1218–1230 (1971).

Kirby, A. C., Hall, E. G., Coackley, W.: Neonatal diarrhea and vomiting outbreaks in the same maternity unit. Lancet **1950 II**, 201–207.

Koch, R.: In: Die Konferenz zur Erörterung der Cholerafrage. Dtsch. med. Wschr. **10**, 499 (1884).

— Über den augenblicklichen Stand der bakteriologischen Choleradiagnose. Z. Hyg. Infect.-Kr. (Lpz.) **14**, 319–338 (1893).

Kohler, E. M.: Studies of *Escherichia coli* in gnotobiotic pigs. IV. Comparison of enteropathogenic and nonenteropathogenic strains. Canad. J. comp. Med. **31**, 277–282 (1967).

— Enterotoxic activity of filtrates of *Escherichia coli* in young pigs. Amer. J. vet. Res. **29**, 2263–2274 (1968).

— Observations on enterotoxins produced by enteropathogenic *Escherichia coli*. Ann. N.Y. Acad. Sci. **176**, 212–219 (1971).

— Bohl, E. H.: Studies of *Escherichia coli* in gnotobiotic pigs. I. Experimental reproduction of *colibacillosis*. Canad. J. comp. Med. **30**, 199–203 (1966a).

— — Studies of Escherichia coli in gnotobiotic pigs. III. Evaluation of orally administered specific antisera. Canad. J. comp. Med. **30**, 233–237 (1966b).

— Cross, R. F.: Studies of *Escherichia coli* in gnotobiotic pigs. VI. Effects of feeding bacteria-free filtrates of broth cultures. Canad. J. comp. Med. **33**, 173–177 (1969).

Koya, G., Kosakai, N., Fukasawa, Y.: Supplementary studies on the multiplications of *Escherichia coli* 0-111 B$_4$ in the intestinal tract of adult volunteers and its relations to manifestation of coli enteritis. Jap. J. med. Sci. Biol. **7**, 655–659 (1954).

KRAFT, A. R., TOMPKINS, R. K., ZOLLINGER, R. M.: Recognition and management of the diarrheal syndrome caused by nonbeta islet cell tumors of the pancreas. Amer. J. Surg. **119**, 163–170 (1970).

KUBOTA, Y., LIU, P. V.: An Enterotoxin of *Pseudomonas Aeruginosa*. J. infect. Dis. **123**, 97–98 (1971).

KUHR, J., BURROWS, W.: Immunity to cholera: Relation of fraction II of type 2 cholera toxin to vibriocidal antibody. J. Bact. **98**, 467–474 (1969).

KURU, M., SUGIHARA, S.: Contributions to the knowledge of bulbar antonomic centres. II. Relationship of the vagal nuclei to the gastrojejunal motility. Appendix: On the vomiting centre. Jap. J. Physiol. **5**, 21–36 (1955).

LABREC, E. H., FORMAL, S. B.: Experimental *shigella* infections. IV. Fluorescent antibody studies of an infection in guinea pigs. J. Immunol. **87**, 562–572 (1961).

— SCHNEIDER, H., MAGNANI, T. J., FORMAL, S. B.: Epithelial cell penetration as an essential step in the pathogenesis of bacillary dysentery. J. Bact. **88**, 1503–1518 (1964).

LANYI, B., SZITA, J., RINGELHANN, B., KOVACH, K.: A water borne outbreak of enteritis associated with *Escherichia coli* serotype 124:72:32. Acta microbiol. Acad. Sci. hung. **6**, 77–84 (1959).

LARSON, C. L., RIBI, E., MILNER, K. C., LIBERMAN, J. E.: A method for titrating endotoxic activity in the skin of rabbits. J. exp. Med. **111**, 1–20 (1960).

LEITCH, G. J., BURROWS, W.: Experimental cholera in the rabbit ligated intestine: Ion and water accumulation in the duodenum, ileum and colon. J. infect. Dis. **118**, 349–359 (1968).

— — STOLLE, L. C.: Experimental cholera in the rabbit intestinal loop: Fluid accumulation and sodium pump inhibition. J. infect. Dis. **117**, 197–202 (1967).

LEVINE, M. M., DUPONT, H. L., FORMAL, S. B., LIBONATI, J. P., GANGAROSA, E. J., SNYDER, M. J., HORNICK, R. B.: An immunologic approach to the control of epidemic shiga dysentery. Clin. Res. **19**, 461 (1971).

LEWIS, A. C., FREEMAN, B. A.: Separation of type 2 toxins of *vibrio cholerae*. Science **165**, 808–809 (1969).

LING, G. N.: Thoughts on the molecular mechanism of the normal intestinal mucosa as a barrier to sodium ion movement and massive fluid loss in cholera. Proc. of the Cholera Research Symposium, Honolulu, 103–106 (1965).

LOSPALLUTO, J., FINKELSTEIN, R. A.: Chemical and physical properties of choleragen and choleragenoid. Fed. Proc. **30**, 304 (1971).

LOVE, A. H. G.: Water and sodium absorption by the intestine in cholera. Gut **10**, 63–67 (1969).

— ROHDE, J. E., VEALL, N.: Studies on bidirectional sodium fluxes across the int estinal mucosa in cholera patients. Gut **11**, 1056–1057 (1970).

MACCHIA, V., BATES, R. W., PASTAN, I.: The Purification and Properties of a Thyroid-Stimulating Factor Isolated from *Clostridium Perfringens*. J. biol. Chem. **242**, 3726–3730 (1967).

MARKUS, Z.: Enterotoxin B synthesis by *staphylococcus aureus* S-6. Bact. Proc. p. 81 (1969).

— SILVERMAN, G. J.: Enterotoxin B. Production by nongrowing cells of *staphylococcus aureus*. J. Bact. **96**, 1446–1447 (1968).

— — Enterotoxin B. Synthesis by replicating and non-replicating cells of *staphylococcus aureus*. J. Bact. **97**, 506–512 (1969).

MARTIN, W. J., MARCUS, S.: Relation of pyrogenic and emetic properties of enterobacteriaceal endotoxin and of staphylococcal enterotoxin. J. Bact. **87**, 1019–1026 (1964).

MCCARTNEY, J. E., OLITSKY, P. K.: Separation of the toxins of *bacillus dysenteriae* shiga. J. exp. Med. **37**, 767–779 (1923).

McLean, R. A., Lilly, H. D., Alford, J. A.: Effects of meat curing salts and temperature on production of staphylococcal enterotoxin B. J. Bact. **95**, 1207–1211 (1968).

McNaught, W., Roberts, G. B. S.: Enteropathogenic effects of strains of *bacterium coli* isolated from cases of gastroenteritis. J. Path. Bact. **76**, 115–158 (1958).

Merrill, T. G., Sprinz, H.: Ultrastructural changes of intestinal capillaries in cholera. Fed. Proc. **25**, 456 (1966).

— — The effect of staphylococcal enterotoxin on the fine structure of the monkey jejunum. Lab. Invest. **18**, 114–123 (1968).

Metchnikoff, E.: Recherches sur le cholera et les vibrions. Ann Inst. Pasteur **8**, 529–589 (1894).

Moon, H. W., Sorensen, D. K., Sautter, J. H.: *Escherichia coli* infection of the ligated intestinal loop of the newborn pig. Amer. J. vet. Res. **27**, 1317–1325 (1966).

— Whipp, S. C.: Systems for testing the enteropathogenicity of *Escherichia coli*. Ann. N.Y. Acad. Sci. **176**, 197–211 (1971).

— — Baetz, A. L.: Response of the intestinal mucosa of pigs and rabbits to *Escherichia coli* enterotoxin: A histologic and ultrastructural study. Unpublished observations cited by Moon and Whipp (1971).

— — Engstrom, G. W., Baetz, A. L.: Response of the rabbit ileal loop to cell free products from *Escherichia coli* enteropathogenic for swine. J. infect. Dis. **121**, 182–187 (1970).

Moritz, M., Iber, F. L., Moore, E. W.: Rabbit cholera: Effects of cycloheximide on net water and ion fluxes and transmural electric potentials. Gastroenterology **60**, 789 (1971).

Morris, E. L., Hodoval, L. F., Beisel, W. R.: The unusual role of the kidney during intoxication of monkeys by intravenous staphylococcal enterotoxin B. J. infect. Dis. **117**, 273–284 (1967).

Morse, S. A., Mah, R. A., Dobrogosz, W. J.: Regulation of staphylococcal enterotoxin B. J. Bact. **98**, 4–9 (1969).

Mosley, W. H., Aziz, K. M. S., Ahmed, A.: Serological evidence for the identity of the vascular permeability factor and ileal loop toxin of *vibrio cholerae*. J. infect. Dis. **121**, 243–250 (1970a).

— Benenson, A. S., Barui, R.: A serological survery for cholera antibodies in rural East Pakistan. 1. The distribution of antibody in the control population of a cholera vaccine field trial area and the relation of antibody titre to the pattern of endemic cholera. Bull. Wld Hlth Org. **38**, 327–334 (1968a).

— — — A serological survey for cholera antibodies in rural East Pakistan. 2. A comparison of antibody titres in the immunized and control populations of a cholera vaccine field trial area and the relation of antibody titre to cholera case rate. Bull. Wld Hlth Org. **38**, 335–346 (1968b).

— Woodward, W. E., Aziz, K. M. A., Mizanur Rahman, A. S. M., Alauddin Chowdhury, A. K. M., Ahmed, A., Feeley, J. C.: The 1968–1969 cholera vaccine field trial in rural East Pakistan. Effectivness of monovalent Ogawa and Inaba vaccines and a purified Inaba antigen with comparative results of serological and animal protection tests. J. infect. Dis. **121** Suppl. S1–S9 (1970b).

Nakanishi, R., Suchi, H., Tajiri, I., Yamasato, M.: An enteropathogenic *Escherichia coli* isolated from patients with ekiri. J. Japan Ass. Infect. Dis. **31**, 169–174 (1956).

Neter, E.: Enteritis due to enteropathogenic *Escherichia coli*. Present day status and unsolved problems. J. Pediat. **55**, 222–239 (1959).

Nielsen, N. O., Sautter, J. H.: Infection of ligated intestinal loops with hemolytic *Escherichia coli* in the pig. Canad. vet. J. **9**, 90–97 (1968).

NORMANN, S. J., JAEGER, R. F., JOHNSEY, R. T.: Pathology of experimental enterotoxemia. The *in vivo* localization of staphylococcal enterotoxin B. Lab. Invest.
20, 17–25 (1969).
NORRIS, H. T., CURRAN, P. F., SCHULTZ, S. G.: Modification of intestinal secretion
in experimental cholera. J. infect. Dis. **119**, 117–125 (1969).
— FINKELSTEIN, R. A., DUTTA, N. K., SPRINZ, H.: Intestinal manifestations of
cholera in infant rabbits. A morphologic study. Lab. Invest. **14**, 1428–1436 (1965).
— MAJNO, G.: On the role of ileal epithelium in the pathogenesis of experimental
cholera. Amer. J. Path. **53**, 263–279 (1968).
— SUMNER, D. S.: Preliminary observations on mucosal blood flow in experimental
cholera. Fed. Proc. **30**, 544 (1971).
NORTHRUP, R. S., BIENENSTOCK, J., TOMASI, T. B., JR.: Immunoglobulins and antibody activity in the intestine and serum in cholera. I. Analysis of immunoglobulins
in cholera stool. J. infect. Dis. **121**, Suppl. S137–S141 (1970).
— HOSSAIN, S. A.: Immunoglobulins and antibody activity in the intestine and
serum in cholera. II. Measurement of antibody activity in jejunal aspirates and
sera of cholera patients by radioimmunidiffusion. J. infect. Dis. **121**, Suppl.
S142–S146 (1970).
NYGREN, B.: Phospholipase C-Producing Bacteria and Food Poisoning. Acta path.
microbiol. scand. (Suppl.) **160**, 1–88 (1962).
OGAWA, H., NAKAMURA, A., SAKAZAKI, R.: Pathogenic properties of "enteropatho-
genic" *Escherichia coli* from diarrheal children and adults. Jap. J. med. Sci.
Biol. **21**, 333–349 (1968).
OLITSKY, P. K., KLIGER, I. J.: Toxins and antitoxins of *bacillus dysenteriae* shiga.
J. exp. Med. **31**, 19–33 (1920).
OMORI, G., KATO, Y.: A staphylococcal food poisoning caused by a coagulase nega-
tive strain. Biken's J. **2**, 92 (1959) (cited by BRECKENRIDGE and BERGDOLL,
1971).
OSEASOHN, R. O., BENENSON, A. S., FAHIMUDDIN, M.: Field trial of cholera vaccine
in rural East Pakistan. Lancet **1965 I**, 450–452.
OZA, N. B., DUTTA, N. K.: Experimental cholera produced by toxin prepared by
ultrasonic disintegration of *vibrio comma*. J. Bact. **85**, 497–498 (1963).
PALMER, E. D.: The morphologic consequences of acute exogenous (staphylococcic)
gastroenteritis on the gastric mucosa. Gastroenterology **19**, 462–475 (1951).
PANSE, M. V., DUTTA, N. K.: Excretion of toxin with stools of cholera patients.
J. infect. Dis. **109**, 81–84 (1961).
PATNAIK, B. K., GHOSH, H. K.: Histopathological studies on experimental cholera.
Brit. J. exp. Path. **47**, 210–214 (1966).
PFEIFFER, R.: Untersuchungen über das Choleragift. Z. Hyg. Infect-Kr. **11**, 393–412
(1892).
PIERCE, N. F., BANWELL, J. G., GORBACH, S. L., MITRA, R. C., MONDAL, A.: Con-
valescent carriers of *vibrio cholerae*. Ann. intern. Med. **72**, 357–364 (1970b).
— — MITRA, R. D., CARANASOS, G. J., KEIMOWITZ, R. I., MONDAL, A., MANJI,
P. M.: Effect of intragastric glucose-electrolyte infusion upon water and electro-
lyte balance in Asiatic cholera. Gastroenterology **55**, 333–343 (1968).
— — SACK, R. B., MITRA, R. C., MONDAL, A.: Magnitude and duration of antitoxic
response to human infection with *vibrio cholerae*. J. infect. Dis. **121**, Suppl.
S31–S35 (1970a).
— CARPENTER, C. C. J., ELLIOTT, H. L., GREENOUGH, W. B. III.: Effects of prostaglandins, theophylline, and cholera exotoxin upon transmucosal water and
electrolyte movement in the canine jejunum. Gastroenterology **60**, 22–32
(1971b).
— GREENOUGH, W. B., CARPENTER, C. C. J.: *Vibrio cholerae* enterotoxin and its
mode of action. Bact. Rev. **35**, 1–13 (1971a).

Pierce, N. F., Hennessey, K. N., Sack, G. H., Jr., Mitra, R. C.: Gastric acidity in cholera. Clin. Res. **19**, 400 (1971 c).
— Sack, R. B., Mitra, R. C., Banwell, J. G., Brigham, K. L., Fedson, D. S., Mondal, A.: Replacement of water and electrolyte losses in cholera by an oral glucose-electrolyte solution. Ann. intern. Med. **70**, 1173–1181 (1969).
Prohaska, J. V.: Role of staphylococcal enterotoxin in the induction of experimental ileitis. Ann. Surg. **158**, 492–497 (1963).
— Development and fate of experimentally induced enteritis. Gastroenterology **51**, 913–925 (1966).
— Jacobson, M. J., Drake, C. T., Tan, T.: Staphylococcus enterotoxin enteritis. Surg. Gynec. Obstet. **109**, 73–77 (1959).
— Long, E. T., Nelson, T. S.: Pseudomembranous enterocolitis; its etiology and mechanism of the disease process. Arch. Surg. **72**, 977–983 (1956).
Raj, H. D., Bergdoll, M. S.: Effect of enterotoxin B on human volunteers. J. Bact. **98**, 833–834 (1969).
Reiser, R. F., Weiss, K. F.: Production of staphylococcal enterotoxins A, B, and C in various media. Appl. Microbiol. **18**, 1041–1043 (1969).
Rhoda, D. A., Elsberry, D. D., Beisel, W. R.: Fluid compartment alterations in the monkey with staphylococcic B enterotoxemia. Amer. J. vet. Res. **31**, 507–514 (1970).
Rosen, O. M., Rosen, S. M.: A bacterial activator of frog erythrocyte adenyl cyclase. Arch. Biochem. **141**, 346–352 (1970).
Rosenwald, A. J., Lincoln, R. E.: Streptomycin inhibition of elaboration of staphylococcal enterotoxic protein. J. Bact. **92**, 279–280 (1966).
Rosner, R.: Antepartum culture findings of mothers in relation to infantile diarrhea. Amer. J. clin. Path. **45**, 732–736 (1966).
Rowe, B., Taylor, J., Bettelheim, K. A.: An investigation of traveller's diarrhea. Lancet **1970 I**, 1–5.
Richardson, S. H.: Inhibition of intestinal ion translocase enzymes by culture filtrates of *vibrio cholerae*. J. Bact. **91**, 1384–1386 (1966).
— Factors influencing *in vitro* skin permeability factor production by *vibrio cholerae*. J. Bact. **100**, 27–34 (1969).
— Evans, D. J., Jr.: Isolation of cholera toxins by dextran sulfate precipitation. J. Bact. **96**, 1443–1445 (1968).
— Noftle, K. A.: Purification and properties of permeability factor/cholera enterotoxin from complex and synthetic media. J. infect. Dis. **121**, Suppl. S73–S79 (1970).
Sack, R. B., Carpenter, C. C. J.: Experimental canine cholera. I. Development of the model. J. infect. Dis. **119**, 138–149 (1969).
— Gorbach, S., Banwell, J. G., Jacobs, B., Chatterjee, B. D.: Enterotoxigenic *Escherichia coli* isolated from patients with severe cholera-like disease. J. infect. Dis. **123**, 378–385 (1971).
Sakazaki, R., Namioka, S.: Studies on a new *Escherichia coli* type. O136:K78 (B22). Jap. J. exp. Med. **27**, 29–36 (1957).
— Tamura, K., Saito, M.: Enteropathogenic *Escherichia coli* associated with diarrhea in children and adults. Jap. J. med. Sci. Biol. **20**, 387–399 (1967).
Salomon, L. L., Tew, R. W.: Assay of staphylococcal enterotoxin B by latex agglutination. Proc. Soc. exp. Biol. (N.Y.) **129**, 539–542 (1968).
Schaeffer, W. I., Gablicks, J., Calitis, R.: Interaction of staphylococcal enterotoxin B with cell cultures of human intestine. J. Bact. **91**, 21–26 (1966).
— — — Interference by trypsin in the interaction of staphylococcal enterotoxin B and cell cultures of human embryonic intestine. J. Bact. **93**, 1489–1492 (1967).

SCHAFER, D. E., BANNERJEE, D., BHARGAVA, U., SENGUPTA, S., SIRCAR, B., THAKUR, A. K.: Rabbit small-bowel response to cell free filtrate of choleraic fluid. Proc. Soc. exp. Biol. (N.Y.) **134**, 90–94 (1970a).
— LUST, W. D., SIRCAR, B., GOLDBERG, M. D.: Elevated concentration of adenosine 3', 5' cyclic monophosphate concentration in intestinal mucosa after treatment with cholera toxin. Proc. nat. Acad. Sci. (Wash.) **67**, 851–856 (1970b).
SCHANTZ, E. J., ROESSLER, W. G., WAGMAN, J., SPERO, L., DUNNERY, D. A., BERGDOLL, M. S.: Purification of staphylococcal enterotoxin B. Biochemistry **4**, 1011–1016 (1965).
SCHROEDER, S. A., CALDWELL, J. R., VERNON, T. M., WHITE, P. C., GRANGER, S. I., BENNETT, J. V.: A waterborne outbreak of gastroenteritis in adults associated with *Escherichia coli*. Lancet **1968I**, 737–740.
SEGALOVE, M.: Effect of penicillin on growth and toxin production by enterotoxic staphylococci. J. infect. Dis. **81**, 228–242 (1947).
SEREBRO, H. A., BAYLESS, T. M., HENDRIX, T. R., IBER, F. L., McGONAGLE, T. M.: Absorption of d-glucose by the rabbit jejunum during cholera toxin-induced diarrhoea. Nature (Lond.) **217**, 1272–1273 (1968b).
— IBER, F. L., YARDLEY, J. H., HENDRIX, T. R.: Inhibition of cholera toxin action in the rabbit by cycloheximide. Gastroenterology **56**, 506–511 (1969).
— McGONAGLE, T. J., IBER, F. L., ROYALL, R., HENDRIX, T. R.: An effect of cholera toxin on small intestine without direct mucosal contact. Johns Hopkins Med. J. **123**, 229–232 (1968a).
SERENEY, B.: Experimental shigella kerato-conjuctivitis. A preliminary report. Acta microbiol.. Acad. Sci. hung. **2**, 293–296 (1955).
SHARP, G. W. G., HYNIE, S.: Stimulation of intestinal adenyl cyclase by cholera toxin. Nature (Lond.) **229**, 266–269 (1971).
SHEAHAN, D. G., JERVIS, H. R., TAKEUCHI, A., SPRINZ, H.: The effect of staphylococcal enterotoxin on the epithelial mucosubstances of the small intestine of rhesus monkeys. Amer. J. Path. **60**, 1–18 (1970).
— SPRINZ, H.: Cholera toxin: Response to intestinal intramural inoculation. Gastroenterology **60**, 716 (1971).
SHEMANO, I., HITCHENS, J. T., BEILER, J. M.: Paradoxical inhibitory effects of staphylococcal enterotoxin. Gastroenterology **53**, 71–77 (1967).
SHERR, H. P., BANWELL, J. G., HENDRIX, T. R.: Pathophysiological characteristics of *E. coli* enterotoxin: A comparison with cholera exotoxin. Clin. Res. **19**, 403 (1971).
SILVERMAN, S. J., ESPESETH, D. A., SCHANTZ, E. J.: Effect of formaldehyde on the immunochemical and biological activity of staphylococcal enterotoxin B. J. Bact. **98**, 437–442 (1969b).
— KNOTT, A. R., HOWARD, M.: Rapid sensitive assay for staphylococcal enterotoxin and a comparison of serological methods. Appl. Microbiol. **16**, 1019–1023 (1968).
— MOORE, G. T., ROESSLER, W. G.: Effect of formaldehyde on the immunogenicity of staphylococcal enterotoxin B for *macaca mulatta*. J. Bact. **98**, 443–446 (1969a).
— SCHANTZ, E. J., ESPESETH, D. A., ROESSLER, W. G.: Effect of formalin on the immunochemical and biological activity of staphylococcal enteroxin. Bact. Proc. p. 43 (1966).
SMITH, D. H.: Salmonella with transferable drug resistance. New Engl. J. Med. **275**, 625–630 (1966).
— ARMOUR, S. E.: Transferable R factors in enteric bacteria causing infections of the genitourinary tract. Lancet **1966II**, 15–18.
SMITH, H. W.: Observations on the aetiology of neonatal diarrhea (Scours) in calves. J. Path. Bact. **84**, 147–168 (1962).
— GYLES, C. L.: *Escherichia coli* enterotoxin. Vet. Rec. **85**, 694 (1969).

SMITH, H. W., GYLES, C. L.: The relationship between two apparently different enterotoxins produced by enteropathogenic strains of *Escherichia coli* of porcine origin. J. Med. Microbiol. **3**, 387–402 (1970a).

— — The effect of cell free fluids prepared from cultures of human and animal enteropathogenic strains of *Escherichia coli* on ligated intestinal segments of rabbits and pigs. J. Med. Microbiol. **3**, 403–409 (1970b).

— HALLS, S.: Observations by the ligated intestinal segment and oral inoculation methods on *Escherichia coli* infections in pigs, calves, lambs and rabbits. J. Path. Bact. **93**, 499–529 (1967a).

— — Studies on *Escherichia coli* enterotoxin. J. Path. Bact. **93**, 531–543 (1967b).

— — The transmissable nature of the genetic factor in *Escherichia coli* that controls enterotoxin production. J. gen. Microbiol. **52**, 319–334 (1968).

— JONES, J. E. T.: Observations on the alimentary tract and its bacterial flora in healthy and diseased pigs. J. Path. Bact. **86**, 387–412 (1963).

SPERO, L., STEFANYE, D., BRECHER, P. I., JACOBY, H. M., DALIDOWICZ, J. E., SCHANTZ, E. J.: Amino acid composition and terminal amino acids of staphylococcal enterotoxin B. Biochemistry **4**, 1024–1030 (1965).

SPRINZ, H.: Morphological response of intestinal mucosa to enteric bacteria and its implication for sprue and Asiatic cholera. Fed. Proc. **21**, 57–64 (1962).

— Pathogenesis of intestinal infections. Arch. Path. **87**, 556–562 (1969).

— Factors influencing intestinal cell renewal. A statement of principles. Cancer (Philad.) **28**, 71–74 (1971).

— SRIBHIBHADH, R., GANGAROSA, E. J., BENYAJATI, C., KUNDEL, D., HALSTEAD, S.: Biopsy of small bowel of Thai people. With special reference to recovery from Asiatic cholera and to an intestinal malabsorption syndrome. Amer. J. clin. Path. **38**, 43–51 (1962).

SPYRIDES, G. J., FEELEY, J. C.: Concentration and purification of cholera exotoxin by absorption on aluminum compound gels. J. infect. Dis. **121**, Suppl. S96–S99 (1970).

STAAB, E. V., NIEDERHUBER, J., RHODA, D. A., FAULKNER, C. S. II, BEISEL, W. R.: Role of the kidney in staphylococcal enterotoxemia. Appl. Microbiol. **17**, 394–398 (1969).

STALEY, T. E., JONES, E. W., CORLEY, L. D.: Intestinal monocontamination in the neonatal pig: Microbiological and microscopic studies in Germfree biology: Experimental and clinical aspects, ed. by E. A. MIRAND and N. BACK, p. 65–73. New York: Plenum Press 1969a.

— — — Attachment and penetretation of *Escherichia coli* into intestinal epithelium of the ileum in newborn pigs. Amer. J. Path. **56**, 371–392 (1969b).

— — — ANDERSON, I. L.: Intestinal permeability of *Escherichia coli* in the foal. Amer. J. vet. Res. **31**, 1481–1483 (1970).

STARK, R. L., MIDDAUGH, P. R.: Immunofluorescent detection of enterotoxin B in food and a culture medium. Appl. Microbiol. **18**, 631–635 (1969).

STEVENS, A. J.: Coliform enteritis in the young pig and a practical approach to the control of enteritis. Vet. Res. **75**, 1241–1246 (1963).

STOERK, O.: Über Cholera. Beitr. path. Anat. **62**, 121–174 (1916).

STRASTERS, K. C., WINKLER, K. C.: Carbohydrate metabolism of *staphylococcus aureus*. J. gen. Microbiol. **33**, 218–229 (1963).

STROMBECK, D. R.: *In vivo* and *in vitro* studies of intestinal fluid production by cholera toxin in the rat. Gastroenterology **60**, 804 (1971).

STULC, J.: The influence of exotoxin *shigella shigae* on the blood brain barrier permeability to inorganic phosphate. Life Sci. **5**, 1801–1808 (1966).

SUGIYAMA, H.: Endotoxin-like responses induced by staphylococcal enterotoxin. J. infect. Dis. **116**, 162–170 (1966).

SUGIYAMA, H., BERGDOLL, M. S., DACK, G. M.: Staphylococcal enterotoxin: increased vomiting incidence in monkeys following subemetic doses of dihydroergotamine. Proc. Soc. exp. Biol. (N.Y.) **97**, 900–903 (1958).
— CHOW, K. L., DRAGSTEDT, L. R. II.: Study of emetic receptor sites for staphylococcal enterotoxin in monkeys. Proc. Soc. exp. Biol. (N.Y.) **108**, 92–95 (1961).
— HAYAMA, T.: Comparative resistance of vagotomised monkeys to intravenous vs. intragastric staphylococcal enterotoxin challenges. Proc. Soc. exp. Biol. (N.Y.) **115**, 243–246 (1964).
— — Abdominal viscera as site of emetic action for staphylococcal enterotoxin in the monkey. J. infect. Dis. **115**, 330–336 (1965).
— McKISSIC, E. M., JR.: Leukocytic response in monkeys challenged with staphylococcal enterotoxin. J. Bact. **92**, 349–352 (1966).
SULLIVAN, R.: Effects of enterotoxin B on intestinal transport *in vitro*. Proc. Soc. exp. Biol. (N.Y.) **131**, 1159–1162 (1969).
SURGALLA, M. J., BERGDOLL, M. S., DACK, G. M.: Some observations on assay of staphylococcal enterotoxin by monkey-feeding test. J. Lab. clin. Med. **41**, 782–788 (1953).
— — — Staphylococcal enterotoxin: neutralization by rabbit antiserum. J. Immunol. **72**, 398–403 (1954).
— DACK, G. M.: Enterotoxin produced by micrococci from cases of enteritis after antibiotic therapy. J. Amer. med. Ass. **158**, 649–650 (1955).
— KADAVY, J. L., BERGDOLL, M. S., DACK, G. M.: Staphylococcal enterotoxin: production methods. J. infect. Dis. **89**, 180–184 (1951).
SUSSMAN, M., RYAN, C., SHIELDS, R.: Effects of staphylococcal enterotoxin upon the intestinal handling of water and electrolytes. Brit. J. Surg. **57**, 391 (1970).
TAKEUCHI, A., FORMAL, S. B., SPRINZ, H.: Experimental acute colitis in the rhesus monkey following peroral infection with *shigella flexneri*. Amer. J. Path. **52**, 503–529 (1968).
— SPRINZ, H., LABREC, E. H., FORMAL, S. B.: Experimental bacillary dysentery. An electron microscopic study of the response of the intestinal mucosa to bacterial invasion. Amer. J. Path. **47**, 1011–1044 (1965).
TAN, T. L., DRAKE, C. T., JACOBSON, M. J., PROHASKA, J. V.: The experimental development of pseudomembranous enterocolitis. Surg. Gynec. Obstet. **108**, 415–420 (1959).
TAYLOR, J.: Host specificity and enteropathogenicity of *Escherichia coli*. J. appl. Bact. **24**, 316–325 (1961).
— Host parasite relations of *Escherichia coli* in man. J. appl. Bact. **29**, 1–12 (1966).
— BETTELHEIM, K. A.: The action of chloroform-killed suspensions of enteropathogenic *Escherichia coli* on ligated rabbit gut segments. J. gen. Microbiol. **42**, 309–313 (1966).
— MALTBY, M. P., PAYNE, J. M.: Factors influencing the response of ligated rabbit gut segments to injected *Escherichia coli*. J. Path. Bact. **76**, 491–499 (1958).
— WILKINS, M. P.: The effect of salmonella and shigella on ligated loops of rabbit gut. Indian J. med. Res. **49**, 544–549 (1961).
— — PAYNE, J. M.: Relation of rabbit gut reaction to enteropathogenic *Escherichia coli*. Brit. J. exp. Path. **42**, 43–52 (1961).
THATCHER, F. S., SIMON, W.: A comparative appraisal of the properties of "staphylococci" isolated from clinical sites and from dairy products. Canad. J. Microbiol. **2**, 703–714 (1956).
THOMLINSON, J. R.: Symposium: Enteritis in pigs. II. Observations on the pathogenesis of gastroenteritis associated with *Escherichia coli*. Vet. Rec. **75**, 1246–1250 (1963).

THOMSON, S.: The numbers of pathogenic bacilli in faeces in intestinal diseases. J. Hyg. (Camb.) **53**, 217–224 (1955a).
— The role of certain varieties of *bacterium coli* in gastroenteritis of babies. J. Hyg. (Camb.) **53**, 357–367 (1955b).
TOLEDO, M. R. F. DE, TRABULSI, L. R.: Enteropathogenicidade e Comportamento Bioquimico do Colibacilo O136:K78 (B22). Rev. Inst. Med. trop. S. Paulo **11**, 425–429 (1969).
TRABULSI, L. R., TOLEDO, M. R. F. DE: *Escherichia coli* serogroup O115 isolated from patients with enteritis. Biochemical characteristics and experimental pathogenicity. Rev. Inst. Med. trop. S. Paulo **11**, 358–362 (1969).
TRIER, J. S.: Studies on small intestinal crypt epithelium. II. Evidence for and mechanisms of secretory activity by undifferentiated crypt cells of the human small intestine. Gastroenterology **47**, 480–495 (1964).
TRUSZCZYNSKI, M., PILASZEK, J.: Effects of injection of enterotoxin, endotoxin or live culture of *Escherichia coli* into the small intestine of pigs. Res. Vet. Sci. **10**, 469–476 (1969).
VAN HEYNINGEN, W. E., GLADSTONE, G. P.: The neurotoxin of *shigella shigae* 1. Production, purification and properties of the toxin. Brit. J. exp. Path. **34**, 202–216 (1953).
VAUGHAN, M., PIERCE, N. F., GREENOUGH, W. B. III.: Stimulation of glycerol production in fat cells by cholera toxin. Nature (Lond.) **226**, 658–659 (1970).
VAUGHAN-WILLIAMS, E. M., DOHADWALLA, A. N.: The appearance of a choleragenic agent in the blood of infant rabbits infected intestinally with *vibrio cholerae*, demonstrated by cross circulation. J. infect. Dis. **120**, 658–663 (1969).
— — DUTTA, N. K.: Diarrhea and accumulation of intestinal fluid in infant rabbits infected with *vibrio cholerae* in an isolated jejunal segment. J. infect. Dis. **120**, 645–651 (1969).
VERBIN, R. S., FARBER, E.: Effect of cycloheximide on the cell cycle of the crypts of the small intestine of the rat. J. Cell Biol. **35**, 649–658 (1967).
VERNON, E.: Food poisoning in England and Wales. Mth. Bull. Minist. Hlth Lab. Serv. **24**, 321–333 (1965).
VERNON, T. M., CRAIG, J. P.: Unpublished observations (1967). Cited by CRAIG, J. P. In: Microbial toxins, vol II A, p. 189–254. New York: Academic Press 1971.
VIOLLE, H., CRENDIROPOULO: Note Sur le Cholera Expérimental. C. R. Soc. Biol. (Paris) **78**, 331–332 (1915).
VIRCHOW, R.: Gesammelte Abhandlungen auf dem Gebiete der Öffentlichen Medizin und der Seuchenlehre, Berlin **1**, 151 (1879).
WAGMAN, J., EDWARDS, R. C., SCHANTZ, E. J.: Molecular size, homogeneity and hydrodynamic properties of purified staphylococcal enterotoxin B. Biochemistry **4**, 1017–1023 (1965).
WARREN, S. E., JACOBSON, M., MIRANY, J., PROHASKA, J. VAN: Acute and chronic enterotoxin enteritis. J. exp. Med. **120**, 561–568 (1964).
— SUGIYAMA, H., PROHASKA, J. VAN: Correlation of staphylococcal enterotoxins with experimentally induced enterocolitis. Surg. Gynec. Obstet. **116**, 29–33 (1963).
WATANABE, Y., VERWEY, W. F.: The preparation and properties of a purified mouse protective lipopolysaccharide from the Ogawa subtype of the El Tor variety of *vibrio cholerae*. In: Proceedings of the Cholera Research Symposium PHS Publication 1328, p. 253–259. Washington, D. C.: U.S. Government Printing Office 1965.
WATTEN, R. H., MORGAN, F. M., SONGKHLA, Y. N., VANIKIATI, B., PHILLIPS, R. A.: Water and electrolyte studies in cholera. J. clin. Invest. **38**, 1879–1889 (1959).
WEAVER, R. H., JOHNSON, M. K., PHILLIPS, R. A.: Biochemical studies of cholera. J. Egypt. publ. Hlth Ass. **23**, 5–14 (1948).

WEISS, K. F., STRONG, D. H., GROOM, R. A.: Mice and monkeys as assay animals for *Clostridium Perfringens* food poisoning. Appl. Microbiol. **14**, 479–485 (1966).

WILLIAMS, E. D.: Diarrhoea and thyroid carcinoma. Proc. roy. Soc. Med. **59**, 602–603 (1966).

— KARIM, S. M. M., SANDLER, M.: Prostaglandin secretion by medullary carcinoma of the thyroid. Lancet **1968I**, 22–23.

WILLIAMS, E. P., CAMERON, K.: Upon general infection by the *Bacillus Pyocyaneus* in children. J. Path. Bact. **3**, 344–351 (1894).

WILSON, B. J.: Comparative susceptibility of chimpanzees and *macaca mulatta* monkeys to oral administration of partially purified staphylococcal enterotoxin. J. Bact. **78**, 240–242 (1959).

YAHAGI, H., GHODA, A., SASAKI, S.: Early features of infection in ligated loops of the rabbit small intestine inoculated with *Shigella flexneri 3a*, enteropathogenic *E. coli*, *Escherichia coli* and *Vibrio parahemolyticus*. Keio J. Med. **16**, 119–132 (1967).

ZAKARIAN, L. M.: Types of hemolysins and enterotoxins in staphylococci isolated from gastrointestinal illnesses in children. Zh. Microbiol. (Mosk.) **44**, 56–58 (1967).

ZIEVE, P. D., PIERCE, N. F., GREENOUGH, W. B. III.: Stimulation of glycogenolysis by purified cholera enterotoxin in disrupted cells. Clin. Res. **28**, 690 (1970).

Author Index

Page numbers in *italics* refer to bibliography

Subject Index

The numbers set in *italics* refer to those pages on which the respective catch-word
is discussed in detail

Index to Volumes 37—55

Ergebnisse der allgemeinen Pathologie und der pathologischen Anatomie

Current Topics in Pathology

Current Topics in Pathology

Ergebnisse der Pathologie

Reprint from   Vol. 56

Ultrastructural Pathology of Parathyroid
Glands

E. Altenähr

With 18 Figures

Springer-Verlag Berlin · Heidelberg · New York 1972

Current Topics in Pathology

Ergebnisse der Pathologie

Vol. 56

Structure of Synovial Membrane in
Rheumatoid Arthritis

F. Huth, A. Soren, W. Klein

With 16 Figures

Springer-Verlag Berlin · Heidelberg · New York 1972

Current Topics in Pathology

Ergebnisse der Pathologie

Reprint from **Vol. 56**

Experimental Thyroid Carcinogenesis

K. Christov, R. Raichev

With 2 Figures

Springer-Verlag Berlin · Heidelberg · New York 1972

Current Topics in
Pathology

Ergebnisse der Pathologie

Reprint from   Vol. 56

Current Aspects of Bacterial Enterotoxins

D. G. Sheahan

Springer-Verlag Berlin · Heidelberg · New York 1972

Brain and Human Behavior

Edited by
Alexander G. Karczmar
and **Sir John C. Eccles**

With 162 figures
X, 475 pages. 1972

Twenty experts in the interdisciplinary field of neurosciences contributed to this book. The contents were structured beforehand to illustrate the status and the problems of the neuroscience. The contributors, who include three Nobel Prize winners, as well as British, American, French, German, Argentinian and Russian scientists, were selected for their ability to cover the wide range of topics. These include molecular and subcellular organization of the neurons their function in field systems and as scanners of the environment, to their involvement in processes of learning and memory, and extend to the behavior of the organism in the light of its genetic and sociological interactions. This leads on to the perennial problems of the relationship of mind to its substrate and of behavior either as a mechanism or as an expression of free will. Examples of advanced techniques in these various areas are presented. This text should help to develop overall understanding of the current state of behavioral theory and practice; moreover, philosophical and sociological implications are emphasized.

Published earlier :

John C. Eccles: The Physiology of Synapses

The subject of this book is the research work for which Professor Eccles was awarded the Nobel prize
With 101 figures. XII, 316 pages. 1964

Studies in Physiology

**Presented to Sir John C. Eccles. Edited by D. R. Curtis
and A. K. McIntyre**
with the collaboration of numerous experts
With 80 figures. VIII, 276 pages. 1965

Brain and Conscious Experience

Study Week September 28 to October 4, 1964, of the Pontificia Academia Scientiarum. **Edited by Sir John C. Eccles**
With 147 figures. XXII, 591 pages. 1966

John C. Eccles: Facing Reality

Philosophical Adventures by a Brain Scientist
With 36 figures. XI, 210 pages. 1970 (Heidelberg Science Library, Vol. 13)
Distribution rights for U.K., Commonwealth, and the Traditional
British Market (excluding Canada): Longman Group Ltd., Harlow/Essex

Experimental Brain Research
Experimentelle Hirnforschung
Expérimentation Cérébrale

Editorial Board: O. Creutzfeldt, D. R. Curtis, P. Dell, J. C. Eccles, R. Jung, D. M. MacKay, D. Ploog, J. Szentágothai, V. P. Whittaker, V. J. Wilson
Subscription Information. 1972, Volumes 15—16 (4 issues each) —
DM 128,—; US $38.40 per volume, plus postage
Sample copy available upon request

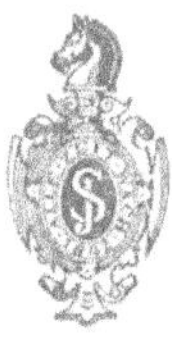

**Springer-Verlag
Berlin
Heidelberg
New York**
London · München · Paris
Sydney · Tokyo · Wien

GPSR Compliance
The European Union's (EU) General Product Safety Regulation (GPSR) is a set
of rules that requires consumer products to be safe and our obligations to
ensure this.

If you have any concerns about our products, you can contact us on

ProductSafety@springernature.com

In case Publisher is established outside the EU, the EU authorized
representative is:

Springer Nature Customer Service Center GmbH
Europaplatz 3
69115 Heidelberg, Germany

www.ingramcontent.com/pod-product-compliance
Ingram Content Group UK Ltd.
Pitfield, Milton Keynes, MK11 3LW, UK
UKHW052345070726
473059UK00009B/2543